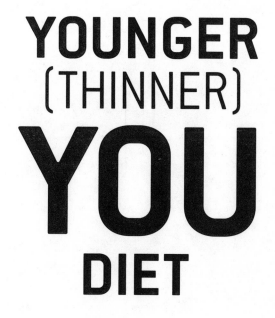

YOUNGER
(THINNER)
YOU
DIET

YOUNGER (THINNER) YOU DIET

How Understanding Your Brain Chemistry Can Help
You Lose Weight, Reverse Aging, and Fight Disease

ERIC R. BRAVERMAN, MD

Author of the *New York Times* Bestseller *Younger You*

RODALE

The information contained in this book is intended to provide helpful and informative material on the subject addressed. It is not intended to serve as a replacement for professional medical advice. Before beginning any diet, exercise, or healthcare program, a healthcare professional should be consulted regarding your specific situation. All nutrient, hormone, and medication recommendations mentioned in this book are not to be taken without the advice of a medical doctor, naturopathic physician, registered dietitian and/or endocrine specialist.

Mention of specific companies, organizations, or authorities in this book does not imply endorsement by the publisher, nor does mention of specific companies, organizations, or authorities imply that they endorse this book. Internet addresses and telephone numbers given in this book were accurate at the time it went to press.

Rodale books may be purchased for business or promotional use or for special sales. For information, please write to: Special Markets Department, Rodale Inc., 733 Third Avenue, New York, NY 10017

Printed in the United States of America
Rodale Inc. makes every effort to use acid-free ♾, recycled paper ♻.

Illustrations by Wesley Bedrosian
Book design by Christina Gaugler

Library of Congress Cataloging-in-Publication Data

Braverman, Eric R.
    Younger (thinner) you diet : how understanding your brain chemistry can help you lose weight, reverse aging, and fight disease / Eric R. Braverman.
        p.   cm.
    Includes bibliographical references and index.
    ISBN-13 978–1–59486–777–4   hardcover
    ISBN-10 1–59486–777–1   hardcover
    1. Reducing diets—Popular works.   2. Aging—Prevention—Popular works.   3. Rejuvenation—Nutritional aspects—Popular works.   I. Title.
    RM222.2.B687   2008
    613.2'5—dc22   2008047363

Distributed to the book trade by Macmillan

2 4 6 8 10 9 7 5 3 1   hardcover

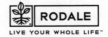

LIVE YOUR WHOLE LIFE™

We inspire and enable people to improve their lives and the world around them
For more of our products visit **rodalestore.com** or call 800-848-4735

For my beloved wife Dasha and my children
Ari, Stevie, Danny, J.J., and Ellie,
who have been my inspiration, my love, and my comfort.
Thank you for all your continued faith in me.

ACKNOWLEDGMENTS

THE CREATION OF THIS BOOK would not have been possible without the help of many individuals. I would like to thank my agent, David Vigliano, my successful team at Rodale, led by Andrea Au Levitt, and my publicist, David Ratner. I would also like to thank my writer, Pamela Liflander, as well as my assistant writer, Monica O'Rourke, for their unique skills, insights, and attentiveness in helping to get my ideas onto these pages.

I am grateful to my colleague Tatiana Karikh, MD, who has always been an invaluable critic of my work.

I am fortunate to have a gifted team of medical and administrative personnel who have helped turn my ideas into successful work. Their skills are unsurpassed and I am lucky to have them: Manpreet Kalra, Mallory Kerner, Victoria Gibbs, Melissa Dispensa, Anish Bajaj, DC, Javier Carbajal, Xudong Fu, and Donna Ruth.

I would also like to thank my medical staff members whose contribution to this book, as well as their loyalty and dedication to helping my patients, cannot go unnoticed: Ellie Capria, RPA-C, Rosina Giaccio-Williams, RPA-C, Stephanie Thornton, RPA-C, Susan Kaplysh, Tina Feldnov, and Tanya Perepada.

And finally to my patients, the greatest teachers of all, who are responsible for providing me with the material for writing this book.

God Bless You All!

CONTENTS

INTRODUCTION

WHAT IF I TOLD YOU that everything you know about dieting is completely wrong? Don't be embarrassed: Most people—including doctors and other "weight loss experts"—are in the same boat. Long before obesity became the number-one medical crisis, we've been taught that controlling your weight begins and ends with the stomach or the digestive tract. We've all heard about the "burning" fuel theory of metabolism, and that dieting is all about creating a better ratio of "calories in versus calories out." But where do you think this metabolism takes place? Is there really some special place in the body that "ignites" your food? The truth is that your stomach doesn't control your weight at all. Neither do your hips, thighs, or your butt. It's not your feet or arms either, even when you move them wildly during exercise. Weight loss occurs *in your brain.*

A healthy brain orchestrates all of the organs and systems of your body. But an unhealthy, aging brain cannot do its job. If you are noticing that losing weight is harder now than ever before, your brain is aging.

Weight gain isn't completely due to the fact that you're eating too much and exercising too little (although that often is a factor). Many of us are eating less and exercising more than ever before. Yet as early as age 30 your brain and body will begin to age, both inside and out. And when this happens, the battle with your weight begins.

You may have found your first gray hairs, or have had a momentary lapse when trying to remember a phone number or someone's name. But these clues aren't really the signs of the beginning stages of aging: By the time they occur, you're already well into the process. Inside your body, greater changes have already started. As you age, you begin to lose brain cells and gain extra weight. Without a full complement of brain cells, the connection between your physical brain and the electricity it produces slows down along with your metabolism, which actually is controlled by your brain! Four critical brain chemicals govern the way the brain processes this electricity, which is the energy your body and brain need to keep

Retrain Your Brain

It is possible to lose weight following any diet—from high-protein to high-fat to low-carb, or even all-grapefruit. But according to the National Eating Disorders Association, 95% of all dieters will regain their lost weight in 1 to 5 years.[1] All diets on the market today are missing the brain component! Until you can retrain your brain, you won't be able to achieve permanent weight loss.

running effectively. If this electricity is not transferred to the brain and body at the right power, speed, rhythm, and synchrony, your brain will create specific food cravings to resolve these issues. You end up unwittingly self-medicating your brain—often to excess—and creating food addictions.

The key to losing weight, and keeping it off forever, is to literally replenish these lost brain cells, rebalance your brain chemistry, and recreate a younger, more vibrant brain. Neurogenesis, the ability to grow new brain cells, is the opposite of aging. Every time you grow new brain cells, not only are you getting smarter, you are raising your metabolism another notch. The goal is to get smarter and thinner as we get older. Smarter brains burn more calories. Smarter brains become more fit, so that you can stop dieting forever.

YOU'RE NOT JUST OVERWEIGHT, YOU'RE AGING

When your brain becomes old, every part of your body begins to slow down. When your body is not functioning properly—whether you are suffering from something as minor as fatigue, insomnia, or allergies, or something major like heart disease, depression, or diabetes—it is a sign that your brain chemistry has been compromised. So not only does a brain chemistry imbalance lead to weight gain, it also leads to aging and disease.

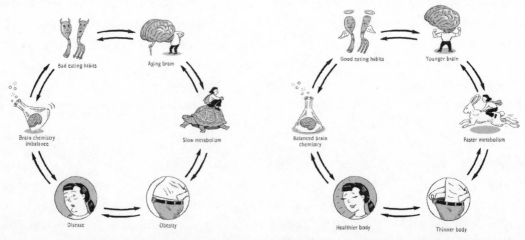

Your health, your weight, and your brain chemistry are intricately linked, creating a cycle that feeds from one to another. For example, the cycle on the left shows how bad eating habits age your brain, which slows your metabolism, leading not only to weight gain but to disease and unbalanced brain chemistry. However, once you reverse the cycle, as shown on the right, any of these starting points will lead to a more balanced brain and a younger, thinner you.

Worse, virtually every organ system is affected by excess weight. Think of it this way: Eating a spoonful of sugar is like dumping a truckload of sugar onto a highway. You can't drive your car through that. And you can't drive your car through honey, even if it is "all-natural" or "unrefined." You need a clean road to travel on, whether you are driving a brand new sports car or a twenty-year-old pickup truck.

As you start gaining weight, this is exactly what's happening to your body:

- Excess weight exerts unnecessary pressure on your muscles and bones, which weakens your muscles and joints, and leads to arthritis and osteoporosis. Excess fat seeps into your bones, making them more brittle and making you less flexible (and making it more difficult for you to exercise).[2]
- Excessive consumption of white sugars and white flours increases the amount of fat circulating in your body and raises your triglycerides, which clog everything from your brain to your arteries, veins, and internal organs, and affect your sexual health as well, according to the Cleveland Clinic.[3,4]
- Excess body fat pours into the brain, leading to Alzheimer's disease and dementia.[5] A July 2006 article in the *Archives of General Psychiatry* reported that excess weight and eating the wrong foods literally messes with your brain, causing depression, social/emotional issues, and stress.[6]
- Bacteria feeds and grows on excess sugars in the body (glucose), leading to some autoimmune disorders.[7]

- Excess sugars in the bloodstream cause insulin resistance, leading to Type 2 diabetes, gestational diabetes (diabetes during pregnancy), chronic yeast infections, and metabolic syndrome, according to a 2002 study appearing in the *Journal of American Medicine*.[8]
- Fat deposits, which contain cholesterol, create plaque that cause coronary artery disease, stroke, heart enlargement, hypertension, congestive heart failure, and other conditions.[9, 10]
- According to *Menopause Insight*, obesity can trigger early-onset menopause as well as menstrual abnormalities throughout the life cycle.[11]
- Increased size literally stretches out your skin, damaging its texture. This can cause stretch marks, darkening and thickening of the skin folds, skin disorders, and fungal infections.

THE PROMISE OF A YOUNGER (THINNER) YOU

In the not-too-distant future, you will be able to go to your local doctor and inexpensively purchase tests that will allow you to uncover your exact genetic predisposition for all facets of your health, including your weight. Then, doctors will be able to prescribe that elusive "diet pill" that will work with your particular genetic makeup. However, until that day comes, we are all resigned to losing weight by making the best choices for our diet and daily lives. The *Younger (Thinner) You Diet* will

Your Aging Metabolism

Your brain metabolism is like a furnace: It needs fuel to keep working. Eating less, or eating foods that are deficient in nutrients (like those 100-calorie snack packs) means less-effective fuel for your metabolic furnace. This will only slow your metabolism down and make you older. Instead, you have the power to choose the right Younger (Thinner) You foods that will keep your furnace burning strong. Once you are eating them in the right proportions, you'll be able to burn excess fat and lose weight.

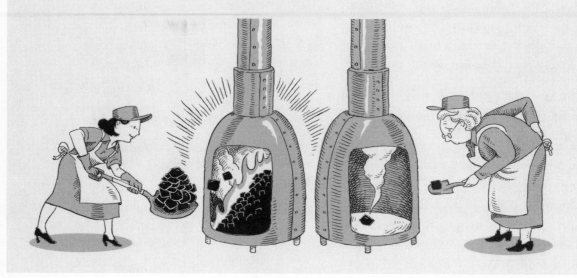

teach you how to compensate for a genetic predisposition to gain weight by teaching you easy ways to change your brain chemistry, that literally enhances your brain so it functions better on every level.

Any brain chemical imbalance is completely reversible once you learn how to address your health headfirst. By retraining your brain, you will be able to get rid of your food addictions and your cravings so you are not self-medicating with fattening, unhealthy foods. By changing the foods you eat to those that enhance brain chemistry, you will increase your metabolism and immediately start to lose weight.

I'm giving you the only diet I know of that has shown dramatic results with thousands of patients. Many men and women came to me when they had abandoned all hope of ever losing weight. They felt tired, lifeless, and older than they wanted to feel. After I evaluated their health, I started with specific weight loss goals and gave them the tools and the training they needed to reach these goals. I taught every patient which foods to choose so they no longer fell into the trap of food addiction. I taught them how to rev up their brain metabolism, which increased their energy and burned more body fat. Within weeks they began to see results . . . and you will too. You'll lose pounds and inches so you can have the body you've always wanted, now and forever.

Not only will you get thinner, you'll look and feel younger. Weight gain does not have to be a "normal" part of aging. When you lose weight and retrain your brain, you can turn back the aging clock by as much as fifteen years. You will begin to feel good about yourself. Your concentration and thinking will sharpen, and your mood will brighten. A better attitude and more physical energy will make staying on a diet easier than ever before. I know that the brain is the great pathway to everything we want. The goal of the *Younger (Thinner) You Diet* is clear: Optimal brain chemistry leads to a great body *and* great health, which leads to an abundant life.

THE DEEP CONNECTION BETWEEN ENHANCING BRAIN CHEMISTRY AND FOOD

The *Younger (Thinner) You Diet* offers you the ability to recondition your brain primarily through the foods you'll eat. Every fruit, vegetable, grain, or source of protein or fat is a precursor to one of the brain chemicals. These foods include lean proteins (meats, fish, poultry, and dairy products), complex carbohydrates (fruits, vegetables, beans, and whole grains), and even fats. They are providing your brain with more power, more speed, more balance, or the ability to rest with every bite. There are hundreds of foods for you to choose from, so you'll have lots of options for every meal, which will increase your ability to stick with this eating plan; rotating your foods will also feed your brain more nutrients.

You will be following a high-protein, low-fat, low-carbohydrate diet, which has been clinically proven to be the best prescription for battling excess weight. It also is proven to be the healthiest diet for body functioning because these foods are loaded with important vitamins, minerals, and antioxidants, which all improve your health. Best of all, you are making the necessary connection between a healthy body and a healthy brain: A better-functioning brain will free you from food addictions, provide you with a stronger metabolism, and ultimately lead to a thinner body.

Take a Good, Hard Look

Start by being honest with yourself. Go to your pantry and refrigerator, and look inside and see what you've been eating. People often underestimate the amount of food they eat in a day, or how quickly small amounts of junk food add up.

If you want to look and feel younger, the first step is to throw away your secret stash of chips, chocolate, and other snacks so you can concentrate on foods that will not only help you lose weight, but improve your overall health so you can look and feel younger.

MAKING CHANGES GETS EASIER

For some of you, switching from eating processed, sugary, or fatty foods to a more natural diet will be a giant life shift. Every day we are faced with a marathon of images, smells, and sounds that test your dieting mettle. That's because your brain makes all your food choices. You may think you are making these choices with your eyes and your nose, but the brain is really guiding you. When your brain is performing as an old brain—confused and malnourished—you will choose the wrong foods, which will ultimately make or keep you fat. Every time you make a bad food choice, the next good choice is harder to grasp.

However, eating good food leads to better choices. Every time you make the right food choice, the next good choice becomes easier. Remember: Losing weight is within your control. You have the power to make change happen. To lose weight, you *must* make the decision to change your brain chemistry. We will work together so you can consistently make better choices and retrain your brain.

If you have had success with other diets but haven't been able to keep the weight off for more than a year, you'll find this plan more effective over the long term. And if other diets have completely failed you, you'll now be retraining your brain so you will achieve weight loss for the first time. No matter how many diets you've been on—and off—this plan will be the one you can stick with forever.

HOW THE BOOK WORKS

Part I explains why the brain is the "furnace" of weight loss, and how this unique brain-based nutrient program is the secret to lasting results. You'll be able to quickly determine if you have a brain chemical imbalance, and learn why this problem is directly affecting your appetite, specific food addictions, or cravings. You'll then learn how to boost these brain chemicals back to normal, healthy levels so you can make permanent changes to your eating patterns and train your brain to help you lose weight.

Part II presents spices, teas, herbs, and colorful foods that are integral to the Younger (Thinner) You Diet. These special foods will enhance your brain chemistry and boost your metabolism. They are the often-missing

What Type of Eater Are You?

- Junk food junkie?
- Emotional eater?
- Gobbler on the go?
- Fast-food feeder?
- Closet consumer?
- Mindless muncher?

Recognizing your vices is half the battle. We're all capable of being each of these types of eaters at different times in our lives. For example, I've been a protein freak, eating steak all the time when I'm low in dopamine; I've been a cheese fanatic when my thinking is slow; I've been a mindless muncher in between my marriages, and I've been a binge eater when I don't get enough sleep, like during my residency.

components that help you burn calories more effectively and efficiently and help you to successfully lose weight and defeat aging. There are shopping lists, meal plans, and dozens of delicious recipes that will make sticking to the program seem effortless. I have provided thirty days of specific meal recommendations, or you can create your own meal plans to support your individual tastes. If you follow these meal plans, there is no need to count calories: My nutritional staff has done the work for you.

The Younger (Thinner) You Exercise Program enhances the diet by providing more opportunities to increase your metabolic rate through aerobic and weight training routines. There's even a journal where you can record your success.

Part III focuses on reversing the aging process in your oldest parts. This section addresses the particular health issues that may be causing premature aging and your inability to lose weight. You will take another quiz that will identify the specific internal systems that may be limiting your weight loss potential. That way you won't

Look at What She's Eating!

The notion that the obese eat more is frequently a myth. Many obese people eat the same, or even less, than non-obese people. You may find while on this diet you'll be eating more than you are used to, and that's a good thing.

chase every weight loss fad for the rest of your life.

The fix for these medical issues is as straightforward as losing weight: Restore your health, restore your brain chemistry. You'll regain your health by concentrating on specific foods, supplements, teas, and spices, and even natural hormones and medicines if necessary. The benefit of brain-based health is undeniable: better bones, better heart, better memory, better sleep patterns, better moods, and better sex. Better *you*.

You'll be able to apply my treatments while working with your own physicians. And best of all, by getting your health back on track, you'll find it even easier to lose the weight you want. Let's get started on the path to understanding how to regain your vitality—and start losing weight.

PART I

How the Diet Works to Reverse Weight Gain and Aging

CHAPTER 1

You Need a Younger Brain for a Younger (Thinner) You

AS I TELL MY PATIENTS, your skin, hair, and nails are repairable and replaceable, and most of your organs can be revitalized. But the brain is the one organ you can't replace (no matter what you've seen in horror movies). The brain is where your life resides. It governs all aspects of your health as well as your emotional state. And while you can't get a new brain, you can improve the one you have. There are many different ways to literally make your brain younger which can enhance every facet of your health.

This chapter will show how you can lose weight permanently once you balance your brain. Without taking the brain into account, you can diet for the rest of your life and never be happy with the results.

DR. BRAVERMAN'S LESSON #1: BRAIN SCIENCE 101

You don't need to be a scientist to understand how the brain works. Simply, the brain is divided into three parts: the cerebrum, the

brain stem, and the cerebellum. The brain stem connects the brain to the rest of the body with hundreds of nerves that branch out from your spinal column. The cerebrum is divided into two equal parts called hemispheres, which are linked by a thick band of nerve fibers called the corpus callosum. These hemispheres, as well as the cerebellum, have designated areas called lobes. Each lobe instructs our bodies to perform unique functions. They control automatic processes, such as digestion and breathing, and manage our internal systems.

Your brain is like the circuit breaker box in your home. When you want to turn a light on, you plug in a lamp and the electricity transfers from the breaker box into the lamp. In much the same way, the brain generates

The Problem with Diets

You "on a diet" is like a hamster racing on a metal wheel: You could run as fast as you can all day long, but without fixing your brain-chemical deficiency, you'll never escape your weight-gain rut.

ABC: Abnormal Brain Chemistry

Abnormal brain chemistry can send you over to the "dark side" of food temptation, which leads to obesity, which leads to illness. Your death certificate will say heart attack, stroke, aneurysm—but the catalyst will really be the brain.

and sends electric currents throughout your body, fueling your internal systems and orchestrating your health. Illness in the body (including weight gain) as well as in the brain (like a decline in memory or attention) is almost always the result of one failing circuit breaker after another.

Now you may be thinking, "All that electricity sounds dangerous." That's where body fat comes in. In some ways, you can think of body fat as nothing more than the insulation surrounding the real you.

Your body's layer of fat provides crucial insulation that keeps the electricity your brain creates safely within the confines of your skin and bones. We all absolutely need some body fat to keep us electrically grounded, as well as warm enough to withstand cold climates. The problem, however, is when your body makes more insulation than it needs.

When you accumulate extra body fat, you're also slowing down every other internal organ system from functioning as they

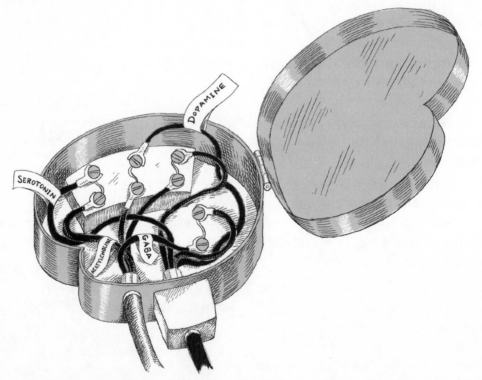

The four brain chemicals—dopamine, acetylcholine, GABA, and serotonin—assist in transferring electricity from the brain to the rest of the body at the correct power, speed, rhythm, and synchrony.

were intended to operate. Your body was perfectly designed to work at your leanest body weight. But when you gain weight, you're not just adding body fat to your existing layer of insulation. Your internal organs are getting bigger, too. That means your heart is becoming enlarged; your veins and arteries are being stretched; your liver fills with fat; your skin is clogged with fat; your sinuses clog and swell, etc. This extra fat literally fills every crevice of the body, which forces each of the affected organs to work harder just to do their "normal" jobs. And when that happens, you are forcing these organs to age faster than they should. You begin to feel sick as your body cannot fight infections or diseases because it needs all of its energy just to keep these fatty organs operating at their minimal levels. And you'll begin to feel old because you actually are accelerating your own aging process: Your organs, muscles, and bones will wear out simply from carrying this extra weight around, and you won't be able to enjoy or even participate in an active life. Adding as little as ten pounds on an average-size frame will begin to disrupt normal body functions for both men and women.

It's not just the added pounds slowing you down: Weight gain contributes to, and is a sign for many of the most common medical illnesses, most of which are aging you prematurely.[1] The following conditions affect your organs and systems and are directly related to weight gain (many of these will be discussed in detail in Part III):

BRAIN

- Alzheimer's disease
- Dementia
- Depression

REGULATORY ORGANS OF METABOLISM (ENDOCRINE) AND THE IMMUNE SYSTEMS

- Allergies
- Autoimmune disorders
- Cancer
- Chronic inflammation
- Diabetes mellitus type 2
- Gestational diabetes
- Growth hormone deficiency
- Hyperlipidemia
- Metabolic syndrome
- Thyroid nodules
- Insulin resistance

MUSCULOSKELETAL SYSTEM

- Decreased ambulation
- Gout
- Muscle weakening
- Orthopedic problems
- Osteoarthritis

CARDIOPULMONARY AND VASCULAR SYSTEMS

- Asthma
- Blood clots
- Congestive heart failure
- Coronary artery disease

- Decreased lung capacity
- Heart enlargement
- Hypertension
- Respiratory infections
- Sleep apnea
- Stroke

DIGESTIVE SYSTEM

- Fatty liver
- Gallstones
- GERD
- Indigestion
- Irritable bowel syndrome
- Malnutrition

SEXUALITY AND REPRODUCTIVE SYSTEM

- Decreased libido
- Decreased sexual functioning
- Chronic yeast infections
- Infertility
- Menstrual abnormalities

KIDNEYS AND URINARY TRACT

- Kidney disease
- Kidney stones
- Protein in the urine
- Urinary incontinence

Obesity and the Brain

The brain's electrical power can only "light" so much space. An obese person's body has hundreds more lights that need power as the circuitry lengthens and stretches throughout the entire body.

SKIN

- Chronic fungal infections
- Darkening and thickening of the skin folds
- Skin disorders
- Stretch marks
- Wrinkles

DR. BRAVERMAN'S LESSON #2: CONTROLLING YOUR INTERNAL ELECTRICITY

Your increasing waistline may be the first indicator there is a problem with one of the four primary biochemicals that is produced in your brain. Each functions differently and determines the brain's effectiveness—or brain age—by controlling a single aspect of the electricity transfer from the brain to the body. These brain chemicals—dopamine, acetylcholine, gamma-aminobutyric acid (GABA), and serotonin—can positively affect your weight in distinct ways, yet a deficiency in any of them can lead to food addictions, which can then lead to obesity.

Scientists used to believe that there was no way to reverse a brain chemical imbalance. They believed that once brain cells were lost, or once your brain chemistry was damaged, you were stuck forever. However, the latest research is finding that these ideas are not only outdated, but untrue. The science of neurogenesis is showing that we each have the capacity to grow new brain cells, and retrain the brain to produce better, enhanced brain chemistry on demand! This means that

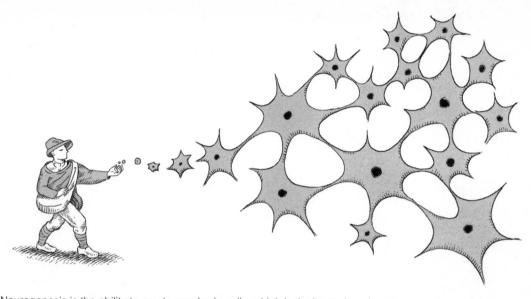

Neurogenesis is the ability to create new brain cells, which is the key to keeping you younger and thinner.

by correcting your brain chemistry through this program, not only can you increase your metabolism so that you will lose weight, you can create a more youthful brain.

Recent data suggests that anywhere from 2 to 10 points of an increase in IQ is associated with brain cell growth. Research also shows that medications, including antidepressants, not only improve your brain chemistry, but they actually build new brain cells. That's why I believe that any modality that can facilitate neurogenesis or brain cell growth—including medications, natural hormone therapies, and specific nutrients and supplements—is not only important, it's vital to living a younger life. Getting fat and senile is not inevitable. Instead, we can age intelligently and gracefully; our brains will stay young, and we'll have more restful sleep, better memory and attention, and a better overall mood. Most of all, new brain cell growth leads to weight loss, so we can stay trim and slim.

Dopamine Creates Brain Power

Voltage is the intensity at which the brain instructs the body to work. This forcefulness is controlled by the brain chemical dopamine, which, in terms of weight loss, is

More on the Brain–Body Connection

Rapid or significant weight gain is one of the hallmarks of a dopamine deficiency. While most doctors recognize that obesity is a metabolic disorder, they miss the point: Metabolism is governed by dopamine. The Younger (Thinner) You program will enhance your body's natural production of dopamine so that you can lose excess weight and keep it off for good.

Who's Your Daddy?

New studies conducted by Brookhaven National Laboratory and the North American Association for the Study of Obesity suggest that many women have impaired dopamine levels, regardless of their age.[2, 3] Many can trace this imbalance back to inheriting a bad set of genes, particularly if they were the daughter of an alcoholic. This genetic deficiency may be the reason why you find yourself eating all the time. Just like an alcoholic, you are suffering from an addiction, only this time the culprit is food. While you can't fix the gene, you can change your destiny by changing your diet.

the most important of the four brain chemicals. Dopamine is your brain's natural power source, which keeps you mentally and physically energized throughout the day. Voltage and dopamine control your metabolism (the ability to turn food into fuel). When your voltage is low, you don't have energy, making your brain and body sluggish. At the same time, without dopamine, your metabolism slows down. When this happens, any unused fuel starts to bulk up in the form of body fat.

If you are always running low on dopamine, you'll gain weight despite your best efforts at dieting. No matter how much you exercise or how little you eat, you will never be able to kick-start your metabolism to burn calories faster and more efficiently. However, you can correct a dopamine deficiency just by teaching your brain to create more of this vital chemical, and I'll show you how you can *train* your brain to make more dopamine. The more dopamine you have, the faster your metabolism will work, which will not only reverse your tendency to gain weight, but provide the fast-burning metabolism you need to lose the weight you want.

The Younger (Thinner) You Diet specifically increases the production of dopamine. You'll be eating foods, herbs, spices, and teas every day at every meal that naturally raise your dopamine. What's more, many of these foods have a thermogenic property: They improve your brain's capacity to increase cell energy and pump fuel to your vital organs. This means that *they improve your metabolism as you are eating them.*

Equally important, dopamine levels directly influence your ability to manage general as well as specific food cravings. Dopamine controls how we quantify the feeling of satisfaction we experience when we are eating a meal. When this brain chemical is balanced we can eat until we feel physically full in our stomachs, and emotionally satisfied in the brain. Dopamine allows us to experience a single, wonderful glass of wine, or one helping of dessert, and then walk away from the table. However, if our dopamine levels are low, we may not ever recognize a sense of satisfaction emotionally or physically. Without the right amount of dopamine, the circuits in our brains do not relay the message that we feel satisfied and full. Instead of walking away from the table, we'll just keep eating and eating and eating: We are never emotionally or physically fulfilled by food, no matter how much we've eaten.

Those with low dopamine levels can finish an entire loaf of bread in a sitting, or eat a pint of ice cream without getting an emotional or physical rush. You can unknowingly develop an addictive relationship with food, in which you'll need ever-larger quantities just to reach some level of reward.

As I said before, low-dopamine individuals often feel sluggish, even cranky. When we feel this way, we experience an instinctive, often unconscious attempt to bring the fire back. Low-dopamine individuals unconsciously crave caffeine, as well as foods that will deliver an energy boost: They tend to choose high sugar, fast-digesting carbohydrates, and they will eat them in copious quantities because they are trying to feel energized. Each of these stimulants actually boost dopamine production, so in effect you are self-medicating a low dopamine level correctly, although dangerously, because these foods are contributing to your weight gain.

You can get your metabolism running better and break the cycle of food addiction largely through choosing to eat foods that are the building blocks for creating dopamine: foods in the lean protein group that are high in phenylalanine and tyrosine. Chapter 3 will give you complete information on the right foods for you to choose. You can also start boosting your dopamine right away by cutting out as much sugary foods and processed "simple" carbs from your diet as possible. By taking both of these steps, you'll immediately begin to get your brain in better shape.

Acetylcholine Controls Brain Speed

Speed measures how fast electrical signals are processed from the brain to the body. It directly affects how we think and how we retain information in the forms of memory and attention. But when the brain loses speed, it loses power (and dopamine), disrupting the flow of electricity and slowing down all bodily functions. When your brain speed slows due to an acetylcholine deficiency, you might become forgetful, and experience a loss of mental and physical quickness. Some people describe this as brain fog. Memory and attention disturbances can cause us to make bad choices, especially with food.

Your speed is governed by the brain chemical acetylcholine, the primary function of which is to provide the lubricants and insulation for our muscles, bones, and other internal systems in the form of fat. This is one of the reasons why foods with healthy fats are an important part of any diet. But when we are running low on acetylcholine, the body

Low on Dopamine?

- Do you recognize when you are full?
- Do you feel happy after eating?
- Can a small snack like a piece of fresh fruit tide you over until the next meal?
- When following other diets, have you found that you were always hungry, even after you finished a meal?
- Do you drink copious amounts of liquid with your meals?

Missing Acetylcholine?

- Have you ever had an eating disorder?
- Do you crave fried foods?
- Do you eat fast food several times per week?
- Do you usually drink at least one serving of alcohol with lunch or dinner?
- Do you eat because you have attention or memory problems?

cannot naturally produce enough internal lubrication, and we literally dry out. You'll recognize this feeling if you begin to crave fat and fatty foods: Your brain is telling you to provide the necessary extra layer of lubrication. But sometimes we get this message and get carried away eating too much fatty food. And then—you know what happens.

The Younger (Thinner) You Diet provides for well-rounded meals with just enough fat to keep your acetylcholine levels stable. Chapter 4 gives complete lists of the right fats to choose, which occur primarily in foods high in omega-3 fatty acids, like freshwater fish. By increasing your brain speed naturally through the foods you eat, you may also experience an improvement in your memory, attention, IQ, and even your behavior. All of these improvements

Need More GABA?

- Do you eat your meals quickly?
- Do you usually help yourself to seconds?
- Do you sample food while you're cooking?
- Do you always have dessert after dinner?
- Do people comment on your ability to "pack it in"?

to your thinking will help you feel younger because your brain fog will naturally dissipate. You'll feel more alert, think faster, and remember where your keys are (well, maybe not your keys, but you get the picture).

GABA Maintains Brain Rhythm

A balanced brain creates and receives electricity in a smooth, even flow, creating a consistent pace, both mentally and physically. The chemical signal that relays your internal pace is transferred to the body by the brain chemical GABA. It determines the pace at which your body and brain function. It also establishes how well you can handle life's stresses. When GABA levels are normal we react appropriately to the daily challenges of life because GABA is also monitoring our dopamine and acetylcholine: Our brain speed is functioning well and with the correct intensity.

However, when GABA is low, we can become unbalanced. We can feel overly emotional and mentally or physically "rocky"; you might be nervous, tense, irritable, or even hungry. When we feel out of sorts, we often have an instinctive yearning for comfort. This often translates into seeking solace in food to resolve our anxiety. We've been taught to call this "emotional eating," and on the most basic levels that diagnosis is correct. However, when we look deeper at the problem, anxiety and stress are linked back to our brain chemicals.

Low levels of GABA are also associated with problems of poor impulse control, often resulting in inappropriate behavior like temper tantrums and overeating. Low-GABA individuals might not recognize particular food cravings, but instead have an issue with portion control.

However, too much GABA can create lethargy. And as our internal energy slows down, we accumulate body fat. This dichotomy makes GABA a difficult brain chemical to keep at the exact right level. Too high, and you become sedated, gaining weight because you aren't interested in moving at all. And when you can't lose the weight you want, you become anxious as your GABA decreases. Soon you'll lose control of portions, and the cycle begins again.

The key to keeping your GABA balanced begins with the foods you eat. The Younger (Thinner) You Diet provides the right raw materials that will create a steady supply of GABA, namely complex carbohydrates that are high in glutamine and inositol. Chapter 5 contains a complete list of foods that will control your GABA. Within a few weeks of following your new GABA diet, you will notice a marked improvement in your physical and emotional health. At the same time, you'll learn how to recognize your emotional eating patterns so that you can break the cycle immediately. You'll see a difference when you can learn to create smaller portions and feel satisfied after eating them, or grab a handful of potato chips instead of scarfing down the entire "price saver" bag.

Serotonin Keeps Your Brain in Sync

The electricity your brain creates moves through your body in waves. There are four types of brain waves,[5] each providing us with a level of consciousness. Synchrony balances the movement of these four kinds of brain waves across the brain. When they are out of sync, you will experience sleep disorders during the night, and depression and fear during the day. Synchrony is determined by levels of the brain chemical serotonin.

Serotonin acts as an "off" switch for the brain and body: It transmits a signal that tells the body when to shut down and when to rest. When serotonin levels are normal, you get the restful sleep you need, and your body is able to recharge for the next day. Good sleep, at least seven hours each night, can reset the brain to improve and enhance every aspect of health, creating high-energy brain metabolism, and a fast-thinking, calm, and steady brain.

We all know how it feels when we don't get enough sleep, or when our sleep is not

Why It's Important to Feed Your Brain

If you're not consuming enough calories every day, you're not giving your brain the fuel it needs.[4] Your skinny friends can stay thin while eating virtually nothing because they are constantly boosting their brain chemicals with cigarettes and coffee. But what you don't see are their poor sleep patterns, mood instability, as well as the inside of their aging body. The Younger (Thinner) You goal is for you to be thin—*not skinny*—and healthy, so you are strong to the core.

Down in Serotonin?

- Do you eat carbohydrates with every meal?
- Do you crave salty snacks like potato chips and pretzels?
- Do you eat pickles and olives?
- Do your cravings get worse around the time of your menstrual cycle?

restful. If our sleep is interrupted during the night, we feel rundown, like we're getting a cold. Our ability to think clearly becomes compromised, and before we know it, we're feeling—and looking—tired and old.

When we're tired, we often make bad food choices, and we reach for simple (refined) carbohydrates, such as pasta, rice, and bread, as well as salt to boost our energy. To be in sync, our cravings for salt and carbs must be in check. The chemical serotonin helps control this.

A tired brain will try to make you eat more to increase energy. This signal is sent by certain hormones, such as ghrelin, that will make you feel hungry. Ghrelin is a protein secreted by the stomach and intestines, which elevates when you haven't eaten in a while, and falls after you eat. Serotonin controls ghrelin levels, so when your serotonin falls, your ghrelin increases. For example, a poor night's sleep has been shown to increase ghrelin levels throughout the following day, according to research conducted by Dr. Shahrad Taheri.[6,7] This would explain why some people experience strong hunger sensations after a disrupted night's sleep.

The Younger (Thinner) You Diet keeps serotonin and ghrelin in check because you will be eating at least three substantial meals each day plus one healthy snack, which is enough calories to keep your stomach and your brain satisfied. By following a serotonin-boosting diet, consisting of foods that are high in the serotonin precursor tryptophan, you will quickly find you are falling asleep easily, and waking rested. You also will lose your cravings for simple carbohydrates and salt, and your overall health will be markedly improved.

DR. BRAVERMAN'S LESSON #3: THE BRAIN AND YOUR PERSONALITY

Brain chemistry not only controls your physical state, but your emotional life as well. The particular distribution of each of the four primary biochemicals affects different aspects of your personality, including your emotional relationship with food. Once you have mastered controlling your unique brain chemistry, you'll find that you are automatically drawn to choosing the foods that are the best for you and your personality. Not only will you understand why you had certain food triggers, you will also be able to see how your personality has dominated your food decision-making skills in the past, and how you can correct this problem right now.

Chapters 3 through 6 deal with the individual brain chemicals, will give you more information on your particular imbalance, including your personality. Once you fully understand your brain chemistry, you'll agree with me that balancing your brain is the single most important aspect for weight loss. Your unbalanced brain is the sole reason why you've been unable to shed those stubborn pounds. What's more, you'll also see how much better you feel about yourself, and how much happier you can be once your brain is perfectly balanced.

THE PERFECTLY BALANCED YOUNGER (THINNER) YOU

When these four brain chemicals are produced at the right levels, your body is able to efficiently run on the energy it takes in through food. When these same brain chemicals are either too high to too low, your ability to control your weight and metabolize food is significantly affected.

What these quick science lessons tell us is fact, not fiction. When you just can't stop eating even after you know you are full, it's not because you're weak. It's not because you're lazy or don't have willpower. It's because you have a brain chemical imbalance. And once we correct that imbalance, once we get your brain running again at full speed, energized, and healed with the proper levels of dopamine, acetylcholine, GABA, and serotonin, only then can you truly experience lasting weight loss.

It's also important to remember that as we age, the production of these same brain chemicals naturally slows down. This is one of the main reasons we gain weight as we get older. The Younger (Thinner) You Diet

Sleep Affects Hunger

To see if a serotonin deficiency is figuring into your hunger equation, keep a food and sleep diary for a week, noting not only what you ate during the day, but specifically what you ate before you went to bed, and how many restful hours of sleep you got. While you thought your hunger might have been due to the small dinner you had the night before, it might really have been caused by your poor sleep patterns.

changes your brain chemistry so you can break the aging code and lose weight.

The core belief of my medical practice is that every illness has a complex brain component. I have seen amazing reversals of chronic, severe pain using medicines that control serotonin; reversals of high blood pressure by controlling GABA; reversal of movement disorders like Parkinson's Disease with agents that control dopamine; reversal of memory loss with agents that control acetylcholine; reversal of heart failure with agents that control dopamine.

The reality is, whatever the health challenge is, it may appear to the person who's

Younger (Thinner) You Diet Mantras

- I can cut my craving for sugar and all foods by raising dopamine.
- I can cut my craving for alcohol or drugs by balancing GABA and dopamine.
- I can cut my confusion-based cravings for fat by raising acetylcholine.
- I can control my anxiety-based cravings by raising GABA.
- I can curb my desire for salts and simple carbohydrates by increasing serotonin.

dieting that they seem to have just a sugar-craving problem. But it's always a four-part component brain problem, and an aging problem: By increasing your dopamine, you'll ramp up your metabolism effortlessly; by increasing acetylcholine, you forego your fat cravings; by increasing GABA, you can get off the obsessive/anxiety–related eating patterns and develop portion control; by increasing serotonin, you can give yourself and your brain the rest you deserve so you will no longer crave carbs and salty foods.

"BRAINLESS" DIETING DOESN'T WORK!

If you're like most Americans, this isn't the first diet book you've ever bought. And if you're dieting again, that means you've been disappointed with your results. Many diet programs can successfully get you to lose some weight, but they do not provide the tools you need to keep the weight off for good.

While there are more diets out there than stars in the sky, traditional medical philosophy regarding weight loss has been

Meet Renee B.: She Said No to Brainless Dieting

Last year, Renee came to see me in tears. She was a 32-year-old executive who said, "I can't lose weight and I don't know why. I'm 160 pounds, yet I exercise all the time. I eat less than my skinniest friends but I can't lose weight. I limit my carbs and salty foods but even when I eat just a little of them I blow up like a balloon. I've strictly followed most of the popular diets, but I'm still 20 pounds heavier than I want to be. I'm exhausted, depressed, and angry with myself all the time. I just want to be thin."

I realized immediately that Renee was a woman with a young, vibrant mind trapped in an old body. I explained that her brain metabolism must be low if she is restricting her food intake but not losing weight. I told her that together we were going to figure out which brain chemicals she was deficient in, and then build a personalized program for success.

After some simple testing, I recognized Renee was low in serotonin and dopamine. I clearly explained that even with all her best intentions, she would never lose weight without addressing her brain chemistry. In fact, every diet she has ever been on has been a failure because they never addressed the brain chemistry component. So I assured Renee it wasn't her fault that she couldn't lose weight.

I put Renee on the Younger (Thinner) You diet, focusing on her dopamine and serotonin deficiencies. Once her sleep was restored and her metabolism kicked in, Renee lost ten pounds almost instantly. Now Renee continues to lose weight, and she looks amazing.

Stop Beating Yourself Up

We've been so conditioned to believe there's blame in weight gain, it's easy to fall into the trap of being disappointed with ourselves. Yet no one has ever proven they can lose weight with talk therapy alone.

As a scientist, I rely on pure data. And the research shows carrying excessive weight is not a purely psychological problem. Once you improve your brain metabolism, you'll see results. This doesn't mean you'll wake up one morning and look like Cinderella, but it does mean that within a few weeks you'll find your jeans are looser and your mood has improved. So stop beating yourself up. I'll teach you how to get your brain back in shape so you will never feel guilty about your weight again.

consistent: "Treat the symptom." If you're overweight or obese, your doctor will tell you to do one of the following: cut calories, count calories, count carbohydrates, cut carbohydrates, stop eating protein, eat nothing but protein, count fat grams, forget fat grams . . . the list goes on and on.

Instead of only treating the symptom—excess weight—I see the bigger picture, which leads us back to the brain. Your excess weight is your aging brain's cry for help. If you don't address your unique brain chemistry deficiencies, you'll still be plagued with hunger and food cravings that will never disappear, no matter how "good" you are.

To my mind, diets that do not address brain chemistry fail for two reasons, which are:

First, when you restrict certain macronutrients (like carbs or fat), your brain isn't

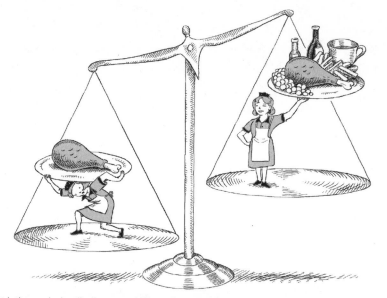

Over time, restricting calories limits your ability to lose weight. Your body will adjust to a reduced caloric intake, and your metabolism will slow. Instead, you need to eat important nutrients all day long to keep your metabolism burning strong. By following this diet, which is high in nutrient-dense fruits, vegetables, teas, and spices, you'll lose weight, even if you eat more.

getting all the nutrients it needs, so the body sends out a hunger signal that results in overeating. Instead, my key to weight management is not found in counting carbohydrates, fat grams, or calories, but in balancing brain chemistry through nutrition—something anyone can do easily and effectively. It is an eating plan you can follow for life.

Second, when we diet, we often deprive ourselves of vital nutrients, our mental state has been taxed and we make bad food choices. We are too fatigued, so we eat to boost our energy. We are too anxious, so we eat to comfort and calm ourselves. Our mental sharpness diminishes, so we forget to eat healthfully. We are depressed, so we eat excessively to force sleep. These mental states are aging you far beyond your chronological age. The good news is that by following a diet that enhances brain chemistry, each of these mental states can be completely reversed naturally. That's what this diet is all about.

On the Younger (Thinner) You Diet, you will not only lose weight because you are increasing your dopamine. As you balance your brain, you will also become more fit as you increase your acetylcholine. You will become calmer as you learn to stabilize your GABA. And you will be happier and sleep better with more serotonin. No other

diet can deliver on this promise. Here is how I think my plan stacks up against some of the diets you might have tried in the past:

- **Low-carb/no-carb, or high protein, or low-fat/no-fat diets** parse macronutrients (fats, carbs, and proteins) so your life feels like an endless high school math final, in which you are constantly figuring out what you can eat and how much. While these programs effectively enhance metabolism by lowering your intake of carbohydrates and increasing exercise, neither one utilizes the ancient powers of spices or teas. What's more, if you have followed one of these diets in the past, you may have felt hungry, especially during the initial phases. That's because these diets don't offer enough volume-based foods. In addition, these diets don't offer the essential brain component, nor do they help you identify your addictive eating patterns that are based on your brain chemical imbalance. And none of these diets focuses on the essential spices that can significantly lower cholesterol.
- **Vegetarian/vegan diets** are too low in protein for the brain to function optimally. And because it doesn't make the

Get on the Metabolism Elevator!

Every change you make following this program will elevate your metabolism. There are cycles of metabolism throughout your life that are triggered by pregnancy, children, family, stress, and so forth. Each one can be impacted through enhancing brain chemistry and the anti-aging techniques described throughout the book.

connection between brain health and physical health, a low protein diet can eventually put you at higher risk for osteoporosis.[8]

- **Low calorie diet programs** offer a host of food choices in particularly small portions. Because virtually anything is allowed, it doesn't teach you how to make good food choices. For example, ice cream and fast-food hamburgers should not be part of anyone's diet. Many followers of this program eventually fall off the diet because the essential component of the brain has not been addressed, so people continue to lose control and fall back on their cravings.

- **Prepackaged meal plans** offer structured programs that are helpful and can be healthy. The problem with these diets is that they don't teach you portion control other than eating everything that's in their box (sometimes leaving you so hungry that you will want to eat the box as well). The prepackaged foods are great while they last, but left to your own devices, you didn't learn to use the tools needed to continue on the right path. Additionally, these plans don't regularly use teas and spices, and don't teach you to enhance your brain chemistry for lasting change.

- **Specific prescriptions** from other doctors may work for some, but not for all dieters. Blood type diets, for instance, are extremely limited, and I don't agree with the logic that there are only four core types of people in the world.

Indulge—It's Fat-Free!

While these foods have lower fat amounts, sometimes they have even *more* calories than their full-fat counterparts. Additionally, these products usually add excessive amounts of sugar, flour, or starch thickeners to compensate for the loss of taste and texture after the fat and additives are removed.

- **Single-food diets**, such as a cabbage soup, grapefruit, or even an all chocolate diet are encouraging to me because I strongly believe that individual foods are powerful weight loss tools. The problem is you can't follow them for very long. You're missing essential nutrients, plus those very necessary spices and teas. Instead, the Younger (Thinner) You Diet harnesses these same foods and combines them in interesting ways so that you can continue to incorporate them into your food choices for the long term.

THE NEXT STEP

Now that you have a basic understanding of how your brain directly affects your ability to lose weight, the next step is to determine which brain chemicals you are currently underproducing. The quiz in Chapter 2 will clearly identify your deficiencies. Then, you can tailor the Younger (Thinner) You Diet to include more of the foods that will increase your unique brain chemistry, and at the same time facilitate your ability to lose weight.

CHAPTER 2

The Younger (Thinner) You Diet Quiz

YOUR BRAIN chemical activity is determining which foods you are compelled to eat, the speed of your metabolism, and your ability to stop eating and recognize when you are full. Restoring or enhancing your dopamine, acetylcholine, GABA, or serotonin, or any combination of them, is the only way you will be able to lose weight effectively and keep it off permanently. Luckily, we have the technology to easily determine which brain chemicals you are deficient in or are not producing efficiently.

BRAIN MAPPING AND 21ST-CENTURY MEDICINE

Doctors and researchers today are more capable than ever at uncovering the mysteries of the brain and the body. For example, studies conducted at Boston University conclusively show that fat cells are really no more than aged cells, and they can be rejuvenated just like well-maintained skin.[1] Your body fat can be restructured and sculpted just like your brain's neurons. In fact, the two are intimately linked. We used to claim that the human body was incapable of creating new brain cells. The theory was that we would lose brain cells as our metabolism deteriorates, and gain fat cells instead. This turned out not to be the case. In fact, this myth was completely debunked by evidence supporting neurogenesis: the growth of new brain cells. We now know that we can grow new brain cells, and as we gain more brain cells, our fat cells actually shrink and change. This means that new brain cells mean smaller fat cells, and even the loss of fat cells, and the alteration of the content of different types of body fat.

This new evidence completely supports what I have been saying all along: The brain is the absolute key to weight loss. When you can increase your brain function, you are literally turning your existing metabolism into a fireball. At the same time, better brain functioning is at the core of neurogenesis, which assists at shrinking your existing body fat. As your brain remodels, your figure remodels.

The twenty-first century has given doctors like me the ability to thoroughly examine the entire body with computers, and we are now able to identify the external markers that are signaling internal health problems. The signs were right in front of us, but now science is confirming what we could only previously hypothesize: Belly fat predicts heart disease,[2] dense breast tissue signals a higher risk for breast cancer,[3] ear creases frequently correlate to a predisposition for heart attacks,[4] and balding men often have prostate problems.[5]

Computers have been integral in helping us unlock the mysteries of the brain. Based on the findings of brain imagery, we can confidently say that the brain controls your carb binging, salt binging, sugar binging, and late night binging. These issues aren't caused from problems with digestion (stomach), cardiovascular health (heart), or a polluted body filled with toxins (liver).

My private medical practice is called PATH Medical—the Place for Achieving Total Health. I like to think of it as Eastern philosophy meeting Western technology. At PATH, we make a definitive diagnosis by starting with a thorough examination of the brain. We consider the whole body when formulating a treatment plan. We use every proven conventional and alternative treatment protocol. I'm proud to say that

Brain Diagnostics 101

Brain electrical activity, which results from chemical reactions, is now easy to assess with quantitative electro-encephalography (QEEG) and is part of brain mapping.

my PATH medical office is considered one of the foremost practices in integrative medicine—the combination of conventional, alternative, and holistic therapies recognized as the new medical paradigm for the twenty-first century.

In my office, I can accurately map the brain, and show my patients their production and expression of brain chemicals, through the use of brain electrical activity mapping, a system known as BEAM™. First developed by researchers at Harvard Medical School in the 1980s, this computer-based technique measures the brain's electrical activity. BEAM technology and research is at the forefront of medical science. Without it, we would not have the data to conclude that obesity is a brain chemical disorder. Because of BEAM, I was able to create the Younger (Thinner) You plan that finally treats excess weight and obesity correctly.

BEAM technology allows us observe the brain at work. This testing assesses electrical transmissions in the brain by measuring the four individual brain waves. It then provides a status report of your power, or metabolism (dopamine); your brain speed (acetylcholine); your rhythm

BEAM Is the Future

Today, there are just a handful of forward-thinking doctors like me who incorporate BEAM into everyday medicine. Yet more and more doctors across the country are starting to use this technology. It's my hope that someday soon everyone will have a BEAM that lights their path to a younger you.

(GABA); and your balance (serotonin). The electrical impulses are converted into pictures showing colored bursts that represent actual brain transmissions: When your brain is in harmony, the image is like a full-spectrum rainbow. From these pictures we can make intelligent decisions about which of the four primary brain chemicals need to be addressed, and then can accurately assess the effectiveness of our treatments.

I believe BEAM testing should be part of every person's comprehensive medical care. It's easy to administer, and takes only about an hour to complete. During the testing you are seated in a comfortable lounge chair, and a cap, similar to a bathing cap, is placed on your head. Electrodes are attached to the cap and connected to a

Your Weight Can Shorten Your Life

If you are obese by age 40, you are shortening your life expectancy by as many as seven years. If you are obese and smoke, deduct fourteen years.[6]

computer via a special interface. At different times during the test you are asked either to rest with your eyes closed or to concentrate on something while a light is flashed or a sound is introduced. You will not feel a thing during the entire test, and there are no side effects.

YOUR CURRENT HEALTH MATTERS

Even with all of the latest technologies, every experienced doctor must first rely on patient information to assess physical conditions. Because not everyone has access to my medical office or BEAM technology, I have developed a simple test that you can take in the privacy of your own home that can also help to identify brain chemical deficiencies. The Younger (Thinner) You Diet Quiz takes just a few minutes to complete.

Blood work as well as additional testing performed at a doctor's office can easily confirm your findings and is recommended once you have taken this quiz. While this book is an important first step, I urge you to seek the care of a physician in terms of making conclusive decisions about your health and weight loss goals. Before you begin the program, make sure to have a full physical with your current physician. Your weight may be a signal there are other medical issues that need to be dealt with. It's not just the added pounds slowing you down:

Weight gain contributes to, and is a sign for, many of the most common medical illnesses, most of which are aging you prematurely.

THE YOUNGER (THINNER) YOU DIET QUIZ

This simple quiz can help you identify your own brain chemical issues that are exacerbating your weight problems. First, you'll be able to determine which of your brain chemicals are deficient, and directly affecting your ability to lose weight. Then, we'll determine how much weight you need to lose. Together, you'll have the information you need to tailor the program specifically to your unique needs.

Define Your Deficiency

Answer each question by circling either T for true or F for false. At the end of each group, record only the total number of True statements in the space provided.

These questions relate to how you feel about the foods you eat as well as your current emotional state. Answer the questions in terms of how you feel most of the time. For example, if you've had a bad night's sleep and feel tired today, answer the questions that pertain to your energy levels based on how you feel on average, not just today.

DOPAMINE

1. At parties I can't control my eating. T/F

2. Caffeinated drinks, like coffee, tea, or sodas,
   put me in a better mood. T/F

3. I am a smoker. T/F

4. I am a very domineering individual. T/F

5. I am eccentric and do things differently than others. T/F

6. I am self-centered. T/F

7. I am very hard on myself. T/F

8. I bloat easily after eating. T/F

9. I crave sugar. T/F

10. I drink more than three alcoholic beverages per week. T/F

11. I eat alone. T/F

12. I eat my lunch while I'm working. T/F

13. I eat only to re-energize my body. T/F

14. I find exercise invigorating. T/F

15. I get easily depressed or blue. T/F

16. I have a temper. T/F

17. I have gained more than 20 pounds since I was 20 years old. T/F

18. I have no energy to exercise. T/F

19. I have trouble getting out of bed in the morning. T/F

20. I know I need to exercise, but I always seem to put it off. T/F

21. I need to have at least one cup of coffee to
    jump-start me in the morning. T/F

22. I overeat when I am stressed. T/F

23. I sometimes experience total exhaustion
    without even exerting myself. T/F

24. I tend to be a loner. T/F

25. I'm hard on myself but I'm harder on my friends and family. T/F

Total # of T responses: _____

ACETYLCHOLINE

1.	Cheese is a large part of my diet.	T / F
2.	I am a person who can't get enough new ideas or experiences.	T / F
3.	I am detail oriented.	T / F
4.	I am flirtatious.	T / F
5.	I can't get enough new drugs or new places.	T / F
6.	I crave fatty foods.	T / F
7.	I don't exercise anymore.	T / F
8.	I eat lots of low-calorie foods, like fresh fruits and vegetables.	T / F
9.	I experience mood swings.	T / F
10.	I find it more comfortable to do things alone rather than in a large group.	T / F
11.	I have had an eating disorder at some point in my life.	T / F
12.	I have lost muscle tone.	T / F
13.	I have tried many alternative remedies.	T / F
14.	I lack imagination.	T / F
15.	I like to talk about what's bothering me.	T / F
16.	I like to try new foods and cuisines.	T / F
17.	I love yoga and stretching my muscles.	T / F
18.	I need a lot of love and nurturing.	T / F
19.	I often feel agitated.	T / F
20.	I tend to see myself in a desirable light.	T / F
21.	Losing weight is a priority for me.	T / F
22.	Lunch or dinner is usually accompanied by at least one glass of wine.	T / F
23.	Some people say I have my head in the clouds.	T / F
24.	Sometimes, by the end of the day, I don't remember what I've eaten.	T / F
25.	When I eat, I love to experience the aromas and the beauty of food.	T / F

Total # of T responses: _____

GABA

1. Caffeine has little effect on me.		T / F
2. Cooking is one way I take care of my family/loved ones.		T / F
3. Dinner is not complete without dessert.		T / F
4. I can create strong, lasting bonds with others.		T / F
5. I can sense that others want to hurt me.		T / F
6. I choose the same things to eat all the time.		T / F
7. I crave bitter foods.		T / F
8. I don't have specific food cravings.		T / F
9. I embarrass easily.		T / F
10. I frequently drink too much.		T / F
11. I have experimented with drugs.		T / F
12. I have fits of rage.		T / F
13. I like yoga because it helps me relax.		T / F
14. I lose my temper easily.		T / F
15. I love to try new things.		T / F
16. I need a lot of food to fill me up.		T / F
17. I often feel fatigued even when I have had a good night's sleep.		T / F
18. I overeat.		T / F
19. I share too much personal information about my life with others.		T / F
20. I eat my meals quickly.		T / F
21. I tend to worry more than I used to.		T / F
22. I'm nervous and jumpy.		T / F
23. I'm afraid of confrontations and altercations.		T / F
24. My thoughts get too confused.		T / F
25. When I make a decision, it's permanent.		T / F

Total # of T responses: _____

SEROTONIN

1. Eating is one of the main ways that I socialize with others. T/F

2. I am a deep-feeling person. T/F

3. I am easily irritated. T/F

4. I am extremely suspicious. T/F

5. I am very artistic. T/F

6. I believe my ideas are superior. T/F

7. I can easily take advantage of others. T/F

8. I can't find meaning in life. T/F

9. I can't relax. T/F

10. I crave carbohydrates. T/F

11. I crave salt. T/F

12. I don't do the activities I used to enjoy. T/F

13. I drain myself giving to others but then fill myself with food. T/F

14. I engage in daring activities such as skydiving, motorcycle riding, and so forth. T/F

15. I've had thoughts of self-destruction or suicide. T/F

16. I find myself thinking about the same things over and over again. T/F

17. I have little energy to exercise. T/F

18. I have many frivolous relationships. T/F

19. I just like to "eat, drink, and be merry." T/F

20. I need an alcoholic drink in order to get a good night's sleep. T/F

21. I need to eat right before going to bed. T/F

22. I rarely stick to a plan or agenda. T/F

23. I usually grab a quick meal on the run. T/F

24. I'm never very hungry, although sometimes I find myself eating more than I should. T/F

25. I'm not as strong as I used to be. T/F

Total # of T responses: _____

RESULTS

Total T Responses: Dopamine Deficiency ____

Total T Responses: Acetylcholine Deficiency ____

Total T Responses: GABA Deficiency ____

Total T Responses: Serotonin Deficiency ____

Assessing Your Results

Circle the highest number. This is your greatest deficiency and is the one most likely to cause your issues with weight control. Any deficiency needs to be adjusted in order to achieve both weight loss and optimal health. Any category with between 1 and 2 true statements is considered a minor deficiency. Any category with between 6 and 8 true statements is considered a moderate deficiency. If you have more than 9 true statements in any one category, it is considered a major deficiency.

Frequently Asked Questions

How does a True–False test reveal brain chemistry?

Your answers to the questions in the Younger (Thinner) You Diet Quiz reveal your thoughts about food and your emotional state. These thoughts and feelings directly represent how your brain is operating, and your brain chemistry. For example, when you have plenty of dopamine, you'll have lots of physical energy, mental energy, intense motivation, quick thinking and mental processing speed, and an ability to fight off cravings. You will not be looking to self-medicate with foods to improve your alertness. However, when you are lacking in all or some of these abilities and behaviors (as the questions in this test asked you), then we have discovered that you most likely have a dopamine deficiency.

Why are there so many questions about my personality?

Besides regulating your health and weight, brain chemistry also governs your personality. Too much or too little of any one chemical can dominate your personality type and emotional state. And because eating is so closely linked to our emotional life, these two areas need to be fully explored to resolve your particular issue. Often I find that when I can balance a person's brain chemistry, their emotions can be stabilized along with their weight. They end up getting their health under control, too, which makes them feel happier about every aspect of their life.

In the next four chapters we'll look more closely at specific personality patterns that are directly linked to deficiencies in each of the different brain chemicals, and how they play out in terms of eating. You'll find that once you balance your brain chemistry, your emotional life will become more balanced.

What happens if I have multiple deficiencies?

Excess weight, like most health conditions, can usually be traced to more than one chemical deficiency. If you've had problems with your weight all your life, it's very likely you are experiencing a dopamine deficiency as well as others. Treatment therefore must address multiple chemical imbalances. If you are showing moderate or major deficiencies in multiple categories, make sure to review each of the next four chapters to get a full picture of your current health. You can incorporate the specific recommendations for treating each brain chemical deficiency at the same time, tailoring the Younger (Thinner) You Diet to get the results you need.

When should I take the quiz again?

I recommend you retake the test whenever you feel markedly different for a week or more, make a major change to your vitamin/medication program, and after every ten pounds you lose. By retaking the test often, and tailoring your diet to the results, you will be able to keep your brain chemistry in perfect balance so that you can continue to lose weight, and then maintain your new younger body once you reach your goal weight.

Determine How Much You Can Lose

When you eat Younger (Thinner) You foods in the right portions, you are learning to correctly feed both your body and your brain. By doing so, you will lose weight, as many as 20–40 pounds in 40 days. This is especially true if you currently weigh more than 300 pounds. The average person who is about 50 pounds overweight will be able to lose 20 pounds in 40 days.

Realistic weight loss goals depend on several factors, including your current metabolism, your physical activity level, and how much weight you need to lose. Typically, I recommend that weight loss should be a steady process. By following the Younger (Thinner) You Diet, you can expect to lose a healthy 2-3 pounds per week.

A conservative, initial goal for weight loss should be to reduce body weight by about 10% of your current baseline. So if you weigh 150 pounds, let's focus on losing the first 15 pounds, then reassess what your next goal should be.

Am I Overweight or Obese?

Results from the 2003 to 2004 National Health and Nutrition Examination Survey (NHANES) indicate that an estimated 66% of U.S. adults are either overweight or obese.[7] While the word "obese" often conjures images of individuals in the 300-plus-pound category; this is not always the case. In fact, many of us can be considered obese without even knowing it.

The clinical definition of obesity is a person whose body mass index (BMI)[8] is greater than 30. BMI is a statistical measure of the weight of a person scaled according to height and closely correlates with excess adipose tissue. Anything higher than 40 is considered extremely obese, which means your weight will likely kill you.

Your ultimate goal should match your BMI range with a healthy waist circumference, which is less than 40 inches for men and 35 inches for women.[9]

To determine how much weight you should lose, you'll need to weigh yourself on a traditional scale, and figure out your total body fat percentage. Normal body fat percentage for men should be 8% to 18% and for women, 16% to 25%.

There are numerous ways to measure the amount of body fat you have. Some of the more popular testing methods include body mass index (BMI), dual-energy X-ray absorptiometry (DEXA), waist-to-hip ratio, skin fold measurement, and hydrostatic weighing (underwater weighing).

DEXA Scan

A far more effective method of determining body fat percentage is by using dual-energy X-ray absorptiometry, more commonly known as a DEXA (or DXA) scan. The DEXA outshines standard BMI charts and formulas and virtually all other methods of weight measurement. Only DEXA can accurately identify your true percentage of body fat.

DEXA involves two different low-dose X-rays and a body scanner that reads bone and soft-tissue mass. This machine is most commonly used by doctors to assess bone mineral density when testing for osteoporosis. The scan itself is like a full body X-ray that lasts about ten minutes. Many hospitals have DEXA scans; we have one in our PATH medical offices. You might also be able to locate one of these machines at a specialized weight loss center.

Many times women come into my office for a DEXA scan, and then are surprised at how much body fat they actually are carrying. For example, if a woman is 5' 3" and weighs 160 pounds, she may realize that she is roughly 45 pounds overweight. But in terms of body fat percentage, it really means that she is carrying as many as 55 extra pounds of body fat. It's not just her weight

The BMI Scale

Your personal BMI may be accurately calculated using the following formula:

$$BMI = 703 \times \frac{weight\ (lbs)}{height^2\ (in^2)}$$

that will have to change in order for this woman to feel younger. What she'll really need to do is add 20 pounds of muscle and lose the 55 pounds of body fat, for a net loss of 45 pounds. Then she'll feel that she has the right amount of body fat for her frame.

Even if we have been relatively good to our bodies by following a healthy diet and exercising, the aging process alone changes our body composition. As we get older, we automatically lose a large amount of muscle mass and replace it with fat. Our job now is to regain our muscle mass, because without it, our metabolism can't burn efficiently all day long. Just like growing new brain cells stimulates metabolism, increasing muscle mass is another important stimulus. So the hidden lesson in knowing your body fat percentage is also learning how much muscle you need in order to reignite your aging metabolism. You'll be able to add muscle by following the diet and exercise suggestions, and by taking basic supplements. The following list of medications, bioidentical hormones, and nutrients have all been shown to add muscle to some degree:

- Growth hormone
- Forteo (which builds bones)
- 7 Keto DHEA
- Tribulus: an herb
- Pregnenolone
- DHEA Sulfate

Skin Fold Testing

On the other end of the spectrum of tests for obesity is the classic skin fold test, which

A *Star Trek* Physical

I use BEAM testing as part of my standard evaluation for everyone who walks into my office. It's part of what I call my Star Trek physical. Instead of relying on my hands, I let the many advances of science give me the most accurate diagnoses. I also use DEXA scans to measure body fat, along with ultrasounds, EKGs, and other advanced diagnostic tools to help me develop the most accurate treatments for each patient.

uses an old-fashioned set of calipers to measure your body fat. A caliper is a handheld instrument that gently squeezes your body fat in various places to determine the thickness, or density, of the fat under your skin. This test can be done at the gym or at a doctor's office. However, the results are only as good as the tester. The test requires someone else to do the measuring. The measurements are then plugged into an equation to determine your body fat percentage.

Bioelectrical Impedance

This is a fancy bathroom scale that can be purchased at home goods stores. However, it can be even less accurate than calipers. It is supposed to provide your current weight as well as determine your body fat percentage.

What's Wrong with BMI?

BMI fails to take into account many other factors in total weight, such as muscle mass. So according to standard BMI charts, a good number of professional athletes would have a high percentage of body fat and would therefore be classified as obese, which of course isn't the case.

Healthy Habits

As you begin to follow the program, you'll find it natural to have spices on your table, to drink plenty of water throughout the day, to load up on herbal teas, and to say no to the foods that cause you to gain weight. Each one of these steps will make your brain metabolism more youthful.

It does this by sending a mild electrical current (which you do not feel) through your body up through the soles of your feet, and measuring the time it takes the current to make the trip upward. The water and lean tissue, such as muscle, in your body are better conductors of this current than fat, so the more fat you have, the slower the current will travel.

SELF-HELP REQUIRES MORE THAN YOU

You'll get the best results and reap the most benefits from the Younger (Thinner) You Diet program if you create a support team. Your physician, physician's assistants, personal trainer, dietician, friends, and family can all help you on your path to permanent weight loss. Tell everyone you know about the details of this diet, and make sure they buy into the ideas and directions you'll be following.

Exploring your spiritual self is another important way for you to increase your support team. It is empowering, and strengthens your mind and personal connections, so you are more equipped to deal with the changes that are going to happen with your body. Consider becoming more involved with your religious institution or developing your spirituality on your own through personal exercises like meditation, chants, or prayer.

ON THE OTHER HAND, WEIGHT LOSS STARTS FROM WITHIN

Brain chemistry may be the culprit behind some of your worst eating habits. But in order for you to lose weight, you'll also need to take responsibility for your actions and become more honest with yourself. You will get better

Moderating Pregnancy Weight Gain

While it's important to gain weight consistently during pregnancy, make sure your doctor is monitoring your monthly increases. Seven categories of infant birth defects have been linked to pregnancy-related obesity. These include abnormal penile openings, limb reduction defects, diaphragmatic hernia, omphalocele hernia (hernia of the belly button), spina bifida, abnormal spines, cleft palate, cleft lip, and gastroschises (advanced intestinal failure).[10] The Younger (Thinner) You Diet is safe for pregnant women to follow because it allows for a balanced approach to nutrition that is high in vitamins and nutrients. Discuss this with your doctor before starting any weight loss program, especially if you are pregnant.

results from this diet if you can change your eating habits as well as address personal limitations that may be holding you back.

There are various personality patterns that lead to certain types of behaviors: Each is directly linked to specific brain chemical deficiencies, and fully discussed in the next four chapters. If you can analyze your behaviors and your thoughts, you will unblock major life obstacles that not only affect your relationship to food, but extend to the way you conduct yourself in everyday life. You

Meet Sarah M.: Young Body, Old Brain

Sarah first came to me when she was 33 and miserable. She weighed 155 pounds, which was a lot of weight for her to carry on a 5' 5" frame. She told me, "I'm so unhappy with how I look. I get anxious every time I walk into a room, because I know people are staring at me. I feel old, even though I should be in the prime of my life. I need to make a change, fast."

Sarah told me that for years she'd been counting on the rush from carbohydrates, salt, and sugar when she felt she wasn't as sharp as she should be. Sarah's BMI was an unhealthy 26. Her girth and her complaints made me think she probably had a brain metabolism imbalance, so I suggested a BEAM mapping. The BEAM results proved me correct. I showed Sarah her test results. What's great about BEAM testing is that the results are clear for interpretation. Each of the brain chemicals appears on a computer screen in different colors, and a physician can compare a balanced brain photo to each patient's particular BEAM results. So it was easy for me to show Sarah that her sluggishness and weight gain was due to a dopamine deficiency, because the area that should have shown lots of dopamine was coming up blank. What's more, Sarah's GABA was also out of balance, which was why she felt lethargic and anxious.

Sarah's personal prescription was easy to determine: we needed to increase her metabolism and decrease her appetite. I started Sarah on the Younger (Thinner) You Diet, heavily emphasizing to her the importance of drinking as many as five cups of tea—either caffeinated or decaffeinated—throughout the day. She also started taking dopamine-enhancing supplements, including thiamine, tyrosine, phenylalanine, and chromium, which would help balance her GABA and keep her on an even keel.

Months later, Sarah came back to my office. She has gone from 34% body fat to 21%, and maintains a healthy weight of 135 pounds. She has a new lease on life. Today Sarah is healthy and active, and feels like she should: 33 and thriving!

might need to eliminate certain behaviors, thoughts, or even people around you who are negatively affecting you in order to lose the weight you want.

Answer these questions as honestly as you can:

● What are your food triggers, and what is your typical response?

● Can you eliminate the triggers, or must you rely on modifying your behaviors?

● Are there other issues that may be contributing to your current weight?

● Is eating the only way you deal with anxiety, or do you have other "nervous habits"?

● Were you ever overweight during childhood?

● Were you ever overweight or obese in the past, even if you aren't now?

● Have you ever lost or gained a significant amount of weight (at least ten pounds) in a short time period (at most two months) with no apparent lifestyle or diet change?

● Does your weight tend to fluctuate?

● Does the media affect your desire to eat? If so, how? Which actions or behaviors trigger your desire to eat?

LET'S GET STARTED

In the next four chapters we will examine each of the brain chemicals more closely. You will be able to see how the results from this quiz can be addressed by personalizing the Younger (Thinner) You Diet. You'll learn to augment your deficiencies naturally with foods you'll eat every day. My program of teas, herbs, and spices are natural ways to supplement specific nutrients, so make sure to follow those directions throughout the course of the diet. If you have a major deficiency, you might want to consider supplementing your diet with nutrients, or talking to your physician about particular brain chemistry enhancing medications or natural hormones.

Regardless of your greatest deficiency, start by reading Chapter 3. Even if you have other brain chemicals that are more out of

Losing Weight Can Be Contagious

An important new study was published in the *New England Journal of Medicine* in July, 2007, which proved that individuals were more likely to become obese when their friends became obese. One explanation to these findings is that weight gain is perceptive to all, and accepted by many.[11,12] When we see our friends put on a few pounds, we might think that it's acceptable to do the same. This may be one reason why obesity has reached epidemic proportions in the United States. As individuals gain weight their friends do as well, doubling and tripling the numbers of obese citizens.

One great dieting tip has always been to diet with a buddy, and this research proves its point. If you have friends who are overweight, get them to try the Younger (Thinner) You Diet, too, and see if everyone you know can turn back the clock and become younger.

balance, I can guarantee you'll get the best results from the diet if you incorporate the lessons regarding a dopamine deficiency. Each

your cravings change, retake the Younger (Thinner) You Diet Quiz again to confirm your thoughts. Then, switch to the plan that focuses on eliminating any new cravings.

Once you begin to balance your brain, you will automatically feel younger. Your brain will be working optimally, and you may experience better moods, better memory retention, and even better sleep. When you are thinking more clearly, and feeling refreshed, as well as better about yourself, you will have a much better attitude toward sticking with the Younger (Thinner) You Diet and finally losing the weight you want.

CHAPTER 3

Get Thin Faster with Dopamine

WITHOUT DOPAMINE, your body and your brain will lose its spark. You'll feel tired all the time, or just plain burned out. Worse, because you are low on energy, the fuel you are taking in as food is not getting metabolized efficiently, so it's just sitting around, accumulating as body fat. If these symptoms describe how you are looking or feeling right now, it is very likely that you have a dopamine deficiency.

A dopamine deficiency can be caused by genetics, illness, aging, or previous weight gain. But in reality, it doesn't matter what the culprit was, because the fix is the same.

The first step to becoming younger and thinner is to enhance your dopamine levels to restore your natural energy. By doing so, not only will you have an increase in your stamina, you'll also see that your excess weight will start falling off your body. I call reaching this high dopamine level the Weight Loss Zone, and I'll show you exactly how to get there.

When you are not in the Weight Loss Zone, and you are low in dopamine, three important changes occur in your brain and body. Each of them has the potential to directly affect your ability to lose weight:

How Much Dopamine Do I Need?

Your four main brain chemicals need to be at a perfect balance that's just right for you, and only you. It's like the story of "Goldilocks and the Three Bears": This chick wasn't happy until she had a chair, a bed, and a bowl of porridge that was *just right* for her. The other chairs, beds, and bowls just wouldn't do.

You'll know when you are producing enough dopamine because you will feel great all the time. In fact, you'll feel younger than you have in years. You will have tons of energy and feel mentally alert. If you aren't producing enough dopamine, then I need to teach you how to enhance your levels, either by creating more dopamine through the Younger (Thinner) You Diet, or by supplementing with medication or natural hormones.

- You start the cycle of food addiction in an attempt to keep your energy up.
- The hormone cortisol is triggered to supplement your waning energy supply, leading to weight gain—especially belly fat. Swollen shoulders (picture a woman with a classic "buffalo hump") and swollen face can also occur with excessive cortisol production.
- Your metabolism slows drastically, and you are no longer properly burning the foods you eat.

THE REAL DEAL ON FOOD ADDICTION

Food addiction is no different than any other type of addiction, including illegal or prescription drugs, cigarette smoking, or drinking. They are all compulsions that are linked to the same underlying disorder: a brain chemical imbalance. In order to treat any of these addictions, you need to rebalance your brain chemistry, remove the addictive substance, and *retrain* the brain to function properly.

All of us are vulnerable to the addiction cycle when there is a loss of dopamine. In fact, my original research team, which included Dr. Kenneth Blum, and Dr. Ernest Noble, the former head of the National Institute on Alcoholism, in connection with Dr. Nora Volkow, showed that dopamine genetics predicts a very high predisposition for various addictions. As I mentioned in chapter 1, personality types are also shaped by brain chemistry. This is why it appears that a person may have an "addictive personality." However, it's not your personality that's making you gain weight. The bottom line is that your health, your personality, and your ability to gain or lose weight all begin with the brain, and aberrations in brain chemistry.

To understand how food addictions can manifest, let's start with a healthy individual who has healthy brain chemistry—meaning plenty of dopamine. Dopamine works like a natural amphetamine, giving us power and controlling our energy. High levels of this brain chemical also help keep us focused. When you see a person you are strongly attracted to, your dopamine production will spike. The same will happen if you are hungry and smell food. Whenever you eat, your dopamine levels increase, which makes you feel really good. For those of us with balanced brains, that "dopamine rush" is recognized as satiety or *satisfaction*. If you can recognize satiety, you're already in the dopamine Weight Loss Zone.

However, when people who are low in dopamine eat, they don't feel full or satisfied as quickly, and when they do, they interpret the dopamine rush as a euphoric experience, instead of an everyday feeling. The low-dopamine person needs more food, or more stimuli to achieve what others would consider to be a "normal" level of satisfaction. And, because they are so turned on by this euphoric sensation, they will seek to replicate the experience over and over again by eating more and more food. This quest for the dopamine rush creates a food addiction.

Any addictive brain seeks the dopamine rush in the form of treasures, or rewards. The specific reward will depend on your personality and what gives you the greatest high. For some, the dopamine rush can come from illegal drugs, sexual encounters, or from something as ethereal as romance. Food is no different; it's just a more fattening reward.

The catch is that the brain and body can't sustain constant euphoria. Instead, it strives to reach homeostasis, or balance. So each time we eat, the brain naturally releases less dopamine, which will disappoint even the most ardent food addict. When this happens, the euphoric feeling won't come back at all, yet low-dopamine people will still continue to eat in the hopes of it returning. In order to break this cycle, low-dopamine people need to be able to increase their dopamine in a more balanced approach, so that food does not become their only source of happiness.

Unbalanced dopamine levels can also create a craving scenario—which occurs when you are consumed with the expectation for a reward. My research into this relationship is along similar lines to what Dr. Nora Volkow has published. Recently, her study, published in the *Journal of Neuroscience*, showed the relationship between dopamine and cocaine use. She used brain scanning to look at the dopamine expressions in eighteen cocaine addicts. When these participants were shown a video of other people using cocaine, their dopamine levels increased: These people achieved a craving and were stimulated enough to produce an increased level of dopamine just from watching the video.[1,2] Their addicted brains didn't need the substance to feel the dopamine rush: They were able to produce it themselves.

The same can be said of food addiction. If your dopamine brain is damaged, it won't matter if you have eaten or not. Once a food trigger is introduced, such as a visual stimulus, you will produce low levels of dopamine, and you'll never feel satisfied after eating. Worse, without the proper levels of dopamine, your metabolism slows down anyway, so all the extra food you eat

Experts Agree that Dopamine Deficiencies Lead to Addiction

Dr. Nora Volkow, head of the National Institute on Drug Abuse, confirms my analysis (as discovered with my colleague, Dr. Kenneth Blum) on the brain dopamine system as the key to addictive behavior. Dr. Volkow reports, "Since eating, like the use of addictive drugs is a highly reinforcing behavior, inducing feelings of gratification and pleasure, we suspect that obese people might have abnormalities in brain dopamine activity. Impaired function of the brain dopamine system could make some people more vulnerable to compulsive eating, which could lead to morbid obesity."[3,4]

is processed at a slower rate, leading to more weight gain.[5]

At the same time, if your dopamine level is low, your brain is also creating fewer dopamine receptors. These receptors act like a baseball glove, catching dopamine as it is fired from the brain, and then transmitting the feeling of excitement that connects dopamine to the rest of the body. When the receptor catches dopamine, it transmits the feeling of happiness to the global brain. These receptors modulate the brain's reward system. When you eat low-nutrient foods that don't produce dopamine, it becomes harder for these receptors to transfer a feeling of reward after eating, so you eat more and more junky foods in search of this reward. The ability to receive stimulus from bad foods decreases as the receptors become more inefficient. Ultimately, the receptors break down completely because of your bad food choices.

Studies I have been involved with indicate that people with few dopamine receptors experience a less intense reward signal, causing them to overindulge in order to feel satisfied. So, if you are low in dopamine, the rest of your brain is less likely to respond with excitement every time you eat a piece of chocolate cake. Instead, the brain will need larger amounts of food to feel rewarded.

We've also discovered obese individuals have lower levels of dopamine receptors than those who are not obese. Interestingly, within a range of obese individuals, the number of dopamine receptors will decrease as the individual gets larger.[6,7] So the heavier you are, the fewer dopamine receptors you are likely to have, which will make you want to eat more.

THE FOOD ADDICTION FIX

Recognizing that food addiction is a true brain disorder completely changes the way we look at obesity. The medical community has finally realized what I have been saying all along, that the brain is affected by food consumption in much the same way it is affected by alcohol and recreational drugs. When a person consumes food in a way that becomes detrimental to his or her health, and when what he or she consumes has the potential for bodily harm, he or she is considered an addict. This person has become reliant upon food to meet both physiological as well as psychological needs.

However, food addictions can be reversed when you balance your brain. That's what the Younger (Thinner) You Diet is all about. First you'll change your brain chemistry by choosing foods that support higher dopamine levels. Then you'll learn to trade in your carb reliance for better, healthier food options that will give you real energy instead of a quick fix. You'll retrain your brain to increase your metabolism through fat-burning, muscle-building exercise as well as diet. By doing so, you'll be free of food addictions once and for all.

FOOD ADDICTION AND YOUR PERSONALITY

When your dopamine levels are balanced, you've got plenty of energy, your day is organized, and you seem to get along with everyone. But when dopamine is low it affects your emotional stability. You may begin to lack the energy to socialize and no longer desire to feel love or joy. In fact, you may be having a hard time feeling much of anything, including sadness, desire, or rage. You might believe you are becoming alienated from the rest of the world, and as a result avoid interacting with others. You may have trouble asking people for help

Low Dopamine Personality Traits

EMOTION/ACTION	WHAT IT MEANS:
Eccentric	• Acts silly or aloof; rarely smiles or nods • No close friends (or only one) outside of family • Unkempt appearance • Suspicious or paranoid • Social anxiety • Odd beliefs or magical thinking (i.e. superstitious, belief in telepathy or sixth sense)
Loner	• No close friends (or only one) outside of family • Indifferent to praise and criticism • Little or no desire for sex • Avoids close relationships, including family • Prefers to be alone • Claims to rarely experience anger • Doesn't care about other people's feelings
Procrastinator	• Puts things off, misses deadlines • Does a bad job on tasks they don't want to do • Complains that others are making unreasonable demands • "Forgets" obligations • Sulks or becomes irritable when asked to do something they don't want to do • Thinks they are doing a much better job than others think they are doing • Resents suggestions of others • Is critical or scornful of persons in authority
Masochist	• Remains in abusive relationships • Rejects help to avoid being a burden • Feels unappreciated and complains about it • Feels undeserving • Pessimistic • Obsesses over worst features and ignores positive features • Sabotages one's own goals • Turns down opportunities for pleasure

because you don't feel worthy. You eat because you're alone, bored, disorganized, and can't establish boundaries. Food becomes a trusted friend and provides comfort.

This pattern is typical of introverted individuals as well as passive-aggressive types. These personality traits are typically common for those who are low on dopamine: They feel negative toward themselves, have trouble building or maintaining relationships, and have difficulty communicating. Loners, eccentrics, shy individuals, procrastinators, those that are codependent, masochists, and obsessive-compulsives are frequently deficient in dopamine.

Once your dopamine levels are restored, not only will you be able to lose weight, you will no longer need to turn to food instead of friendship. These negative traits often lessen—and even vanish—when your brain chemistry is repaired.

THE CORTISOL EQUATION: LOW DOPAMINE = BIG BELLY FAT

For every brain chemical that becomes deficient, a hormone usually takes its place. In the case of dopamine, the body naturally increases production of the hormone cortisol when there is a dopamine imbalance.[8] Cortisol is the backup energy hormone: it provides us with additional power so the brain and body can continue to function without the right levels of dopamine. Cortisol is also released when you are under stress, whether or not your dopamine is low. In fact, when you are stressed, you naturally burn more dopamine, which is why the cortisol is released.

While cortisol can be plenty helpful, I call it the obesity hormone. Even though it effectively keeps your brain running, it does not improve dopamine levels.[9] It actually forces your metabolism to slow down, adding insult to injury. This happens because when brain energy falters (low dopamine), the body is forced to send up to the brain its reserve units to pick up the slack, in the form of steroid hormones (cortisol) from the adrenal glands. The cortisol increases the effectiveness of catecholamines like adrenaline and creates the necessary energy, while conveying a feeling of happiness. However, this dopamine substitute is supposed to be a temporary safety mechanism. But when your brain is continually turning to cortisol for energy, it becomes a way of life. Then, excess cortisol is released, you get puffy, round-faced, your blood pressure rises, and your appetite increases. Worse, excess cortisol also causes bloating and weight gain, especially around your midsection.

It has been linked as a direct cause of belly fat in both men and women: It causes fat to be deposited in the abdominal area where there are the most cortisol receptors. So if you are a "high energy" individual but are stuck with an apple body shape, chances are your cortisol levels, instead of your

Meet Lauren T.: Diary of a Food Addict

Lauren T. was 28 when she first came to my office. She stood 5' 7" and weighed close to 270 pounds. Lauren's body scan showed she had a 42% body fat, which is considered extremely obese. Her blood pressure was elevated, and blood sugars showed she was prediabetic. She was clearly in denial about her food addiction, but that began to change when I asked her to keep a food diary for a week before she came to see me for our next appointment.

Initially she said to me, "I've tried every diet imaginable. I exercise, though not as much as I should. I have a small appetite but I can't seem to lose any weight." When I asked her what a typical day's food was like, she shrugged. "I usually skip breakfast. Lunch is maybe a light salad from the deli."

That "salad" turned out to be anything but light. Lauren wrote down in her food diary that her "salad" often consisted of a plate spilling over with pasta salads loaded with mayonnaise, and hot foods like fried chicken and barbecued ribs. Even when she filled her plate with greens, she often doused them with salad dressings that were loaded with fat and sugar. Her daily salad was weighing her down. Lauren discovered that she was creating a vicious cycle every time she sat down for lunch. Her excessive carb-laden meals often led to overeating at lunch and the desire to continuously consume even more unhealthy carbs throughout the day. When I pointed this out to her, Lauren realized she was not only addicted to food, but was thwarting her own attempts to lose weight.

I started her on the Younger (Thinner) You Diet, and taught Lauren how to increase her dopamine levels simply by choosing foods that were the building blocks to this brain chemical. Once she was making better food choices, Lauren was also able to control the quantity of foods she was eating and end her food addiction. I also showed Lauren how to eat slowly, savoring every bite. Eating slowly allows the dopamine satiety signals to reach the brain before overeating occurs, which trains the brain to need less food to feel satisfied.

Within two weeks, Lauren started dropping weight. Adding breakfast to her day gave her the nutrients and energy she needed to start right. Eating protein at breakfast filled her until lunch, so she was able to avoid sugary midmorning indulgences. Within a month, Lauren no longer had food cravings, and the pounds continued to melt away.

dopamine, are supporting your body's energy needs.[10]

A big belly is also an indicator that you are at high risk for metabolic syndrome, which you'll learn more about later in the book. When you see someone with a big belly, think of brain burnout. It is often accompanied by a poor attention span, poor sleep patterns and attention deficit problems.

Cortisol also boosts adrenaline, which can make you feel restless: When your adrenaline is pumping, you might be anxious during the day and not able to sleep at night. These two factors also contribute to weight gain: Your anxiety causes you to self medicate with "comfort foods," and a lack of sleep prevents your brain from resetting its other chemicals to the right levels. Eight or nine hours of restful sleep are crucial for weight loss because proper amounts of sleep increase your metabolism and lower cortisol levels.[11,12]

Reducing Stress Naturally Increases Dopamine

I'm the father of five kids, so believe me, I know stress. I also know how difficult it can be to reduce stress. For me, I've found that exercise is a great stress-reduction technique. And, it also helps increase my levels of dopamine, giving me the extra energy I need to keep up with my family.

I know it's hard to fit exercise into everyone's busy schedule, but it *is* doable, and it should be a mandatory part of your day. Even fifteen minutes a day can make a profound difference. Best of all, exercise increases your metabolism, so you'll lose weight as you de-stress.

Just like food addiction, this low-dopamine problem can be reversed. By increasing dopamine, your body will no longer rely on cortisol to support its energy needs. You'll break the cortisol cycle once and for all, and your belly fat will diminish.

Cortisol Addicts Are Fat and Unhappy

The cortisol/adrenaline connection is directly related to a loss of dopamine. If you can't get your "high" from your brain, you'll push your adrenal glands in the rush of action and success. Many people trade their health to work harder and make more money. They push their brain and body beyond normal limits and end up getting older, heavier, and sicker. They burn out their dopamine by pushing themselves too hard, and when the body replaces it with cortisol, the feeling of extra energy lets them continue to live their aggressive lifestyle. But as their cortisol levels out, they turn to even more caffeine and more bagels and more sugar, seeking that energy: Basically they are looking for their "steroid high." The bad news is they've just aged themselves prematurely and become internal steroid addicts. The Younger (Thinner) You Diet breaks cortisol addiction by enhancing brain chemistry and teaching you to slow down, rest up, and move forward with your life with healthier long-term goals.

Meet Janet K.: Stressed and High on Cortisol

Janet was a 43-year-old mother of four who came to see me because she suspected she had a thyroid condition: No matter what she tried, she just couldn't lose weight. She was having trouble sleeping at night and spent her day eating on the run. Her youngest child was only four, and he kept Janet going at a frantic pace, on her toes all day long. Janet was still having a difficult time shedding her pregnancy pounds, so she was sure that her health was failing her.

It was apparent the moment she stepped into my office that Janet was facing health issues, but I wasn't sure her diagnosis was correct. To me, Janet looked like she had a problem with excess cortisol: Her face was round and bloated, her complexion flushed. She was overweight by about 30 pounds, and most of it was concentrated around her midsection. I did a complete physical, including BEAM testing. We found out Janet was very low in dopamine, and she was also hyperglycemic and had elevated blood pressure. We did a bone density scan and she didn't fare well: Janet was osteoporotic. Her thyroid function, however, was normal.

In order to get Janet to lose weight, we needed to raise Janet's dopamine levels so we could increase her metabolism. It was also important that she attempt to diminish the stress in her life so her cortisol levels would naturally reduce, so I recommended exercise, especially yoga. I explained to her that even fifteen minutes a day of quiet yoga or meditation would make a profound difference.

I also encouraged her to make sure she got more sleep every night. Janet hadn't slept well in years, and promised me she would at least give it a try. She realized she would need help, and told me she would enlist her husband to help out more with the children so she could get the rest she needed.

Janet began following the Younger (Thinner) You Diet. She began to eat more healthfully, and so did her family. She switched her breakfast routine to include more protein, which is the food group that is the precursor to dopamine. I encouraged her to get rid of the sugary breakfast cereals her kids were so fond of. Janet got more rest when she could, and started taking yoga classes three nights a week. She kept a food and exercise journal and began to experiment with teas.

Within the first ten days of Janet's new program, she lost seven pounds. Within four months she had reached her goal weight. And after two years, Janet has kept the weight off.

DOPAMINE AND METABOLISM

As you get older, your metabolism naturally slows down. Your metabolism is determined by a massive genetic equation, which takes into account your age and your current health. This equation looks like:

Rate of Metabolism =
Your hormones (growth hormones, estrogen, testosterone)
×
your bone strength, muscle strength, and active neurons (working brain chemistry),
÷
the number of diseases you currently have

As you age, your hormones drop, muscle is lost, bone density is lost, and your brain cells fizzle. At the same time you accumulate illnesses. All of these factor into your metabolic rate. However, by reversing these individual health issues, you can increase your metabolism, feel younger, and lose weight.

When you were young, the food you ate supported your growing brain and body. Yet once you reached your final adult height, you may have experienced weight gain even when you were eating the exact same foods in the same quantities. The problem: Your metabolism weakened over time. To compensate, you need more voltage, or dopamine, to jump-start your fat-burning furnace. Without it, you'll just continue to accumulate body fat.

If you follow my dopamine-enhancing suggestions in this chapter, regardless of whether you have a dopamine deficiency or not, you will experience weight loss, because you will be increasing the strength of your own metabolism by concentrating on foods that increase your dopamine. These foods and nutrients will increase your metabolism now while boosting your dopamine levels to the point where eventually, you will retrain your brain to create more dopamine on its own.

Your metabolism works as an automatic system that is set by the fuel you throw at it. If you've been eating junk, your metabolism is working like a low-burning fire. However, when you provide it lots of dopamine, this brain chemical acts like a pile of wood, and ignites your metabolism to burn off your calories.

Get Over Yourself

Some people will always have great metabolism, even as they age. I know women who can survive on six olives a day and not lose weight, while others can eat a cow and still stay thin. The people who can eat a lot without gaining weight have high-dopamine levels. If you don't, you need to get over it. Instead of sulking, get with the program: the Younger (Thinner) You program, which includes nutrient-dense foods that are the building blocks to dopamine, as well as the right medications and natural hormones, if necessary. The more dopamine you produce, the faster your metabolism works, which makes it possible for you to burn more calories and turn less food into body fat.

Meet Tara F.: Tired of Weighing Too Much

Tara, a 45-year-old overweight mother of two first came to see me in 2005. She told me she was having difficulty losing weight. At 5' 5", Tara weighed 150 pounds. Her body composition showed her body fat was 25%. Her BEAM testing confirmed a 68% decline in dopamine. The reason why Tara couldn't lose weight was because low dopamine levels had slowed her metabolism.

I started Tara on the Younger (Thinner) You Diet to increase her metabolism. Luckily for me, Tara had a great disposition, and she took to the plan with much enthusiasm and determination. When she checked in a few weeks later, I could see she was being compliant with my recommendations.

By the following year, Tara showed a 28-pound weight loss, and her body fat composition had dropped to 20.5%. She also reported she was able to have deeper, more consistent sleep, as well as increased energy and self-confidence throughout the day. Best of all, a childhood friend remarked that she looked just as beautiful and even more radiant at 46 than she did on her wedding day.

WHAT DOES A DOPAMINE DEFICIENCY FEEL LIKE?

Without dopamine you are not in the thin zone: You've got no juice; no fire. A dopamine deficiency will not only affect your weight, it will affect your overall health. If you are dopamine deficient, you may find that it takes more time and effort to get things done. Your concentration may wander, your thinking and decision-making may not be as quick, and your intensity at work diminishes. You may even sleep a little longer but still wake up tired. Every time you feel tired, it usually means a loss of one of the brain chemicals. In the case of low dopamine, your brain chemistry will react by searching for a stimulant, like coffee or another caffeinated beverage, just to get you going. The coffee supplies the energy fix you need to feel like yourself, but the effect is temporary. So you reach for more throughout the day, because otherwise you can't sustain your usual level of performance. Your energy seems to spike after lunch, so you learn to snack throughout the day because food seems to help keep your concentration and focus high.

In the evening, you may pour yourself a couple of drinks to settle down from the day's roller-coaster ride, not realizing you are self-medicating to calm your brain down after all the coffee or other stimulants you might be taking. You may notice your sexual performance is compromised. Every night you go to sleep thinking that by tomorrow you'll be back to normal. But tomorrow isn't any better. You begin to create a self-medicating cyclical response to your own unique rhythm: Your low dopamine brain is dragging you down, and you respond by pulling yourself up with foods and stimulants.

REMOVE FOODS THAT DEPLETE DOPAMINE

Many common foods actually can deplete your levels of dopamine. These foods are not allowed on the Younger (Thinner) You Diet:

Sugar and its many hidden forms—high fructose corn syrup, fructose, dextrose, sucralose, molasses, syrup, and others—should be avoided. Sugar substitutes like aspartame and saccharin are recommended (aspartame in particular, because it contains phenylalanine), but sorbitol should be avoided because of its potential negative effect on your system.[13] Or substitute agave nectar, honey, or maple syrup instead of sugar. These alternatives contain additional vitamins, minerals and antioxidants that may benefit your health.

Stevia[14] is another natural sugar substitute. It comes from a plant, *Stevia rebaudiana*, which is native to Brazil and Paraguay and has been used for thousands of years. It's 200 to 300 times sweeter than sugar, so just a tiny amount will do the trick, and it contains 0 calories. Stevia can be used for anything you might use sugar in, including baking. In the United States, Stevia can only be sold as a "dietary supplement" instead of a "sweetener," and can be found in most health-food stores.

Simple carbohydrates and high glycemic foods are the foods you crave if you are dealing with a dopamine deficiency, because they give you the feeling of increased energy in the short term. Foods in this category include:

- Cakes
- Corn
- Crackers
- Chips
- Pasta
- Pastries
- Pies
- Potatoes
- Processed foods
- Puddings
- Tapioca
- White breads or foods made from white flour
- White rice

Instead of these "white" foods, choose more colorful versions that have more nutrients. Whole grain, colorful carbs provide lots of energy without being instantly converted into body fat. While they won't

Stop Messing with Your Dopamine

These are the "simple carbs" that you need to stop eating right now:

- All white flour products
- Anything with the words "high fructose corn syrup" in the ingredients
- Candy and sweets
- Sweetened coffee drinks and full-calorie sodas
- Foods that contain lots of sugar, honey, or other "natural" sweeteners

create more dopamine, they won't feed into the addiction cycle:

- Instead of white rice, choose brown rice
- Instead of white potatoes, choose sweet potatoes or yams
- Instead of white flour, choose whole wheat flour

THE YOUNGER (THINNER) YOU DIET IS THE DOPAMINE FIX

In order to break the cycles of food addiction and cortisol elevation we need to find the best ways to increase dopamine production. Most doctors will look to medicine to "cure" the problem. However, the drugs that have been proven to alter dopamine levels are highly addictive and not the preferred method of treating this deficiency. However, eating the right foods that will stimulate the brain to produce higher levels of dopamine is the only way to get your brain healthier and younger. By doing so, I know you will finally be able to reduce your tendency to overeat.

The Younger (Thinner) You Diet is a dopamine-enhancing diet and by following it you can break the cycle of cravings and weight gain once and for all. More important, the Younger (Thinner) You Diet is a lifestyle diet: Even after you lose all the weight you want, you can continue to follow this eating plan for the rest of your life.

That way, you are constantly making sure that your dopamine levels do not fall.

By raising your dopamine, you are also raising your body's metabolism. This means you will not only be balancing your brain, you will be teaching the rest of your body how to use the food you eat more efficiently. The teas, spices, and herbs that complement all of the foods you will eat help to increase your metabolism at every meal. Exercise, particularly strength training, will also raise your metabolism so you will burn more fuel throughout the entire day.

INCREASING DOPAMINE NATURALLY

On the Younger (Thinner) You Diet you will be following a balanced, high-protein, healthy-fat eating plan that will ensure the body has enough raw materials for a steady supply of dopamine. The building blocks of dopamine are the amino acids phenylalanine and tyrosine. These are found in protein-rich meats, poultry, fish, and many vegetables.

However, keep in mind that anything you eat should be consumed in moderation. No matter the food, it's easy to overindulge and wind up consuming more calories than your body needs, resulting in no weight loss, or worse, weight gain. Dopamine enhancing foods are by nature calorically dense, so make sure you consume them in the amounts prescribed.

Phenylalanine: Fatigue and Pain Reliever

Phenylalanine can be a fatigue and pain reliever. It is an essential amino acid found in high-protein foods, such as meats and poultry, dairy products, and wheat germ. Phenylalanine can also be found in the sugar substitute aspartame, which is packaged as either NutraSweet or Equal. These artificial sweeteners are safe and nutritious. Aspartame has been the subject of more than 200 research studies over 30 years, in which its safety continues to be demonstrated.[15]

Increasing your phenylalanine levels will boost your metabolism, which is why everyone on the Younger (Thinner) You Diet should get plenty of it. Use the following food lists to increase your total phenylalanine intake to between 8 and 11 grams a day. You'll need to include protein in each of your three main meals to keep your dopamine high throughout the day.

PHENYLALANINE-RICH FOODS INCLUDE:

- Beef
- Chicken
- Cottage cheese, low-fat
- Duck
- Eggs
- Granola
- Oat flakes
- Pork
- Ricotta cheese, low-fat
- Turkey
- Wheat germ
- Whole milk
- Wild game
- Yogurt

Tyrosine: Dopamine Builder

The amino acid tyrosine is another precursor to dopamine. In abundance, it increases your resistance to stress and acts as one of the body's natural pain relievers.[16,17] Most important, tyrosine is an adrenaline builder: Tyrosine can give you the increased energy you may be lacking, and the ability to burn calories more efficiently. The minimum daily requirement is about 1000 mg. Use the following food lists to increase your total tyrosine consumption in order to balance your dopamine deficiency.

TYROSINE-RICH FOODS INCLUDE:

- Beef
- Chicken
- Cottage cheese, low-fat
- Duck
- Eggs
- Granola
- Oat flakes
- Pork
- Ricotta Cheese
- Turkey
- Wheat germ
- Whole milk
- Wild game
- Yogurt

By increasing your consumption of phenylalanine and tyrosine, you can reverse your dopamine deficiency. Your body will be getting the energy it needs from these amino acids—ending your dependency on sugar and caffeine. You will find that you are no longer craving foods that will give you energy, because your body will be producing enough on its own.

An Energy-Boosting Eating Plan

Your body needs lot of protein so you will feel full and satisfied and not binge on the easy-to-eat carbs you crave. Your body will be getting the energy it needs from amino acids in proteins—not from sugar and caffeine. Foods high in calcium and vitamin D are also effective obesity busters.[18] By combining these categories, your energy level will rise, your concentration and thinking will sharpen, and your sleep will be more restful.

One of the goals of the Younger (Thinner) You Diet is to eliminate as much sugar as possible because using sugar will continue to slow down your metabolism, even when you are eating high-dopamine foods. You can continue to use caffeine, which is a metabolic stimulant. However, most of the caffeine you'll be getting is through drinking a variety of teas, which are also rich in nutrients.

LEAP INTO WEIGHT LOSS: ENHANCE YOUR LEPTIN

Leptin is a hormone secreted by your body's fat tissue. It is known to regulate the appetite: Its production is integral for becoming younger and thinner, because the more leptin present, the less hungry we are.[19] Leptin is also connected to dopamine because when leptin is released, dopamine production also increases, which is why you'll feel satisfied sooner and eat less.

On the Younger (Thinner) You Diet, these foods are incorporated into the meal plan every day because they stimulate leptin production. But if you were only going to choose one, go for broccoli: It is the best dopamine-enhancing food. It's high in fiber and contains leptin-enhancers. Steamed in the microwave, roasted, or raw, eat as much broccoli as you can.

LEPTIN-RICH FOODS INCLUDE:

- Broccoli
- Apples
- Unsalted almonds
- Pomegranate juice
- Spinach
- Carrots
- Egg whites
- Salmon

Cottage Cheese

Methionine, an essential amino acid, can help relieve the anxiety that comes with acutely stressful situations when you take it in conjunction with tyrosine. A single serving of cottage cheese (½ cup) contains one whole gram of methionine, as well as tyrosine. So if you find yourself stressing about what to have for lunch, cottage cheese is a great choice on the Younger (Thinner) You Diet.

SPICES BOOST YOUR METABOLISM

Spices are nutrient dense: Each one can provide between twenty to eighty different nutrients. By adding them to your foods, you bring important vitamins, minerals, and even antioxidants to every meal. These nutrients allow your foods to be better metabolized, because calories are handled

Beef It Up

One reason many people fall off the diet wagon is because they get bored eating a restricted menu. On the Younger (Thinner) You Diet you'll find there are tons of delicious options, including many of the foods that you thought were "off limits." Take beef, for instance. We've been told to stay away from red meats because they were too fatty. However, beef is still loaded with nutrients, including dopamine-producing tyrosine and phenyl-alanine. What's more, beef is now produced so that it is leaner than ever before. While you can't indulge in beef every day, you can have it occasionally, and in the right serving sizes.

There are twenty-nine different cuts of beef that meet United States government guidelines to be considered lean:[20] These are low in total fat, saturated fat, and bad cholesterol. These cuts usually have only one more gram of saturated fat than a skinless chicken breast. So choose your beef carefully, watch portion sizes, trim off all visible fat before cooking, and indulge. You'll feel younger with each meal because you are feeding your brain and body exactly what it needs to increase your metabolism. Choose from this list when you are at the grocer or eating out:

- 95 percent lean ground beef
- Bottom round roast
- Bottom round steak
- Brisket
- Chuck shoulder pot roast
- Chuck shoulder steak
- Eye round roast
- Eye round steak
- Flank steak
- Round steak
- Round tip roast
- Round tip steak
- Shank cross cuts
- Shoulder medallions
- Shoulder center steak
- Shoulder petite tender
- Sirloin tip center roast
- Sirloin tip center steak
- Sirloin tip side steak
- Strip steak
- T-bone steak
- Tenderloin roast
- Tenderloin steak
- Top round roast
- Top round steak
- Top sirloin steak
- Tri-tip roast
- Tri-tip steak
- Western griller steak

more efficiently when they are accompa-nied by nutrients. That's why your body can burn through the proteins, good fats, and healthy whole grain carbs you eat, and doesn't metabolize the junky foods that are low in nutrients. By adding spices to all your meals, you are then guaranteeing that you'll burn all calories at a higher rate.

You'll learn more about the power of spices in Chapter 7, but here is a quick list of spices that can boost your weight loss and your dopamine (a more complete list can be found in Appendix A):

- Basil
- Bay leaves
- Black pepper
- Cayenne
- Cumin
- Fennel
- Flaxseed
- Garlic
- Ginger
- Mustard seed
- Rosemary
- Savory
- Sesame seeds
- Tarragon
- Turmeric

CRAVING COFFEE?

Coffee provides a jump start to your brain and body, especially when you're tired. A 2005 study from the University of Scranton[22] shows that for most Americans, coffee is the number one source of antioxidants. And it facilitates weight loss, acting as a diuretic to relieve you of excess water weight. Each cup contains lots of soluble dietary fiber, which is why it loosens your bowels and prevents constipation. It may also improve your short-term memory, so you not only look younger but think younger, too.[23]

But like everything else, it's only good for you in moderation. Top off with no more than two to four cups per day; 300 mg is more than enough, depending on the size of your cup. Make sure to check with your doctor about your caffeine consumption. And be careful not to drink too much caffeine too late in the day, or you'll disrupt your sleep patterns.

Unfortunately, the higher phenylalanine levels your body needs to increase dopamine are actually *lowered* with every cup of coffee or can of Coke, Pepsi, or Jolt you drink. So while you'll feel more powerful and awake, the end result is negative. You are unintentionally creating a low-dopamine spiral that's making you older, sicker, and fatter: The instant fix to combat your low-dopamine levels is to drink more coffee, which then lowers your dopamine further.

BOOST YOUR DOPAMINE POWER WITH TEA

Teas are a healthier caffeinated choice than sodas or coffee because they are also high in nutrients and antioxidants. Teas contain caffeine but don't have the same stimulant effect as the caffeine in coffee or soft drinks. Tea contains L-theanine, which actually helps to relax you.

Black and green teas are metabolic enhancers that can help you burn calories and body fat. But choose your teas wisely. Fresh brewed tea from loose tea leaves has far more nutrients than tea made from processed tea bags. Bottled tea beverages may also be sweetened, adding unnecessary calories. You'll learn more about teas in chapter 7.

YOUNGER (THINNER) YOU FOODS THAT REDUCE FATIGUE

High-octane foods provide lots of energy:

- Brown rice
- Dates
- Kelp
- Legumes
- Lentils
- Quinoa
- Soy (when combined with citrus fruit, peppers, strawberries, cauliflower, parsley, or watercress)
- Split peas
- Whole wheat bread

DOPAMINE-BOOSTING SUPPLEMENTS

Modern farming techniques are certainly efficient, but they do not allow the maximum amount of nutrients to absorb into many types of produce. So even when we are eating lots of fruits and vegetables, we are only getting a fraction of the nutrients these foods should contain. That's why supplementation is becoming more important than ever.

Readily available vitamins and nutrient supplements are an excellent way to ensure a steady supply of dopamine. Because the supplements that boost dopamine are energy-related, they are best taken on a full stomach after you've eaten breakfast or lunch—you wouldn't want an extra charge in the evening when it's time to relax.

Curb Your Cravings for Sweets

If you're a sugar binger, make sure you always have something nutritious on hand to curb your cravings so you don't reach for the wrong foods. Raw vegetables neutralize your palate and keep cravings for sweets at bay. Another strategy is to feed your need with any variety of apple, which is naturally sweet, packed with nutrients, and is low in calories. On the Younger (Thinner) You Diet you can have an apple whenever you feel the need to eat something. Start with half, wait twenty minutes, and see if you need to eat the other half. Within the first week you may find that half an apple is all it takes to curb your cravings.

Retrain Your Brain for a Younger You

The benefits of your dopamine diet will be evident after a few weeks. You may find constipation or other digestive problems will ease, as well as your food cravings. What's happening is that your brain has been reprogrammed so it is no longer looking for the rush that accompanied foods: Instead, it's being supplied by better nutrition, which supports better brain functioning.

For example, at age 58, my patient Jocelyn started the Younger (Thinner) You Diet with skepticism, because she thought it seemed too easy. She changed her mind after she lost nine pounds in the first few weeks and completely lost her cravings for sweets and processed carbohydrates. Ultimately, she shed 27 pounds and was able to keep them off.

There are a large range of dopamine supplements available. Taken on a daily basis, each of these supplements can help increase your metabolism, and break your craving cycle for carbohydrates and sugar. Often, these nutrients are sold in combinations. Or you may want to take these nutrients individually, depending on your specific needs. Refer to the chart below to see how each one can positively affect your weight loss. As always, talk with your physician before starting a supplement program.

Boost Your Brain Power— Natural Supplements That Create Internal Energy

NATURAL TREATMENTS	SUGGESTED DAILY DOSAGE	HOW IT AFFECTS YOUR WEIGHT
Tyrosine	500–4000 mg	Stimulates the body's ability to burn up regular adipose tissue, and releases the hormone CCK-PZ that increases satiety
Phenylalanine	500–4000 mg	Stimulates the body's ability to burn up regular adipose tissue, and releases the hormone CCK-PZ that increases satiety
Rhodiola rosea	50–750 mg	Promotes physical and mental energy; improves endurance exercise performance so that you can expend more calories
Thiamine (Vitamin B$_1$)	10–500 mg	A B$_1$ deficiency can cause fatigue, reducing physical activity and calorie expenditure
Chromium	100–1000 mcg	Helps stabilize blood sugar levels, reducing sugar cravings
Folic acid	200–1000 mcg	Improves exercise tolerance and increases amount of calories burned
Yohimbine	200–400 mg	May increase thermogenesis, with an effect of increased weight loss below the waist
Methionine	500–2000 mg	Elevates mood which may increase desire to exercise
Hydroxycitric acid (HCA) (Garcinia cambogia; common name brindle berry)	500–2000 mg	Makes it harder for the body to convert excess calories from carbohydrates into fat; suppresses appetite and induces weight loss
Calcium	500–1000 mg	Increasing calcium results in significant reduction in adipose tissue and helps speed up weight loss
Vitamin D Magnesium	400–2000 IU 200–500 mg	Controls metabolic syndrome and helps with weight loss
Phosphatidylserine	200–400 mg	Can increase dopamine levels and lower cortisol levels; cortisol and DA can work together to promote feelings of satisfaction

FOR MANY WOMEN, A DIET WITHOUT NATURAL HORMONE SUPPLEMENTATION IS A LIE

Our body's natural levels of hormones decline as we age in much the same way as our brain chemistry does. We simply do not produce the amount of hormones we had when we were younger, and this loss of hormones is an integral part of aging. In order to look and feel younger, and in many instances lose excess weight that is associated with aging, you may need to increase your hormone levels. This alone may provide the kick start you need to make this diet more effective. That's because each of us loses different hormones at different times and at different rates, and any hormonal imbalance will lead to weight gain. The good news is that a decline of any hormone is neither irreparable nor permanent. In fact, it's often an easy and painless fix.

Unfortunately, hormones cannot be reproduced through foods or nutrient supplementation. The only way to safely increase your hormones to younger levels is to take hormone supplements. These hormone supplements work as nutrients to feed your aging brain, increasing specific biochemicals, including dopamine. Increased levels of hormones can boost your metabolism, or work on any of the other biochemicals so that you can become more aware and focused (acetylcholine), decrease anxi-

| Reducing Stress Increases Dopamine |

The following are some examples of stress-busting activities that allow the brain to re-sync and rebalance, producing more dopamine:

- For half an hour each day, try to set aside time for quiet relaxation, which can include nonwork-related reading, nonviolent TV programs, or even a competitive game such as chess.
- Anaerobic exercise, such as weight lifting, as well as aerobic exercises like running or swimming, are great ways to relieve stress and increase your metabolism at the same time.

ety (GABA), or get better sleep (serotonin). But before you get scared off the subject, you might want to know a bit more about hormone supplementation other than what you have been reading in the newspapers.

First, natural, bioidentical hormones are generally safe. Most of these hormones are not new on the market; they have been available for more than twenty years and are so lacking in side effects they are frequently sold over the counter as supplements, including Vitamin D_2, D_3, pregnenolone, progesterone, DHEA, and melatonin. Others require a doctor's prescription. Bioidentical hormones are often plant-based hormone supplements with the same molecular structure as those that come from the human body, and have the same effect on our body as the ones we naturally produce. They are far safer than traditional hormone therapies, and offer great results.

STAY AWAY FROM NON-BIOIDENTICAL HORMONES:

- Methyl testosterone (such as Android, Testred, Virilon)
- Conjugated estrogens (Prempro, Premarin)
- Medroxyprogesterone (Provera)
- Cadaver growth hormones (cadaver-GH)
- Birth control pills

REVERSE AGING AND LOSE WEIGHT WITH THESE BIOIDENTICAL HORMONES

Increasing your hormone levels will improve your ability to lose weight in many ways. Some of the hormones will also be discussed in later chapters as they relate to specific health conditions and brain chemicals. Use this comprehensive list of bioidentical hormone therapies to begin a discussion with your physician about how they can be used to enhance weight loss:

- **Androstenedione** is a precursor for sex hormones.
- **Calcitonin** is produced by the thyroid gland and affects bone growth and calcium regulation. It is generally administered as a nasal spray or through injection. It reduces bone loss in the spine and the risk of spinal fractures. This can be obtained with a doctor's prescription.
- **DHEA** is produced in the adrenal cortex and testes (in men) and converted to other sex hormones (estrogen and testosterone). DHEA facilitates weight loss as it increases the body's metabolism, inhibits body fat storage, and reduces appetite for dietary fats. It is also used for chronic fatigue syndrome, depression, erectile dysfunction, memory loss, menopause, osteoporosis, and to increase skin thickness. This can be purchased over the counter as a supplement.
- **Erythropoietin (EPO)** is produced by the kidneys and is the hormone regulating red blood cell production in the bone marrow. It is used in treating anemia. This can be obtained with a doctor's prescription.
- **Estradiol (E2)** is a sex hormone produced by ovaries, testes, and adrenal cortex. Estradiol has critical impact on reproductive and sexual functioning, is responsible for changes in the body shape affecting bones, joints, fat deposition, improves arterial blood flow in coronary arteries, has favorable effect on lipid profiles, and as an antioxidant it protects brain chemistry. It is also used as an antidepressant. This can be obtained with a doctor's prescription.
- **Estrone** deficiency can make women particularly choose the wrong foods and crave sugar. This hormone can be applied topically for vaginal use. This can be obtained with a doctor's prescription.
- **Human growth hormone** is produced by the pituitary gland. Growth hormone is critical for tissue repair, muscle growth, healing, brain function, immune system function, physical and mental health, as

well as bone strength. It is integral for the conversion of body fat to muscle mass, and it reduces visceral and subcutaneous fats and inhibits the formation of body fat. This can be obtained with a doctor's prescription.

- **Incretin** is a naturally occurring hormone secreted from the intestines in response to food intake. It is used for diabetes mellitus type 2 sufferers and helps to ensure an appropriate insulin response following ingestion of a meal, suppressing inappropriately elevated glucagon levels, promoting satiety and reducing food intake, and slowing the rate of gastric emptying. This can be obtained with a doctor's prescription.

- **Insulin** is an anabolic hormone that regulates carbohydrate metabolism. It is used for diabetes mellitus type 1 and type 2, and has effects on fat metabolism, changing the liver's activity in storing or releasing glucose and in processing blood lipids, and in other tissues such as fat and muscle. This can be obtained with a doctor's prescription.

- **Melatonin** is produced by the pineal gland, it plays a role in the body's circadian rhythm, helps regulate sleep patterns, changes in body temperature, blood pressure, and heart rate. It also has antioxidant properties. It is used for treating prostate cancer, epilepsy, fibromyalgia, insomnia, jet lag, and headaches. Avoid if pregnant. This can be purchased over the counter as a supplement.

- **Pregnenolone** is a naturally occurring hormone that is produced in your body from cholesterol. It is called the "grandmother of hormones" because the body uses it to create many other hormones, including testosterone, cortisone, progesterone, estrogen, DHEA, and others. While pregnenolone levels do not decline with age, its byproducts do, leading to illnesses and conditions like menopause. Taking pregnenolone supplements allows you to keep all your hormones at more youthful levels.[24]

Pregnenolone also appears to block the effects of cortisol, preventing stress and abdominal fat buildup while producing a calming effect. I have found that pregnenolone supplementation is a very effective weight loss tool, especially if you are deficient in dopamine. It keeps the brain healthy, and the metabolism stays high. It also increases testosterone levels for both men and women, which is important because testosterone helps to maintain an aggressive metabolism. Pregnenolone is prescribed by a doctor, so discuss this option with your physician before starting the Younger (Thinner) You Diet. They may likely agree with me that it is a good way to kick-start a healthy eating plan, so that you see increased weight loss over the first few weeks of the diet. This can be purchased over the counter as a supplement.

- **Progesterone** is a sex hormone that, when imbalanced, makes women crave too much food and overeat. It is used as a part of hormone replacement therapy in women. Progesterone may be useful for treating excessive weight as it facilitates the utilization of stored body fat as energy. This can be obtained with a doctor's prescription and is also sometimes available as a supplement.

- **Testosterone** is a sex hormone produced by both the ovaries and testes. Testosterone drops cause sugar cravings and can lead to insulin resistance. It is used for increasing sexual desire and ability, as well as combating extreme tiredness, low energy, depression, brittle bones, and loss of certain male characteristics such as muscular build and deep voice. Testosterone is also used in weight management as it facilitates weight loss by inhibiting body fat storage, especially in the abdomen. This can be obtained with a doctor's prescription.

- **Thyroid (T_3, T_4)** is produced by the thyroid gland. It is used for hypothyroidism, nodular goiter, and helps reverse obesity in individuals who are low in this particular hormone. This can be obtained with a doctor's prescription.
- **Vitamins D_2, D_3** are essential for formation of normal bones and teeth, and influences absorption and metabolism of phosphorus and calcium. These are used for treatment of cancer, multiple sclerosis, and osteoporosis. This can be obtained with a doctor's prescription and is also sometimes available as a supplement.

DOPAMINE-ENHANCING HORMONES

Each of these hormones are directly related to dopamine, and may prove beneficial in enhancing your metabolism and creating more of this vital biochemical:

- Testosterone/ estrogen
- Vasopressin
- DHEA
- Thyroid
- Cortisol
- HGH
- Erythropoietin
- Calcitonin
- Insulin
- TRH

THE LAST RESORT: DOPAMINE-RELATED WEIGHT LOSS MEDICATIONS

These weight loss medications work by directly boosting your dopamine. They should be considered a last resort instead of a first choice option. **Stick with the Younger (Thinner) You Diet for at least three months before talking with your doctor about taking any of these medications. Consult with your medical doctor regarding all issues related to your weight loss regimen, especially if you have other existing medical conditions.**

- **Diethylpropion** (Tenuate, Tenuate Dospan) stimulates the central nervous system, which increases your heart rate and blood pressure and decreases your appetite.
- **Phentermine** (Adipex-P, Fastin, Ionamin) suppresses your appetite so you feel less hungry, and may also increase the rate at which your body burns calories.
- **Mazindol** (Sanorex) stimulates the central nervous system.

CHANGE YOUR WEIGHT BY CHANGING YOUR BRAIN

You will not be able to make a permanent change in your weight without enhancing your brain chemistry. This is why other diets have failed you in the past. Now that you've committed to the Younger (Thinner) You Diet, and learned how to increase your dopamine, you've taken another important step towards losing weight and becoming a Younger (Thinner) You.

CHAPTER 4

Increase Your Weight Loss with Acetylcholine

ACETYLCHOLINE monitors our brain speed, another important requirement to keeping your brain metabolism powerful. Like dopamine, acetylcholine is one of the brain's "on" switches; it controls the speed at which the electrical signals from the brain are sent throughout the body. It also regulates the rate at which we process sensory input and access stored information. Acetylcholine provides the body and the brain with an internal lubrication. A healthy, high acetylcholine brain is fast-moving, quick-thinking, and moist, so information can pass easily from the brain into the body.

While the dopamine brain is all about seeking reward, acetylcholine is your key to awareness. With it, you have lots of wonderfully creative ideas and long-lasting relationships based on fond memories. Without it, you won't be able to remember the last time you ate, so you'll eat again and again and again.

Just as you may reach for sugar and caffeine for that burst of energy to compensate for a dopamine deficiency, you might reach for fatty foods to eat your way into thinking better. An acetylcholine deficiency can make you crave foods high in fat, like those found in greasy fast foods, fried foods, ice cream, pizza, or pastries. That's because fat is a main source of choline, the building block of this brain chemical. When you eat foods high in fat, they deliver an instant acetylcholine boost. However, this strategy works against you in two distinct ways. First, bad fats literally clog your brain and circumvent its natural mechanism for the production of acetylcholine. When the brain can't produce acetylcholine on its own, and the fats you are feeding it aren't helping the situation, the brain will further deplete its stores, creating an even larger deficiency.

Second, foods that are high in fat are both calorie-dense and low in nutrients, so they are not helping to improve your overall health. You already know that the body and brain can only burn so many calories a day, and excess calories are stored as body fat. So as you pack on the pounds with bad fats, not only are you getting heavier, you are getting older. You are aging your body by increasing your likelihood of developing type 2 diabetes and other diseases associated with obesity. Worse, you are also aging your brain by changing its functionality. Without acetylcholine, your brain will literally dry out, increasing your tendency to develop memory and attention issues, including Alzheimer's disease. These are just a few of the reasons why the fat cycle needs to be broken.

WEIGHT GAIN ISN'T DOING YOUR BRAIN ANY FAVORS EITHER

Just as brain chemical deficiencies can cause weight gain, weight gain itself can injure the brain, making it older and slower than it should be. The process is a form of apoptosis, in which obesity and insulin resistance cause cellular death in the brain.[1,2] A healthy brain is filled with fats and oils—it actually contains more than 60% fat. However, inside the obese brain, cell membranes become damaged when even more fat accumulates.

When you gain weight, you see it on your torso, arms, legs, and even your face. What you don't see is that body fat is also accumulating inside your organs, and even in your brain. As you add weight to every part of your body, you are also adding excess fat to the brain, forcing it to work harder to keep the body and itself functioning.

However, there is a surprising catch. When the brain is filled with excess fat, the brain's white matter actually expands. This white matter is the part of the brain that contains myelinated nerve fibers that are made of acetylcholine.[3] Myelin is essential to a healthy brain because it lines, protects, and insulates nerve fibers.[4] It also aids in the quick and accurate transmission of electrical currents that are carrying data from one nerve cell to the next. When the myelin expands, you may experience increased intellectual benefits, where your brain can actually function faster. This means that carrying excess weight can make you feel more mentally alert. This may be one of the reasons why you crave fats: Your brain is subconsciously telling you to support its intellectual functioning by creating more myelin from acetylcholine.

Yet while we all should want a faster brain, obesity is not the way to get there. Carrying extra pounds by supplying your brain with choline will make your mind stronger, but the remaining health risks are taking their toll.

At the same time, excess fat can fill up other areas of the brain in the form of cholesterol. Normally, cholesterol is converted into hormones, including estrogen, testosterone, DHEA, pregnenolone, and others. However, as you get older and your brain slows down, your can no longer make this conversion efficiently, and excess cholesterol accumulates, causing degenerative diseases. The brain's response is simple: It recognizes that it is being starved of hormones as it is choked by the growing cholesterol, and sends a signal for you to eat more.[5]

The good news is that even a damaged brain can be healed. As you lose weight, you'll lose some of the excess fat that has been stored in the brain, leaving more room for new cellular growth as well as better brain functioning. By increasing your acetylcholine in healthy, effective ways, you can get the faster brain you want; one that will increase your metabolism for rapid weight loss. The secret is in choosing which fats will support, not thwart, a Younger (Thinner) You.

WHAT DOES AN ACETYLCHOLINE DEFICIENCY FEEL LIKE?

Early symptoms of an acetylcholine deficiency include memory lapses, increasing paranoia, frequent urination and bowel movements, sexual dysfunction (men and women), as well as dry skin and dry mouth. If you are experiencing a more advanced acetylcholine deficiency, you may find yourself avoiding contact with others, because there is a noticeable tension in your relationships. Your ability to get into a routine gets totally out of hand, and you can't manage your daily schedule. Where you used to move rapidly from one idea to another, from one activity to another, you may start to obsess on a single thought.

You find solace in high-fat "comfort foods" like rich meals (macaroni and cheese) and fried foods, and you pacify yourself with ice cream. As your forgetfulness increases, so do your cravings, and you will probably find that the diets you've tried can't help you squelch these cravings.

ACETYLCHOLINE AND YOUR PERSONALITY, OR "WHERE DO THE REAL SKINNY BITCHES FIT IN?"

The skinny bitches of the world are the women (and once in a while men) you can't help but hate. They eat all day long and do not seem to ever gain a pound. I'm not talking about the gals who wrote the best-selling diet book that recommends eating organically. Instead, I'm referring to your polar opposites: They're full of acetylcholine, and have the ability to flit from one project, or boyfriend, or meal to the next. These people have a high acetylcholine personality, and are often drama queens with agendas even the paparazzi can't keep up with.

Instead, with an acetylcholine deficit, you end up worrying about everyone except yourself. The following table indicates an acetylcholine deficiency. Interestingly, nurturing, dependant women tend to have the highest rates of obesity. One 220-pound patient recently stopped by my office. Her acetylcholine levels had tanked. She said to

Low Acetylcholine Personality Traits

EMOTION/ACTION	WHAT IT MEANS:
Nurturer	● Lets others make her major life decisions ● Fears being alone ● Always agrees with people to avoid an argument ● Little or no initiative ● Volunteers to get other people to like her ● Feels helpless or uncomfortable being alone ● Fears being abandoned ● Easily hurt by criticism or disapproval ● Constantly seeking reassurance, approval, or praise
Perfectionist	● Trouble expressing warm and tender emotions ● Lack of generosity ● Unable to complete tasks because of obsession over perfection ● The major point of an activity is lost due to preoccupation with details ● Insists others do things their way ● Excessive devotion to work and productivity, sacrificing social functions ● Cannot make a decision because of inability to prioritize ● Collects worthless objects ● Inflexible

me, "As soon as I start thinking of taking care of myself, I start getting tense and anxious, and I start eating again."

MORE ACETYLCHOLINE KEEPS YOU THINKING

We can also stimulate acetylcholine production by increasing our intellectual stimulation: mastering physical and mental skills, reading books, magazines, newspapers, completing word or number puzzles, engaging in debates, or creating artwork. Keeping your brain young and constantly engaging your mind is one of the keys to becoming a Younger (Thinner) You. As you exercise your brain, you are increasing its ability for attention and retention, therefore creating more "brain memory." And by increasing your acetylcholine, you are creating a faster, more fluid brain, which will ultimately facilitate an increase in your metabolism.

Dr. Braverman's Vanity Quotient

Add together all the hours you spend shopping, fixing your hair, selecting your jewelry, shoes, and purses, tweezing and manicuring to get that perfect look. For the average American woman the time it takes to do all this comes to around fifteen to twenty hours per week.

Now add together all the hours you spend exercising that body you just preened and pampered and dressed. All I'm asking you for is three and a half hours a week of exercise. If you can't fit exercise into your busy schedule, but you can do all the rest, be prepared to pay the price for being vain, which is your health. Your health will be "in vain" as well.

Cigar, Cigarette?

It's true the nicotine found in cigarettes increases your acetylcholine production and kills your appetite. While it sounds like the perfect diet aid, it's still going to kill you. Don't replace a bad habit with a worse one: Increase your acetylcholine naturally with the right foods and nutrients.

How intellectually stimulated are you? Rate yourself on a scale from 1 to 5, with 1 being completely bored and 5 being constant intellectual stimulation, like reading the newspaper cover to cover or attempting a crossword puzzle every single day. The higher your score the younger your brain will be. Then, look for ways to boost your score every day. Remember, good choices today promote better choices tomorrow. By choosing to engage in a mental workout, you'll be benefiting your brain and your body. And, you'll understand why people get hooked on Sudoku.

THE LINK BETWEEN ACETYLCHOLINE AND DIABETES, DEMENTIA, AND ALZHEIMER'S

Diabetes begins when the body can no longer correctly process the sugar it takes in from carbohydrate-dense foods like white rice, white flour, and white potatoes. A healthy body—attached to a healthy brain—should be able to metabolize, or break down, these foods into simple sugars, or glucose, to use as fuel. The hormone insulin transports the glucose to the cells. However, when the pancreas does not produce enough insulin, the glucose builds in the blood stream, resulting in hyperglycemia or high blood sugar. If you have had this condition from a young age, you suffer from type 1 (juvenile-onset) diabetes. However, if you have developed this pattern later in life, you are suffering from type 2 (adult-onset) diabetes.

A sedentary lifestyle paired with excess weight caused by the overconsumption of

Are You Forgetting to Eat?

An acetylcholine deficiency may be affecting your memory and attention now, causing that familiar feeling of midlife "brain fog." Have you ever been so busy that you "forgot" to eat? Or, have you found yourself sitting around doing nothing all day, unmotivated to cook or prepare healthy meals? This mental fatigue can cause you to make the wrong food choices, especially if you are "forgetting" to eat breakfast or lunch. Your quick fix may have been to grab something "fast and easy" like a bagel or a muffin to make up for a missed meal when you're on the run. Unfortunately, these carb-rich feasts, as well as your typical fast food meals, are full of all the things you shouldn't be eating: tons of simple carbs and bad fats.

carbohydrate-rich foods creates insulin resistance, further exacerbating the problem. Insulin is produced in different regions of the brain as well as the pancreas. The highest production is found in the hippocampus, the region associated with memory, learning, and other cognitive functions. Insulin is also created in the hypothalamus, another area of the brain that regulates emotions and involuntary functions. If this is beginning to sound familiar, you're right: Both of these areas are where acetylcholine is most active.

The latest brain research links both diabetes and dementia to the brain chemical acetylcholine. Low levels of acetylcholine are directly linked to a loss of insulin and insulin-like growth factor function in the brain. A 2005 study from Brown University Medical School, and a more recent 2008 study out of Sweden found that insulin production in the brain declines as Alzheimer's disease advances. The study showed that many of the unexplained features of Alzheimer's, such as cell death and tangles in the brain, appear to be linked to abnormalities in insulin signaling. This demonstrates that the disease is most likely a neuroendocrine disorder, or another type of diabetes. The brain levels of insulin fall precipitously during the early stages of Alzheimer's, and continue to drop progressively as the disease becomes more severe. This finding has lead to the suggestion that Alzheimer's disease should be referred to as type 3 diabetes.

Alzheimer's Is Not a Thin Man's Disease

The majority of people with Alzheimer's disease or dementia tend to be thin because the typical overweight person who is low in acetylcholine will probably die from heart disease or other obesity-related illnesses before their memory is too far gone. It's not that Alzheimer's is innately a thin person's illness; it's just that almost everyone overweight is dead by age 75 or 80, before this ravaging disease usually begins.

One of the most devastating illnesses related to acetylcholine is Alzheimer's disease. Recent studies are showing that low acetylcholine levels, like those that may have been highlighted in your results from the Younger (Thinner) You Quiz, not only affect your weight and health now, but can have a cumulative effect that could be related to this destructive illness. Researchers at Case Western Reserve University found that obesity in midlife may predispose a person to developing Alzheimer's years later. The study compared a group of 72 people with Alzheimer's with 232 people who did not have the disease. It found that people who consumed the highest fat diets had a seven-fold higher risk of developing Alzheimer's disease than people with the same genetic predisposition who had lower-fat diets.

What's more, a second study from Case Western University in 2000 posited that a high-fat diet during early and mid-adulthood could be associated with an increased risk of

Am I Becoming Diabetic?

Diabetes is easily confirmed by measuring your blood glucose levels. But be on the lookout for these symptoms:

- Blurred vision
- Excessive thirst
- Extreme hunger
- Increased urination
- Increased fatigue
- Irritability
- Neuropathy
- Weakness
- Weight gain

developing Alzheimer's later in life. In people aged 20 to 39, the combination of a genetic predisposition and a diet with more than 40 percent of calories from fat raised the risk of Alzheimer's by almost 23 times.[6]

I believe these two diseases are connected in a cycle. Obesity, combined with a low level of acetylcholine, leads to diabetes, which leads to dementia. Said another way, type 2 diabetes begins with food cravings, binge eating, and weight gain, which leads to obesity, which leads to dementia, and further overeating. An estimated 18.2 million Americans have diabetes.[7] What's more, one-third of these people are walking around with this disease and have yet to be diagnosed.

Insulin resistance is a major health problem that can rapidly age you. However, it is completely treatable and reversible. What's more, type 2 diabetes is also preventable and very often reversible. In order to treat insulin resistance and reverse premature aging you need to rebalance your brain chemistry, replace your overconsumption of bad fats with healthy fats, and retrain the

brain to function properly. The Younger (Thinner) You Diet program will help, as it will teach you to eat less of the foods that cause insulin resistance, along with exercise recommendations that will meet your specific health concerns.

CHOOSE FOODS HIGH IN CHOLINE

One of the easiest ways for you to keep your acetylcholine levels balanced is by making better food choices when you eat. In order to rebalance your acetylcholine, you'll need to choose lots of healthy, acetylcholine-producing foods each day. Your body needs more choline, a nutrient that begins as a B vitamin and is converted through digestion to acetylcholine. Choline serves various functions in our bodies, such as helping protect our livers from fat accumulation. The body is capable of making some of its own choline stores, but dietary choline is essential.[8] Adding choline-rich foods that include good fats to your diet will help eliminate cravings for really fattening fried or greasy foods because your acetylcholine will be boosted in a healthier manner.

Choline is so important to brain functioning that food manufacturers are now adding it to a wide variety of products. The government has established a 55 mg per portion requirement for manufacturers to claim their food is "a good source of choline" on the label. Experts agree that an adequate amount of choline per day would be 425 mg for women and 550 mg for men. One hard-boiled egg alone has 125 mg of choline, more than 20% of your daily supply.[9]

Choline is always plentiful in foods that contain fats, like plant oils such as olive oil, lean meats, dairy products, eggs, avocados, and nuts. Other good fats would include safflower oil, olives, fish oil, and seeds: All are excellent choices and can even help you lose weight. Choline can also be found in

Meet Anita H.: Anita Stopped Type 2 Diabetes in Its Tracks and Lost 45 Pounds

Anita was a gentle, sweet-faced woman. At 47 years old and 5' 5", Anita weighed 198 pounds and had been diagnosed with diabetes. With a BMI of 33, she was obese. Her son prompted her to seek help. He'd just graduated from college and told her he wanted her around to dance at his wedding—and baby-sit her future grandkids.

Anita wiped away her tears as she told me how difficult it was living with her excess weight. "I can barely climb a flight of stairs. My ankles and knees hurt. I feel more like 90 than 47!"

After a complete assessment, including BEAM testing as well as taking the Younger (Thinner) You Diet Quiz, I determined Anita had an acetylcholine imbalance. Her blood sugar levels were also too high. I told Anita that her elevated blood sugar can have a deadly impact on her health. But I reassured her that health problems caused by diabetes—even the diabetes itself—can be treated and even reversed.

I started by boosting her acetylcholine through the Younger (Thinner) You Diet, which increased her metabolism and decreased her appetite. I recommended additional spices, like cinnamon, garlic, and turmeric, which are terrific at decreasing insulin resistance, improving blood sugar levels, and have anti-inflammatory properties. In Anita's case, because her blood sugars were dangerously high, we changed her current diabetes medication to one that would more effectively lower her sugars to a normal level. I assured Anita that when she took off the excess weight, chances were excellent she would no longer need the medication at all.

Anita lost 45 pounds in the first six months of the program, which she continues to follow. She lowered her cholesterol from 221 to 186, and as I had predicted, was able to stop taking diabetes medication. Today, Anita is fitter, healthier, and younger than she was when she first walked in my door. Better still, she has a new outlook on life.

certain fruits and vegetables. Healthy foods naturally high in choline include these Younger (Thinner) You choices:

- Almonds
- Beef
- Blueberries
- Broccoli
- Cabbage
- Cauliflower
- Caviar
- Celery
- Chicken
- Cod Roe
- Coffee
- Eggs
- Fava beans
- Fish
- Grape juice
- Hazelnuts
- Lettuce
- Oranges
- Peanuts/peanut butter
- Soybeans
- Tofu
- Wheat germ

BREAKING DOWN YOUR FAT CHOICES

Despite what you may have learned from other fad diets, fat consumption is integral to good health. Eating the perfect quantities of the right fats will crank up metabolism and increase the amount of body fat burned during exercise. When you replace carbohydrates with good sources of fat, your body increases the enzymes that help turn body fat into an energy source. This dietary exchange also prevents the body from storing more body fat. Adding fat to meals also helps us feel satisfied and keeps us feeling full longer. Combine these reasons with the ability to create more acetylcholine and improve your memory and attention, and you can clearly see why adding good fats to your diet is an important part of becoming younger.

You need to choose the best fats in order to get the choline you need without the detriments you don't. But choosing fats isn't as easy as you think, because the bad fat culprits aren't always the ones you've been told to avoid. For example, **saturated fats**, which become solid at room temperature (think butter), are the ones we've been told to limit. However, the latest research shows these fats are actually not so bad.[10],[11] A small amount of saturated fat is not unhealthy or fattening as long as it is combined with the other types of fats. This doesn't mean that you should eat bars of butter at a time; it just means saturated fats are not dangerous in small amounts. It also means you don't have to drink only skim milk or avoid red meat to lose weight. I tell my patients to choose low-fat (1% or 2%) milk instead of fat-free, and to choose low-fat yogurt instead of fat-free. But you still can't pour a pitcher full of cream on your breakfast cereal.

- **Monounsaturated fatty acids** are liquid or soft at room temperature, and are the best fats to choose. They are found in foods like olive oil, avocados, nuts, seeds, and egg yolks. Monounsaturated fats are a featured part of a Mediterranean diet that is thought to keep people healthy and slim. Monounsaturated fats are easy for our body to use as energy.

- **Polyunsaturated fatty acids** are also a good source of fat, and are found in many plant and animal foods. There are two types of polyunsaturated fats, the omega-3s and the omega-6s. Omega-3 fats play a pivotal role in maintaining good health, and can also help control and reduce body fat. This happens because omega-3 fats have the ability to increase blood flow so fats are more easily delivered, where they can stimulate metabolism.[12]

Omega-3 fats are only found naturally in a few plant foods like flax, a few fish like salmon and shrimp, and specially raised eggs. Fish oil is rich in two omega-3 polyunsaturated fatty acids called EPA and DHA and is the best source of omega-3 essential fatty acids. Cutting out saturated fats worsens your omega-3 status, which is one reason why not to go completely fat-free.

The omega-6 polyunsaturated fatty acids are found in highest quantities in vegetable oils like corn, soybean, and safflower oil. The omega-6s also make up all the polyunsaturated fat found in land-based animals such as chicken, beef, and pork. Because omega-6s are found in so many of the foods we normally eat, we usually get enough of these fats to meet our dietary needs. Omega-3 fats are called "essential" because they have to be supplied from outside of the body. The Younger (Thinner) You Diet contains an almost equal ratio of the omega-6s and omega-3s. You will be eating lots of fish, flaxseed, and walnuts and will use canola or olive oil for salad dressings and when cooking.

You can also supplement omega-3 fish oil in capsule form, which I highly recommend. You'll need to take at least 3 grams a

I'm Cool with Olive Oil

Olive oil is one of the healthiest fats around. It is mostly made of good fats that actually lower your levels of LDL (bad) cholesterol as well as blood fats called triglycerides. It is also rich in antioxidants and phytonutrients that help prevent heart disease, can reduce high blood pressure, and lower inflammation.

A number of weight loss studies have shown that when people concentrated their fat intake on fats like olive oil, they ate less food and either maintained their weight or lost weight. One study from Boston's Brigham and Women's Hospital[13] showed a diet based on fats from olive oil, nuts, and other natural foods promoted weight loss, as well as the ability to keep weight off. Researchers noted these dieters felt that it was easier to stick to this plan because they didn't feel as if they were dieting.

You need to consume two tablespoons of olive oil each day. One easy way to do this is by dipping a slice of whole grain bread into a single serving. I like to add a little touch of balsamic vinegar and cayenne pepper, or rosemary and basil for a little extra flavor as well as a nutrient boost. Mix up this treat and have it on hand—it will become an important part of your weight loss regimen.

On the Younger (Thinner) You Diet you'll get the most benefits from olive oil when you use it at room temperature. For cooking, I recommend using safflower oil, another good fat that is high in omega-3s.

Reconsider Shrimp

In the early 1990s shrimp was shunned for its high cholesterol levels. But by 1996, a study published in the *American Journal of Clinical Nutrition* found that although high in cholesterol, shrimp did not adversely affect the production of cholesterol in the body.

The American Heart Association has since acknowledged that shrimp had been wrongly accused, but lots of people—including many doctors—still keep shrimp on the "no" list for dieters.

I feel that the benefits of shrimp far outweigh its negative history. Shrimp is low in fat and calories; offers beneficial doses of omega-3 fatty acids; and contains nutrients like vitamin B_{12} and niacin. So it's completely endorsed for the Younger (Thinner) You Diet.

day to get the amount of omega 3 you'll need, but 6 grams is the recommended dose that has been shown to help with fat-loss.

Last and certainly least desirable are the dreaded **trans fats**. These types of fats do occur in nature in small amounts[14] and are usually added to foods like baked goods and packaged snack foods. Food manufacturers use trans fats because they are cheap and were thought to be better than the much-maligned saturated fats. But they turned out to be much worse: Trans fats are so bad for your health that they have been banned from use at restaurants in certain states. Avoid these fats by making sure you check

Younger (Thinner) You Tip to Help You Remember

If you have trouble controlling your fat intake, your brain might not be getting enough omega-3s and omega-6s. You can easily supplement your diet with fish oil capsules. I also recommend a great-tasting fish oil cream that even kids love. It's called Coromega Omega-3 fatty acids supplement.[15] It comes in single-serving packets and has the consistency of a pudding. You can squeeze it directly into your mouth from the packet, or stir it into your daily yogurt.

food labels for the words "hydrogenated" or even "partially hydrogenated" before a particular oil, like soybean oil.

MERCURY RISING

To increase acetylcholine, you need to eat lots of healthy fats, like those in fish. However, some fish have high levels of mercury. As many as a third of all my patients are testing positively for elevated levels of mercury in their blood. Mercury is a known poisonous element, and it accumulates in fish as it falls from our atmosphere into bodies of water. Women who can become pregnant and those with kidney disorders are most at risk for mercury contamination. Choose from this list of fish that are high in omega-3s and low in mercury. Each portion should be about 3.5 ounces[16,17]:

LEVEL OF OMEGA-3 IN FISH

- Salmon (fresh)   1.8 g
- Mackerel (fresh)   1.0 g
- Rainbow Trout (fresh)   1.0 g

DAIRY FOODS BOOST METABOLISM

Researchers at the University of Knoxville revealed that dietary calcium plays a pivotal role in the regulation of metabolism and reduces obesity.[18] High-calcium foods, notably dairy sources, have been shown to increase body fat breakdown and preserve metabolism during dieting, making them one of the Younger (Thinner) You superfoods. That's because dairy foods contain dietary fat, which is a precursor to acetylcholine. And, high levels of calcium will also help you get younger by building strong bones, and may help to break down your stubborn belly fat. The study suggested eating three servings of dairy products a day to get the most benefit.

However, foods that contain calcium in large quantities are high in fat as well as calories, making them prohibitive to eat on a weight loss regimen. There is also a high instance of cellulite-producing effects from cheese and fat. Because of this, I find most people who are overweight cannot afford to increase their dairy consumption at all. Yet I still want you to benefit from these new research findings.

I've figured out a way for you to get your calcium in the foods you eat as well as the right quantities of good fats each day. On the Younger (Thinner) You Diet, you'll be getting most of your calcium from plain, unsweetened low-fat yogurt, which has the necessary levels of this vital nutrient without tons of added calories. You'll learn more about the importance of yogurt in Chapter 7.

Or, you can choose foods that are high in calcium that are not dairy products, such as:

- Sardines
- Soymilk (all flavors), enriched
- Blackstrap molasses
- Almonds, blanched
- Spinach, fresh or frozen
- Tofu, firm
- Brazil nuts, dried, unblanched
- Soy nuts, dry roasted
- Collard greens, fresh or frozen

YOU NEED MORE LECITHIN

A second goal of an acetylcholine-balancing diet is to ensure that you have enough lecithin, a nutrient used by the body to synthesize choline. When your diet is healthy and balanced, your body produces enough lecithin on its own. However, if your

Eggs Are Brain Food

Eggs are a Younger (Thinner) You superfood. They are a perfect protein, low in fat, and keep your acetylcholine high so that your thinking is sharp and fast. I recommend you eat eggs every day on the Younger (Thinner) You Diet. But I know eggs can get boring. Liven them up by seasoning with coriander seeds, sesame seeds, and a range of your favorite spices. My favorite combination is a well-seasoned hard-boiled egg sprinkled with thyme, parsley, and coriander.

Try Choline Powder for a Power Breakfast

Choline powder is another way to create a metabolism-boosting breakfast. Add choline powder, which can be bought at a health food store, and mix it in with cinnamon and wheat germ, and a touch of maple syrup. Top plain yogurt with this mixture to create a super yogurt. You can also find lecithin granules to sprinkle into your foods: They may be even easier to use.

acetylcholine levels are out of whack, you need to focus on foods that provide this vital nutrient.

Lecithin can be produced by the liver: It is a fat-like substance that feeds every cell in the body. Lecithin protects cells from oxidation and largely comprises the protective sheaths surrounding the brain. Although it is a fatty substance, it is also a fat emulsifier, which supports the circulatory system. Lecithin is believed to improve cardiovascular health, physical performance, healthy hair and skin, liver function, memory and learning, arthritis, gallstones, and fat metabolism.[19]

Only a limited number of foods contain sufficient amounts of lecithin, so if you are acetylcholine deficient, you'll need to work these into your personalized Younger

Boost Your Acetylcholine with Asparagus

This delicious green vegetable has been showed to stop the production of acetylcholinesterase, an enzyme that destroys acetylcholine. If you are acetylcholine deficient, substitute asparagus for any other green vegetable on the meal plan at least twice a week.

(Thinner) You Diet every day. Choose at least one serving of the following daily:

- Cauliflower
- Egg yolks
- Liver
- Milk
- Peanuts
- Soybeans
- Wheat germ

SPICE UP YOUR MEMORY

I call turmeric the spice of life. Turmeric stimulates the production of acetylcholine, and it has been proven to help unclog amyloid, the garbage that mucks up the pathways of the brain.[20] Without amyloid, your thinking is much clearer.

Brain-accelerating spices include:

- Allspice
- Basil
- Cumin
- Peppermint
- Sage
- Thyme
- Turmeric

A WOMAN'S LOW ACETYLCHOLINE DOUBLE WHAMMY

Sometimes diabetes and the larger issue of metabolic syndrome can show up at the same time as the beginning of cognitive impairment, because both are related to a loss of acetylcholine. Many overweight women begin to experience this mind-body combination during menopause, because both estrogen and testosterone are hormones as well as acetylcholine stimulants.

Pay Attention when You Eat Out

It may be easy to remember to put coriander and cumin on your hard-boiled eggs when you are at home, but will you remember to ask for these spices when you are eating out? On the Younger (Thinner) You Diet, you need spices every day, no matter where you are. For example, you'll need to remember to put 2 teaspoons of cinnamon in your coffee or yogurt. So don't be embarrassed to ask for what you need when you are eating out. Our society hasn't learned yet how to make you thin: Restaurants stock their tables with life-shortening salt and useless ground pepper, which is mostly dust and not very beneficial. Until they start putting spice racks on the table, your job is to remember what you need and speak up when you need it.

Women rely on these important hormones for cognitive quickness and mental alertness. Without them, many women will begin to feel more forgetful, and begin to eat their way back to a stronger brain.

For some women, menopause can look and feel like a march into "shrinkhood": They literally begin to shrink as they lose height, get weaker, notice drying and wrinkled skin, and end up seeking the advice of a real shrink because they think they're going crazy as they experience the emotional–hormonal roller coaster, or are upset at their increasing forgetfulness because of a lack of acetylcholine. However, you don't have to be older than 50 to be invited to the menopause party. We're finding women as young as 30 are beginning to feel the symptoms of this life change.

Are You in Perimenopause?

Conventional medicine offered women suffering from symptoms of hormonal change little hope. Until a woman was deemed officially in menopause, she was often told her symptoms were all in her head. Even today,

women struggling with hormonal imbalance are frequently sent home with a prescription for antidepressants, rather than being offered real solutions for a very real condition. Antidepressants are not a *wrong* treatment for hot flashes, they address only one problem.

In integrative medical circles, there has long been recognition that a transitional period of time exists before menopause, which is different for each woman, when fluctuating hormones may cause her serious distress. Thankfully, conventional medicine has caught up and we now have an official name for this passage in medical textbooks: *Perimenopause*—defined as a transition period that precedes menopause, as in "premenopause"—which is symptomatic of hormonal imbalances and fluctuations in a woman's body.[21] Between the ages of 30 and 40, most woman experience perimenopause—with multiple-hormone drops, a slowing down of brain speed and function—and consequently achieve weight gain.

During perimenopause your ovaries start to shut down, making less estrogen and progesterone, which then instructs the brain to make less dopamine and acetylcholine. The average length of perimenopause is four years, but for some women it may last only a few months or can continue for ten years. Full menopause is typically reached between the ages of 40 and 60, with the average being age 50.

Symptoms and their severity vary from woman to woman. Some experience almost no symptoms, while others may experience any combination of the following:

● Breast tenderness
● Confusion
● Decreased libido
● Facial hair
● Fatigue
● Hot flashes
● Insomnia or other sleep disorders
● Memory loss
● Menstrual cycle changes (lighter or heavier, shorter or longer, more or less frequent)
● Mood swings
● Night sweats
● Thinning hair or hair loss
● Urinary incontinence or changes in frequency
● Vaginal dryness
● Weakness
● Weight gain

The Perimenopause Fix

Some women are prescribed oral contraceptives (birth control pills) to ease perimeno-pausal symptoms, but I don't recommend this. Instead, I recommend women take bioidentical hormones, such as a compound of progesterone, estradiol, and testosterone (PET), or DHEA. Bioidentical hormones are natural and safe, an effective way to alleviate symptoms of menopause and peri-menopause without adding dangerous, synthetic toxins to your already taxed body. At the same time, these bioidentical hormones will jump-start your brain chemical production, especially of dopamine and acetylcholine.

Following the Younger (Thinner) You Diet, which focuses on herbs, spices, and teas, is essential for women between ages 30 and 50. Foods that increase acetylcholine will keep your mind sharp, and at the same time strengthen your bones to prevent osteoporosis, another low acetylcholine–related disease. I also suggest you avoid alcohol, which can trigger hot flashes in some women. While this doesn't affect your brain chemical balance, it's simply good medical advice.

OTHER IMPORTANT ACETYLCHOLINE-BOOSTING HORMONES

These natural hormones will boost acetyl-choline, and may also help with weight loss as they support a younger, faster brain, which can increase metabolism. One very important hormone is arginine vasopressin, which can be prescribed to inhibit or repair memory loss. Again, discuss each of these options with your physician:

- HGH
- Arginine vasopressin
- DHEA
- Calcitonin
- Parathyroid
- Estrogen

NUTRIENTS THAT AUGMENT ACETYLCHOLINE

One of the easiest ways for you to boost your acetylcholine is by supplementing your diet. Read through the following list and see which ones are best for your particular needs. You can tell which ones to try by reading their descriptions, or discussing their attributes with your physician.

THE LAST RESORT: ACETYLCHOLINE MEDICATIONS

Some weight loss medications work by directly changing the levels of your acetylcholine production. The following may be considered as a last resort instead of a first choice option. Stick with the Younger

NATURAL TREATMENTS	SUGGESTED DAILY DOSAGE	HOW IT AFFECTS WEIGHT LOSS
Choline	200–3000 mg	Improves physical performance over extended periods of time, thus burning more calories
Dimethylamino-ethanol (DMAE)	100–3000 mg	When combined with ginseng, reduces heart rate and lactic acid levels, resulting in increased total workload capacity and maximal aerobic capacity
Acetyl-l-carnitine	500–5000 mg	Aids in burning fat, improves athletic performance and memory function.
Phosphatidyl serine	100–300 mg	Increases stamina and improves memory function
Fish oils (omega-3)	500–3000 mg	Facilitates loss of adipose tissue, decreases appetite, can improve athletic performance; increases ability to burn more calories
Glycerol phosphor-ylcholine (GPC)	200–1000 mg	May increase human growth hormone, which can increase energy production and reduce fat stores
Conjugated linoleic acid (CLA)	1–6 g	Facilitates weight loss and reduces the deposition of additional fat cells in existing body fat
Piracetam (derivative of GABA)	2000–5000 mg	May reduce fatigue, allowing one to exercise more and lose weight

(Thinner) You Diet for at least three months before talking to your doctor about any of these medications. Consult with your medical doctor regarding all issues related to your weight loss regimen, especially if you have other existing medical conditions.

- **Exenatide** (Byetta) is prescribed for type 2 diabetes but has been an effective method of weight loss in diabetic patients.
- **Calcitonin** is known as a satiety hormone, meaning it produces feelings of fullness and prevents overeating by decreasing appetite.
- **Varenicline** (Chantix) is currently available as a smoking cessation medication but has not yet been approved for weight loss by the FDA. It has anecdotally been proven effective for weight loss. As a nicotinic drug, varenicline affects acetylcholine levels.

MOVING FORWARD WITH A BETTER BALANCED BRAIN

Once you balance your brain chemistry by augmenting your acetylcholine, you will be able to make a permanent change in your weight. If you haven't addressed your brain chemistry before, you can now see why other diets have failed you in the past. If you were low in acetylcholine, other so-called low-fat diets were not providing you with the nutrients your brain desperately needs. And other diets that let you eat high-fat foods to compensate for the loss of other single nutrients were not helping, either.

The only way to achieve lasting weight loss is to determine your unique deficiency, and then follow a diet that is customized to your needs. Now that you understand your acetylcholine deficit, you can see how to improve your brain and your total health. Take these lessons and customize the Younger (Thinner) You Diet in Chapter 7 for the best results.

CHAPTER 5

Break the Cycle of Emotional Eating with GABA

GAMMA-AMINOBUTYRIC ACID, OR GABA, is a naturally produced chemical that functions as your brain's calming agent. It helps to regulate the nervous system and keeps all other brain chemicals connected. It also controls the brain's rhythm so that electrical signals can travel from the brain to the body in a steady flow. GABA is the opposite of dopamine and acetylcholine, working as an electrical "off" switch to the electrical system. Along with serotonin, it creates a sense of calm and order, what I call the "Zen" of the brain. In order to lose weight, you need to have a calm, stable brain chemistry supported by exactly the right amount of GABA.

When you have too little GABA, you lose your Zen. It can cause you to feel anxious, overwhelmed, unwell, and even shaky, because your electrical signals are being sent in pulses instead of in a steady stream. That's why migraines, mood swings, sleep problems, anxiety, and panic attacks are all related to a GABA imbalance. Too much GABA stretches out the electrical signals so that it can slowly put you in a coma.

The results of the Younger (Thinner) You Diet Quiz in Chapter 2 may have pointed toward a GABA deficit. If so, your anxiousness might be impairing your ability to lose weight. Living in a state of anxiety often results in losing your sense of boundaries, so that you crave large amounts of food, or choose the wrong foods to eat. Often, my first course of action with overweight patients is to get them to calm down: I relieve their anxiety by increasing their GABA levels through various treatment options, including nutrients, diet, exercise, and medications. Once they are on a more even keel, they no longer rely on comfort foods or binging to relieve the stress in their lives. And when stress is under control, they can concentrate on dieting properly and instantly begin to feel younger.

Studies have long shown that stress can increase your desire for food. Stress alters the way the brain works, particularly in the way it contemplates the consequences of actions. When we are placed in a stressful situation, the brain tunes out everything except what was frightening you. This is called the fight-or-flight mode.[1] When you are stressed, you stop thinking about the consequences of eating. Your judgment is busted, you resort to panic eating, and eat whatever will calm you down.

Without GABA, we cannot soothe ourselves out of this mindset. So we rely on foods to soothe us. The more anxious we become, the more unhealthy food choices we'll make. This is the GABA emotional eating cycle that needs to be broken.

Recent scientific advances have been able to unlock the mysteries behind the relationship between GABA and weight gain, and their findings fall exactly in line with the same treatment protocols I have been using for years. Researchers like me are particularly interested in GABA and its relationship to food addiction. Some hypothesize that the dopamine-addictive craving cycle is also affected by a GABA deficiency. For instance, people

with alcohol and cocaine addictions have been shown to have less GABA in their brains, and medications that increase GABA have shown some effectiveness in treating these addictions.[2] This is why I believe normalizing GABA levels will assist in breaking food addictions along with the craving and anxiety cycles that are aging you.

A GABA deficiency is connected to overeating and lack of portion control. I often share this analogy with my patients: Imagine your body is a car. The dopamine receptors in your brain are the gas and GABA is the brakes. If you are suffering from a food addiction, it's like driving a car with the pedal to the floor, only to find out the brakes don't work. Without the brakes, you may be eating large quantities of food without ever getting the signal from your brain or your stomach to stop. In essence, the brain never gets satisfied.

These findings show that losing weight is not primarily connected to willpower, love, God, discipline, family support, or any twelve-step program. It's about an aging brain, genetic tendencies, and bad habits we've developed. In order to restore your GABA to the proper levels, so you can control your portions and stop eating when you are anxious, you need to reevaluate your food choices, retrain your brain, and learn other effective and less fattening ways to relax.

Pain and Overeating

Chronic pain can make people eat more. GABA plays an important role in pain management, so if you are experiencing chronic pain, you most likely have a GABA deficiency. It doesn't matter whether the pain drains your GABA, or if your low GABA creates the pain: A brain in perpetual GABA deficiency ends up as an overweight body in pain.

ANXIOUS AND HUNGRY

If you constantly feel on edge or have trouble sleeping, these problems can be huge roadblocks to weight loss. Anxiety triggers the release of the stress hormone cortisol. It counteracts all your other good hormones, increasing your pain, anxiety, and mood swings. Chronically elevated cortisol, which we discussed in Chapter 2, causes an increase in belly fat along with a decrease in insulin sensitivity and, most important, an increase in appetite: yet another reason why so many of us eat when we are anxious or under stress. Many of my patients who are battling obesity are also dealing with controlling their moods. But when they begin to ease their anxiety, their mood swings dissipate and they feel relaxed enough to be able to follow the program and achieve the successful weight loss they desire.

On the Younger (Thinner) You Diet, your mood and emotions will be kept in check, largely due to the food choices you will be making. Many of the foods on the diet will balance your GABA so you have just the right amount. By doing so, you may feel your life take on a Zenlike quality: Your mind is at peace, and your body is at its peak. Best of all, you won't even feel the need to overeat.

HOW STRESSED ARE YOU?

One way to see if stress is controlling your life as well as your waistline is to take this stress challenge. Check off each event that you have experienced this year.

EVENT	STRESS SCORES
____ Death of spouse/significant other	100
____ Divorce	73
____ Marital separation	65
____ Jail term	63
____ Death of close family member	63
____ Personal injury or illness	53
____ Marriage	50
____ Fired from work	47
____ Marital reconciliation	45
____ Retirement	45

EVENT	STRESS SCORES
____ Change in family member's health	44
____ Pregnancy	40
____ Sex difficulties	39
____ Addition to family	39
____ Business readjustment	39
____ Change in financial status	38
____ Death of close friend	37
____ Change to a different line of work	36
____ Change in number of marital arguments	35
____ Outstanding mortgage or loan over $500,000	31
____ Foreclosure of mortgage or loan	30
____ Change in work responsibilities	29
____ Trouble with in-laws	29
____ Outstanding personal achievement	28
____ Spouse begins or stops work	26
____ Starting or finishing school	26
____ Change in living conditions	25
____ Revision of personal habits	24
____ Trouble with boss	23
____ Change in work hours, conditions	20
____ Change in residence	20
____ Change in schools	20
____ Change in recreational habits	19
____ Change in church activities	19
____ Change in social activities	18
____ Outstanding mortgage or loan under $250,000	17
____ Change in sleeping habits	16
____ Change in number of family gatherings	15
____ Change in eating habits	15
____ Vacation	13
____ Difficulty coping during the holiday season	12
____ Minor violation of the law	11

Assessing Your Score:

Add up the points you've accumulated.

0–50: Low susceptibility to obesity or weight gain

51–100: Medium susceptibility to obesity or weight gain

101+: High susceptibility to obesity or weight gain

> ### Did You Know . . .
>
> Junk food binges and opiate drugs, like heroin or morphine, set off the same pleasure receptors in the brain. That's why Harvard Medical School professor Harrison Pope, Jr., MD, believes that binge eating is more than just a bad habit: It's a genuine psychiatric disorder. In the extreme, he's found that a single binge can rack up as many as 20,000 calories.[3] Although it sounds unbelievable, I can easily see it happening, especially if you have binged on junk foods, fast foods, whole pizzas, or can sit down and eat an entire cake, pie, or gallon of ice cream.

WHAT DOES A GABA DEFICIENCY FEEL LIKE?

Compared to some of the other brain chemical deficiencies, low GABA symptoms are relatively minor. When your GABA levels first begin to falter you might feel fine, but you can't seem to shake a nagging headache. You're annoyed by the constant burping that follows every meal. Your sleep can be disturbed by night sweats. You might even experience occasional dizzy spells, clammy hands, or forget what your best friend asked you to do for her. And you might ask yourself why daily tasks are suddenly such a chore.

If your GABA levels continue to drop off, you might find that much too frequently your day ends with tasks left undone, which makes the next day problematic. Those close to you may begin to remark how you haven't been your usual self. Meanwhile, your constant anxiety accelerates weight gain and depression, and can cause you to withdraw completely—from your work, your community, and your family. With all this wor-

rying, you will literally grow old right before your eyes.

So you eat and eat to stop your feelings of panic. You help yourself to seconds at every meal. You binge at buffets. You can eat an entire box of cookies in a sitting, or pick at other's plates when you are out to dinner. And even if you've had your fill, when it's time to order dessert, you'll order one "just to taste."

BINGE-EATING DISORDER

GABA and serotonin deficiencies are the primary reasons behind your desire for binge eating. But binging is also a psychological disorder. A recent study in the journal *Biological Psychiatry* suggests more than 3% of women suffer from binge-eating disorder, more than double the incidence of bulimia and four times that of anorexia.[4]

You may not even realize your eating patterns are considered binging, or you may not think you are binging as often as you are. A typical binger will eat carefully all day, eat a normal dinner, and a few hours later will go back to the kitchen for a single cookie and end up eating the whole bag. Then they might move on to eating something salty, so they polish off a bag of pretzels.

When I bring this topic up with my overweight patients, I'm constantly surprised by their need to define and quantify binge eating. For example, one woman once told me that she wasn't a binge eater because she only felt the urge to indulge in eating an entire chocolate cake on the weekends. Another patient told me that she binges on cheese, but didn't think that was a problem because she thought it was a "healthy choice." So let me put it straight: Binging is a problem because it is a sign of *food abuse*. If you are binging once a week and not carrying extra weight because of it, you are lucky. If you are binging and the weight is creeping up, then you have a bigger problem. And if you are reading this book and worrying about your binging, then I guess you can answer the question for yourself.

Your reasons for binge eating are as individual as you are. However, researchers find that certain characteristics commonly affect binge eating:

Depression or "blues": As many as half of all people with binge-eating disorder are currently depressed or have been depressed in the past. Most bingers actually feel "blue," which begins as feelings of anxiety. Feeling "blue" is far more common than being clinically depressed.

Dieting: Some people binge after skipping meals, not eating enough food each day, or avoiding certain kinds of food for long periods of time. For example, if you were following a no-carb diet, you might find yourself craving pizza, and then you'll eat an entire pie instead of stopping after a single slice.

Coping skills: Studies suggest people with binge-eating disorder have trouble handling their emotions. Many people who are binge eaters say being angry, sad, bored, worried, or stressed can cause them to binge eat.

Biology: Researchers suggest genes may be involved in binge eating, since the disorder often occurs in several members of the same family. But does this argument support nature or nurture? If you come from a family of bingers, are you modeling their behavior, or do you have a

Are You a Binge Eater?

My patients with binge-eating disorder often eat large amounts of food and feel out of control while they are eating. The medical description of this syndrome uses these qualifiers. You may be suffering from a binge-eating disorder if you:

- Eat more quickly than usual during binge episodes
- Eat until you are uncomfortably full
- Eat when you are not hungry
- Eat alone because of embarrassment
- Feel disgusted, depressed, or guilty after overeating

biological trigger to eat compulsively? Research also supports certain behaviors and emotional problems are more common in people with binge-eating disorder. These include abusing alcohol, acting quickly without thinking (impulsive behavior), and not feeling in charge of themselves. Sounds like a GABA imbalance to me.

How to Stop Binging

Whether you have been binging all your life or just started this habit following an extremely restricting diet, binge eating may require professional help to resolve. If you follow the Younger (Thinner) You Diet but still find yourself raiding the fridge when you are upset, seek the help of a professional therapist who practices cognitive behavior therapy, or interpersonal psychotherapy. Both of these treatment modalities can get to the root of your problem and give you a unique set of tools so you can stop this behavior. Professional therapy can also address your thoughts and behaviors about eating and self-image, and will help identify if there are any underlying rifts in your current relationships that may be at the heart of the problem. Experts find that treating personal problems often has a positive effect on weight loss, so don't disregard this advice.

Outside of the psychological realm, here are a few techniques I share with my patients to get them off binging:

- Don't over-caffeinate during the day: Switch to a coffee with chicory (a favorite in New Orleans), which will help ease your anxiety and may also help with weight loss.
- Don't overstimulate during the day. Overly excitable people tend to binge at night.
- Make sure your bowels are adequately cleansed by consuming high-fiber foods such as apricots or berries.
- Meditate for a few minutes before you walk into a kitchen. This will allow you to relax so you won't have to rely on foods to improve your mood.
- Stop taking on the emotional burdens of others.
- Focus on what you can do to change a bad situation instead of letting anger fester.

Mindless Munchers

Many people find it hard to express their true feelings, and try to hold their world together without "getting all emotional." Their goal is to control their environment and everyone around them. But when their GABA is low, they can no longer keep their feelings bottled up inside, and they look to food to provide the comfort and order they crave. Food provides the chemical substitute for the emotional connection they are lacking. They need food just to keep their mind going in a singular direction, in effect to stay "on task."

EATING TRENDS AND YOUR PERSONALITY

A GABA deficiency affects your personality, and can change the way food fits into your world. For example, aside from the way you deal with stress, GABA-deficient people tend to gain weight because they are open to new experiences, like tasting new foods, but have poor boundaries. This means they don't know when to stop doing anything: giving too much, taking too much, and thinking too much. In the case of food, they don't know when to stop eating. So it's not just that they lack boundaries in the food component of their life; they lack boundaries in every aspect of their life.

By enhancing your GABA, you'll find it easier to establish proper boundaries, and you'll start to feel like you fit in better with the rest of your community. As you learn to understand your own boundaries, you'll understand the boundaries of others. You will find you are in better control not only in your life but in how and what you eat. You suddenly won't feel controlled by food—you will be in control.

The following are frequent personality components for low-GABA individuals. See if any resemble how you are feeling about yourself right now.

- **Have you been neglecting your weight and your personal care?** The feeling of losing control leads to feelings of hopelessness and ultimately leads to just giving in, asking yourself why you should even bother grooming, dressing up, or caring about your appearance. Enhancing your GABA will calm your nerves, and will enable you to see how others perceive you. When you feel better about yourself, you'll want to take care of your body and health, including improving your personal care.
- **Is your weight affecting long-term relationships?** Again, it boils down to a matter of control and boundaries. You feel bad because you are out of control, and it's affecting your relationships because you are not sharing with others how you really feel. By enhancing your GABA, you'll be calmer, happier, and it will have a positive effect on the other people in your life.

Consistency Creates Calmness

Some say change is good. But in order for you to get control of your weight, you need structure. One way to do so is to create and maintain a daily schedule. Write in the times that pertain to your list of daily tasks below. See if there are items that differ on a daily basis (consider only working days, and at least one hour differences qualify for "differing"). If you have inconsistencies with more than one item on this list, you are setting yourself up for weight loss failure.

- _____ Wake-up time
- _____ Breakfast time
- _____ Work time
- _____ Lunch time
- _____ Exercise time
- _____ Bedtime

● **Has dieting always been hard for you?** Do you find yourself cheating on diets, or not being able to stick with a program for long? Do you have inconsistent meal patterns, fitting in food whenever you can? I find my low-GABA patients are usually not hungry in the morning and rarely take time to plan meals. Then they are surprised when they don't lose weight, but tell me, "I eat whatever, whenever I want." By enhancing your GABA, you'll be able to stick with the Younger (Thinner) You Diet. You'll be able to set limits on the times you eat so you can limit the amount of food you eat. And then you'll lose weight.

GABA Deficient Personality Types:

EMOTION/ACTION	WHAT IT MEANS:
Painfully shy and anxious	● Feelings easily hurt ● Avoids social activities ● Fearful of new experiences ● Puts others in control ● Avoids activities for fear of physical discomfort
Drama queen	● Speech is exaggerated ● Constantly seeks reassurance, approval, or praise ● Inappropriately sexually seductive appearance or behavior ● Overly concerned with physical appearance ● Exaggerated expression of emotions (embraces acquaintances, cries over nothing, has temper tantrums) ● Must always be the center of attention ● Shallow and lacking in genuine emotion ● Egocentric and self-indulgent
Unstable	● Poor sense of boundaries ● Most relationships are unstable ● Constantly feels "out of control"
Self-absorbed	● Feels rage, shame, or humiliation at criticism ● Takes credit for others' work ● Exaggerates self-importance ● Preoccupied with fantasies of success, power, brilliance, beauty, or love ● Requires constant attention and admiration ● Expects of special favors ● Indifferent to the feelings of others ● Feels envious
Aggressive	● Likes to intimidate and humiliate others ● Recklessly daring, thick-skinned, and is seemingly undeterred by pain ● Verbally abusive ● Detached from the impact of own destructive acts ● Lacks sentimental memories, tender feelings ● Provokes conflict, shame, and guilt ● Temper quickly flares

Meet Jessica W: She's Got the Gift of GABA

Jessica is 50 years old, stands 5' 3", and weighs 185 pounds. About a year ago, she'd had enough. When she came into my office, she complained about her weight, but she also told me she was having trouble concentrating at work. She was upset because she had held the same high-powered job for more than twenty years, but suddenly she felt she wasn't good at it. This loyal, giving soul felt she had less energy every day to accomplish the demands of her job. She heard, saw, and understood what her tasks and duties were, but lacked the resources to complete them. She was desperate to keep up with her genius memory, but found her lack of energy impossible as well as frustrating. When she found herself feeling out of control, she ate bagels, cookies, and other junk food in large quantities in an attempt to feel some sort of energy rush. Now she was heavier than ever before.

Every doctor Jessica saw had a different opinion, yet none was able to help. One was sure she was hypothyroid; another tested to see if her leptin levels were elevated. She was prescribed medication for depression and chronic inflammation.

While some of these issues might have been real, resolving them did not allow her to lose weight or regain her concentration. Instead, I decided to work with Jessica using my "headfirst" approach. I gave her a complete physical, BEAM, and memory testing, and found that while she had a 99th-percentile memory, her ability to concentrate had deteriorated to 50%. I told Jessica her weight was accelerating her perimenopause, and that if she didn't take control of her eating, she was looking at a further increase of 40 pounds over the next decade.

I had Jessica start the Younger (Thinner) You Diet, with an emphasis on dopamine- and GABA-producing foods and nutrients. I made sure she drank lots of tea, which contains theanine, to help enhance her attention and focus. The results were instant and long-lasting. Her dopamine brain chemistry was boosted, her GABA chemistry was stabilized, and her weight began to peel off, like the skin of an orange, strip by strip. Now when Jessica comes in, she's got a determined look on her face and a spring in her step. This is not only because she's lighter, but because her internal energy has returned, so she knows where she's headed.

Stick with What's Good for You

You might be thinking that there have been times a candy bar did the trick to calm you down. And you're right. Simple (refined) carbs will calm the brain, but create an imbalance over the long run. Snacking on a candy bar, for example, might provide a quick fix for GABA anxiety, but it's temporary. Within a couple of hours your GABA imbalance will be back. So if you have a GABA deficiency, you should avoid simple sugars, white flours, and most refined wheat products, like pasta, crackers, and pancakes.

- **Do you think bigger is better?** Low-GABA individuals are often narcissistic and have grandiose thoughts. Sometimes they overeat in attempt to literally make themselves larger, thinking that eating big and being big means they are important, and that the size of what one eats and the size of the body is significant to one's character. For example, short men never want to lose a lot of weight. They figure if they have to walk into a room, they don't want to look like a skinny little thing as well as a short thing. They find that girth gives them a sense of presence. While you might not be an opera star, you might think that looking like one—and behaving like one—is a fine way to get attention. But the only person you'll be attracting is your nearest cardiologist.

- **Are you unwilling to take hold of your life?** Low-GABA individuals are often highly excitable and have difficulty facing reality. Very excitable people have a tendency to remain overly wound up well into the evening, and then find themselves overeating in their search for an outlet. By taking a deep breath and reflecting on what is happening in your life, you will be able to relax, and ultimately regain control of your life, your eating, and your moods.

GABA FOODS ARE COMPLEX CARBOHYDRATES

GABA deficiencies can be treated by making better food choices. The more GABA-producing foods you eat, the more GABA you will be able to create. The goal of a high-GABA diet is to ensure the body has enough raw materials for creating a steady supply of glutamine, the amino acid that is the precursor to GABA. The benefits of a high-GABA diet will be evident after a few weeks as your body gets an adequate supply of glutamine to keep its GABA flowing. Daily anxiety symptoms such as headache and irritable bowel syndrome will dissipate. If you've been having trouble sleeping, you'll be amazed at how calm and relaxed you are at the end of the day. You'll fall asleep easily, sleep undisturbed, and wake fully rested.

Glutamine is found in abundance in fiber-rich foods and complex carbohydrates.

Complex carbohydrates are different than the simple, refined carbohydrates I've told you to avoid. Unlike simple carbs, complex carbs will not fit into the definition of "white foods." Instead, complex carbs are found in whole grain form such as whole wheat or whole grain breads, oats, muesli, and brown rice.

All carbohydrates are broken down into glucose during digestion. Simple carbs are easily digested, so you can eat lots of them. In contrast, complex carbs are broken down into glucose more slowly and will provide you with a gradual, steady stream of energy throughout the day. This will help you control mood fluctuations as well as help your GABA send its electrical signals in more even and steady flows.

Most natural, complex carbohydrate sources provide many of the vitamins and minerals we need and are an excellent source of fiber. So when we eat complex carbs, the foods are broken down and used to support the functioning of different parts of the body: The fiber cleanses our internal organs and the vitamins are sent through the bloodstream to be used as needed. On the other hand, simple, refined carbs found in many processed foods tend to be devoid of fiber and other nutrients. When these foods are eaten, the digestive process can't use any of its raw materials, so most of it will simply be converted into body fat. This is often the case even if the calorie content of the simple carb is lower than the calories in a similar complex carbohydrate source, such as comparing the calories in a slice of white bread with a similar-sized slice of whole wheat bread.[4]

Besides being a good source of glutamine, complex carbohydrates will fill you up and keep you full longer. Choose foods from this list every day:

- Beans
- Bran
- Brown rice
- Cassava (yuca)
- Corn
- High-fiber breakfast cereals
- Lentils
- Oatmeal
- Peas
- Root vegetables (such as carrots, beets, rutabagas, turnips)
- Whole wheat or whole meal breads
- Yams (sweet potatoes)

Glutamine can also be found in:

- Dairy products (although most are not allowed on this diet)
- Fish
- Meats
- Poultry

Foods for Thought

Figs, spinach, and kale all contain magnesium, which is a great agent for calming nervousness and irritability and augmenting GABA.

BOOST GABA WITH VITAMIN B FOODS

You'll also need to choose a variety of foods that are high in vitamin B. In particular, bananas, broccoli, and brown rice are all packed with inositol, a B-complex vitamin that boosts GABA production. Try to incorporate at least two of these foods into your meal plan every day. Swap these for other suggested fruits and vegetables on the meal plans to boost your particular brain chemistry needs:

- Bananas
- Beans
- Beef liver
- Beets
- Broccoli
- Cantaloupe
- Figs
- Grapefruit
- Halibut
- Kale
- Lentils
- Mangoes
- Nuts
- Oats
- Oranges
- Spinach
- Wheat and wheat bran

STOP A PANIC ATTACK WITH A SPICY MEAL

Generously sprinkling any of these spices on your favorite vegetables can provide some mental relief when you are stressed. Eat slowly, savor the flavor, and you'll find you can calm down. Remember, no one ever binges on too much broccoli, especially when it's spicy and delicious.

- Caraway
- Cardamom
- Cilantro
- Cinnamon
- Cloves
- Coriander
- Lemongrass
- Oregano
- Paprika
- Poppy seeds

NUTRIENTS THAT INCREASE GABA FOR A YOUNGER, CALMER BRAIN

Proper supplementation will guarantee that you reverse your GABA deficiency, especially at the beginning of this diet, which will be your key to success. There are many readily available vitamins and supplements that can ensure a steady supply of GABA. They are best taken in the late afternoon through the early evening; these supplements will help you relax, and you don't want to slow down in the morning when you need to approach the day with vigor.

Binge Repair

Ate something you know you shouldn't have? Now what do you do? Flush it out. Choose one of the following remedies to get you back on track and reset your metabolism.

- Mix a glass of pomegranate juice with 4 teaspoons of Benefiber (I like the magnesium formula).
- Eat ½ cup blackberries or blueberries.
- Drink two glasses of water.
- A half-day fast can help correct calorie overextension.
- Drink one to four cups of green tea.

Inositol Creates More GABA

Inositol produces a calming and relaxing effect by activating GABA, so foods rich in inositol are essential for the Younger (Thinner) You Diet.

The natural treatments below will not only help your weight loss efforts, but will promote more brain stability and less anxiety. I have created a GABA-balancing nutrient program that I call Brain Calm. It contains valine, isoleucine, leucine, inositol, and B-complex vitamins. Working together, these nutrients convert to a natural "Valium" that can calm the brain. I find that with many of my patients who are dieting, their stress levels skyrocket. Brain Calm is almost always prescribed.

THE POWER OF TEAS

I cannot stress enough the healing and weight loss power of teas. Tea is a calorie-free beverage. Nothing is more relaxing to me than a hot cup of tea on a cold winter day. I drink iced teas throughout the spring and summer for a dose of refreshment. On the Younger (Thinner) You Diet you will be drinking tea with every meal. You'll learn more about tea varieties in Chapter 7.

Tea is great for calming an anxious mind. That's because tea contains an amino acid called theanine.[5] Recent research has shown theanine may play an important role in the stimulatory effects of tea. Several studies have found that L-theanine, the predominant form of theanine found in tea, stimulates alpha brain waves, which are associated with a relaxed but alert mental state of mind. Theanine appears to work quickly and is most effective when someone is stressed, which is why it supports GABA production. Theanine may also help enhance your attention and focus. Because theanine helps the mind stop racing it also seems to help promote a more restful, sound sleep, which will not be interrupted by random thoughts.

NATURAL TREATMENTS	SUGGESTED DAILY DOSAGE	WHAT IT DOES
Nutritional		
Inositol	100–10000 mcg	Produces a calming and relaxing effect by activating GABA
Branched chain amino acids	5–20 g	Works as a fuel source for muscles, helps with physical exertion
GABA	500–3000 mg	Controls anxiety that leads to overeating
Taurine	500–10000 mg	May inhibit weight gain
Magnesium	300–1000 mg	Increases energy production
Theanine	100–500 mg	Reduces mental and physical stress and may produce feelings of relaxation

What about Hoodia?

You may have seen this supplement at your local pharmacy or advertised in a magazine. Hoodia comes from the cactus-like plant of the same name (*Hoodia gordonii*) that is native to African deserts. It may be useful for the prevention and treatment of obesity due to its ability to suppress appetite. It has been used by the Bushmen of the Kalahari for hundreds of years for this purpose. However, there is not much scientific data available about this plant extract.

Hoodia contains a mixture of active ingredients called P57, which acts on glucose-sensing cells in the hypothalamus, suppressing hunger and thirst signals.[6] Check with your doctor to see if it will have any adverse interactions with other medications you may be taking.

LEARN TO RELAX

The greatest lesson of this chapter is that there are many ways of dealing with anxiety that don't involve food. By learning how to recognize your anxiety, and then dealing with the situation instead of literally feeding it, you will keep yourself from falling into the emotional eating trap again.

First, you need to realize your life doesn't have to be defined in terms of someone else. Doing something solely for your immediate enjoyment is healthy. In fact, you'll be much better at taking care of others once you learn to take care of yourself. Listening to music, quietly reading, taking solitary walks, exercising, or praying are all ways to spend time alone without the rest of the world getting in the way. You may need to take an hour a day just to unwind until you feel significantly less stressed. As your body adjusts to the foods on the diet, you may find you don't need as much time to relax. But don't let go of this hour. Everyone deserves alone time to do the things they like to do. Once you carve out this time, keep it.

Visual Meditation

For my patients who can't seem to relax on their own, I have them do the following exercise:

Gaze at your favorite photograph. Choose one that features one of your loved ones, a place you have enjoyed visiting, or even a landscape, still life, or a personally significant work of fine art. If you are looking at a photograph of a religious object, you may find it will help you create a spiritual connection. Whatever you choose, gaze at the image for a few moments, and then close your eyes and calmly try to re-create this image in your mind. Take your time as you redraw the vision in your head. Try to conceptualize what makes this image important to you, and why you have a unique relationship with it. When you feel you are fully connected to the image, open your eyes and see if your mental image matches the actual object.

BIOIDENTICAL HORMONES HELP KICK-START A GABA PROGRAM

Discuss these hormone therapies with your doctor to see if they can help increase your GABA to appropriate levels:

- Progesterone
- Pregnenolone
- GHRH
- Oxytocin

THE LAST RESORT: MEDICATION

GABA agents are medications that will calm you down and may help facilitate weight loss. But medications should be your last resort instead of your first course of action. You can discuss these medicines with your doctor if you have been on the Younger (Thinner) You Diet for more than three months without any weight loss.

- **Topamax:** This medication was originally produced as an antiseizure or bipolar disorder medication. It can be an effective medication for obesity because GABA controls the anxiety of overeating.
- **Campral:** This GABA medication was originally produced to help with alcohol addiction, and some people with obesity have had great results with this drug's ability to control food cravings. It has been shown to counteract sugar and carb cravings to some degree. Campral can be an important adjunct in your fight against obesity, especially if there are other addictions involved in your personal struggle.

CONTROLLING GABA MAKES BRAIN CHEMISTRY WORK BETTER

Even though dopamine is thought to be the most important brain chemical related to weight loss, the reality is that without enough GABA, you will never lose weight. It doesn't matter how strong your metabolism is if you can't stop eating.

In the long run, too much stress stemming from too little GABA burns out your dopamine, acetylcholine, and serotonin. So when you are anxious, you can't eat right, you can't think clearly, and you can't sleep. Basically, you fall from rhythmic balance and you feel older.

This is why it is so vitally important to keep your GABA in check—not only for your weight but for becoming a younger you. With the help of the Younger (Thinner) You Diet, you'll be able to do just that.

You Don't Have to See Your Doctor to Kick-Start GABA

With pregnenolone's neurogenesis power and ability to grow new brain cells, it needs to be increasingly explored as a method of weight loss. It is simple, safe, sold over the counter, and in very high dosages, it has been shown to improve memory as well as help people feel better.

CHAPTER 6

Control Cravings and Find Happiness with Serotonin

SEROTONIN is the brain chemical that allows you to experience pleasure and feel good about yourself. When your serotonin levels are strong, you feel alive and excited about taking on new challenges. At night, serotonin allows the brain to recharge and rebalance as you experience deep, restful sleep, so every morning you begin with a fresh start. That's why I equate balanced serotonin to complete serenity. And when your brain is balanced and refreshed, you'll find it a whole lot easier to lose weight.

Yet as we get older, serotonin levels begin to wane. You may notice that your mood is the first aspect of your overall health that has changed. While dopamine and GABA deficiencies affect our emotional life, serotonin deficiencies are markedly different, and even more pronounced. Instead of feeling fatigued (low dopamine) or anxious (low GABA), without serotonin we don't feel much of anything. That's why the stereotypical aged person is often portrayed as crotchety or withdrawn: This is an

example of someone who has burned out their serotonin.

The results of the Younger (Thinner) You Diet Quiz in Chapter 2 may have indicated you have a serotonin deficiency. You might have noticed that you just don't feel like yourself. You may be less willing to take chances, and you can't get a restful night's sleep no matter what you try. You may even feel depressed, or find yourself in a blue mood that you can't seem to shake.

Both sleep disturbances and depression can influence weight gain, because either instance of low serotonin levels will alter your thinking, which can then cause a host of food-related problems. Emotional upheavals can subliminally lead you to self-medicate through food, fostering specific food cravings that when satisfied, can temporarily change your mood. For example, have you ever told anyone "I eat when I'm depressed"? If so, think about the foods you choose when you are in a funk. If you are low in serotonin, chances are very good that you are a "salty snack" binger: simple carbs and salty foods actually provide more energy to combat fatigue, and actually help to release stored serotonin.[1] Multiple studies have shown that serotonin deficiency leads to salt craving, which then rebalances the serotonin system.

But even though highly salted carbs, like potato chips, provide the lift you are looking for, they don't provide the nutrition your body desperately needs. Worse, salty foods make you retain water, so you are constantly bloated. Those are real pounds you will shed almost immediately once you give up excess salt. The harder-to-shed pounds come from the excess carbs you're gorging on, which are the same ones that become instant body fat when you overload.

You don't have to become a caricature of the typical nursing home patient. Instead, you can boost your serotonin levels in a variety of healthy ways and become younger. By following the suggestions in this chapter, you will be able to increase your serotonin and retrain your brain. You will learn how to get out of a black mood without the help of fattening foods so you can reverse your bad and often dangerous eating habits. At the same time, you'll learn the tricks you need to get a better night's sleep so your brain can rest, allowing you to make better food choices the next day. By doing so, you will finally be able to lose weight permanently and feel better about yourself.

THE BAD NEWS ABOUT SEROTONIN AND SALT

Even though salty foods promote the release of serotonin and can improve your blue mood, too much sodium is extremely bad for the body, especially if you have high blood pressure. Salt causes blood vessels and organs to swell and bloat, and interferes with metabolism by slowing it down. At the same time, increased salt consumption leads to making more bad food choices, because the more salty foods you eat, the more powerful cravings will be. And if you're a smoker, you are probably adding more salt to your food than the average person because you've fried your taste buds (yet another great reason to quit).

Some foods are surprisingly loaded with salt, and if you are low in serotonin, put these on your Stay Out of My Kitchen List.

- Canned vegetables
- Smoked fish (smoked salmon, trout)
- Cured meats (hot dogs, luncheon meats, ham, bacon, sausage)

Low Serotonin Is a Flavor Bust

Have you ever kept eating even after you realized you were full because you weren't satisfied, or searched for an elusive flavor or texture in your favorite foods? When you are low in serotonin, your connection with your five senses declines. Often, you can't taste your food so you compensate lack of flavor with quantity or load your food with salt. Try loading your food with spices instead.

- Sauerkraut
- Fast food
- Desserts containing baking soda, baking powder, salt, or buttermilk
- Soy sauce
- Worcestershire sauce
- Salted snack foods, crackers, or nuts
- Pickles
- Olives

SLEEP IS THE EASIEST WAY TO BECOME YOUNGER AND THINNER

Lack of sleep is one of the great age accelerators, prematurely aging your brain as well as your body. That's because as you age, the quality of your sleep deteriorates, even if you are getting the same amount of sleep as you always did. When your serotonin levels fall, you won't get as much REM (rapid eye movement) sleep, which is the deepest, most restorative sleep phase.[2] Poor sleep affects every aspect of your health, including your:

- **Brain and nervous system:** Poor sleep affects your thinking and response time, and creates attention disturbances and impaired memory. Mental and emotional problems linked to a lack of deep sleep include irritability, anxiety, and depression.
- **Cardiovascular system:** The body senses sleep loss as a "stress-inducing" state, which raises levels of stress hormones such as adrenaline and cortisol, which leave you bloated. These hormones also regulate blood pressure. When these hormone levels are chronically elevated, blood pressure becomes more difficult to control, leading to a higher risk for heart disease. Lack of sleep seems to affect women more than men. Researchers at Warwick Medical School in Canada found that women who slept five or fewer hours per night were at an increased risk for hypertension as compared to men who slept five or fewer hours.[3]
- **Immune system:** During times of elevated physical, emotional, and mental stress, such as illness or emotional upset, the mind and body need greater amounts of sleep to support healing. Your body and immune system do most of its repairs and rejuvenation while you sleep, so if you are not getting enough sleep, you are limiting your body's natural ability to repair itself.

CONTROLLING HUNGER WITH BETTER SLEEP

Have you ever had a restless night's sleep and feel famished in the morning? The cause of your hunger is actually too little sleep. And the result from being overtired is that your body and your brain are primed to make two distinct but equally bad decisions. First, when you wake up starving, you might reach for something easy and quick to eat.

No Sleep = No Motivation to Make Good Choices

A recent study by psychologist Dr. Dean Cruess at the University of Pennsylvania shows that people who get less sleep are more likely to choose foods the next day that will put on extra pounds.[4] That's because people are less motivated to make healthy food choices when they're tired. They are also less motivated to exercise. The no sleep = no motivation equation directly affects your metabolism, which is now at a simmer instead of a full-flamed burn.

The typical American breakfast of cold cereals, toast, or a bagel will provide an energy burst as well as satisfy your hunger. But literally feeding your energy needs this way will only slow you down. When you reach for any of these carbs, your body will turn them directly into body fat. The next carb-heavy meal will do the same thing, and eventually you will train your body to store all carbs and never burn them. This leaves you more tired and ultimately heavier. As a result, chronic sleep deprivation may not only lead to weight gain, but to an increased risk for diabetes.

Poor sleep can also affect your internal chemistry. Researchers are now discovering that sleep directly influences two key hormones that regulate satiety and hunger: ghrelin and leptin. Elevated levels of ghrelin increase feelings of hunger, while leptin acts to suppress appetite. Interestingly, serotonin is vital to regulating the brain's response to both of these hormones.

The hormone leptin is found in our body fat. Its job is to communicate with the brain about your energy stores by sending signals to the brain when the body has had enough to eat.[6] If serotonin levels are low, leptin levels will become low as well, and the message that you are full will never reach the brain. So you eat really large quantities of food and, not surprisingly, gain weight. If you've ever heard someone say, "I'm really big so I need a lot of food to fill me up," chances are they are low in serotonin and leptin. In fact, the amount of food

Are You Losing Sleep over Your Meds?

A serotonin deficiency may not be the only reason you aren't sleeping. If you are taking any of the following medications, they may be affecting your ability to get restful sleep, which is disturbing your ability to lose weight:[5]

- Anticholinergics
- Antidepressants
- Beta blockers
- Bronchodilators
- Clonidine
- Central nervous system (CNS) stimulants
- Corticosteroids
- Decongestants
- Levodopa (L-dopa)
- Oral contraceptives
- Phenytoin
- Quinidine
- Smoking cessation medications
- Thyroid preparations

you need to eat has nothing to do with your current size, but has everything to do with a balanced brain.

Insufficient sleep—caused by low serotonin—can also affect your leptin levels. When you suffer from sleep deprivation, your body's levels of leptin and ghrelin fall, creating that "hungry but never satisfied" feeling. One study suggested that individuals who sleep fewer than five hours a night were found to have significantly more ghrelin and significantly less leptin than those who sleep at least eight hours. Another study put it more bluntly: Researchers at Columbia University found people who get less than four hours of sleep per night were 73% more likely to be obese than those who get seven to nine hours of shut-eye.[7]

A third hormone affected by sleep deprivation is growth hormone. Just one week of recurring nights of poor sleep can inhibit your natural production of growth hormone. This hormone is vital for controlling the body's proportion of muscle to fat. Without proper levels of growth hormone, you increase the tendency for the body to store fat instead of building metabolism-enhancing muscle.

The Younger (Thinner) You Diet is not necessarily a low-carb diet, but it does require you to choose more complex carbs that provide nutrition as well as the building blocks of serotonin. These carbs are slower to digest, so you feel full longer, and the body has more time to use them as fuel. That way, you're burning more and storing less: You are retraining your body, which will facilitate weight loss. With more serotonin, you'll also get more sleep, so you can produce more ghrelin, which then boosts growth hormone levels and cuts your carbohydrate cravings.

DEPRESSION, BLUES, AND BODY WEIGHT

As many as 35 million people suffer from depression,[8] an emotional state that can be caused by a hormonal imbalance, nervous system disorders, infection, medications, poor diet, genetics, or age. Mild depression may last for only a day or two, and can send you on an eating binge that you may be able to snap out of once your mood lifts. However, a major depression may last many months or years, and can cause significant weight gain when your binges won't end.

Many in the medical community are aware of the connection between depression and obesity. Yet it is still unclear which condition comes first. Researchers have found evidence for both mechanisms. For example, we know increased appetite and weight gain are common symptoms of depression. On the other hand, depressed individuals are also more likely to binge eat and less likely to exercise. Some antidepressants actually lead to weight gain, and the social stigma attached to obesity may lead to depression.[9]

It really doesn't matter which is the proverbial chicken or egg. Depression and obesity are triggered by a brain chemical imbalance. When they occur together, the brain chemical that is missing is likely to be serotonin. I believe that because of the direct connection between a serotonin deficiency and depression, the symptoms of a low mood probably precede significant weight gain: The excess weight occurs in an effort to self-medicate toward a state of happiness. And while food is a powerful tool that can improve mood, my goal is to teach you the other techniques that will make you even happier, without the unhealthy side effect of weight gain and its associated illnesses and conditions.

AM I UNHAPPY ABOUT MY WEIGHT OR AM I TRULY DEPRESSED?

It's natural to be unhappy about certain aspects of your life from time to time, especially if you are focused on your weight. But when you are unhappy about every aspect of your life it may be time to get professional help. If you find that you are pervasively sad most days, you might have a serotonin deficiency. Many physical and mental symptoms are linked. If you have any of the following symptoms, you may benefit from professional therapy, prescription medications, or both.[10,11] The following list of mental and physical conditions are sure signs of a serotonin deficiency.

- Recent bouts of aggression/drastic change in temperament
- Reliance on alcohol or recreational drugs to improve mood
- Frequent anxiety/irritability
- Unexplained aches and pains
- Persistent fatigue
- Gastrointestinal disturbances
- Pervasive feeling of guilt for no apparent reason
- Headaches/migraines
- Feeling of hopelessness unattached to a particular situation
- Insomnia
- Change in your self-esteem
- Obsessive-compulsive disorder
- Overeating
- Poor impulse control
- Problems thinking or making decisions
- Recurrent sadness and tearfulness
- Suicidal thoughts

Don't Wait Until You're Happy to Lose Weight

Increasing your serotonin is easy, and will certainly help you to lose weight and feel better about yourself. That's why starting the Younger (Thinner) You Diet, which focuses on rebalancing your brain chemistry, is critical. You don't have to wait until you are "emotionally stable" to lose weight. In fact, there is no clinical evidence that ever proved that you cannot lose weight while you are feeling low. Weight loss success might be just the thing you need to lift your black mood.

FOOD, SEROTONIN, AND YOUR PERSONALITY

Your brain chemistry directly affects your psychological profile. Many people who have a serotonin deficiency can be considered to be "self-absorbed." They have lost their sensitivity to, or interest in, others and instead focus on themselves and meeting their own needs. This directly affects their relationship to food and to eating. For example, in the case of an extreme serotonin deficiency, many people find themselves lying around the house all day and spend their energy checking out YouTube instead of putting in the time for thoughtful meal planning. They'll end up eating whatever is on hand and easy to fix, instead of what they know is good for them.

Another common trait among those low in serotonin is that they consider themselves to be outlaws or rule-breakers. They become overly impulsive and shortsighted, proceeding rashly without considering

Serotonin-Deficient Personality Profile

EMOTION/ACTION	WHAT IT MEANS:
Suspicious	• Expects to be exploited or harmed by others • Questions the loyalty of friends • Reads hidden threats in benign remarks • Suspicious of significant other's fidelity • Believes personal information will be used against them and refuses to confide • Easily feels slighted and quick to counterattack • Carries grudges
Self-absorbed	• Feels rage, shame, or humiliation at criticism • Takes credit for others' work • Exaggerates self-importance • Most relationships are unstable • Preoccupied with fantasies of success, power, brilliance, beauty, or love • Requires constant attention and admiration • Expects special favors • Indifferent to the feelings of others • Feels envious
Rule-breaker	• Breaks the law • Irritable and aggressive • Constantly getting into physical fights • Fails to honor financial obligations on a regular basis • Fails to plan ahead • Disregard for the truth • Reckless • Has never sustained a totally monogamous relationship for more than one year • Lack of remorse

consequences. When they think about food, they rationalize that living "off the grid" means that they don't have to follow an eating plan. They eat whatever they want, whenever they want.

The following list indicates other ways that a serotonin deficiency can affect your relationship with food.

- You don't feel full until it's too late, and then you feel sick to your stomach. With a serotonin deficiency, you might not feel any of your internal triggers. So you end up eating blindly and numbly.
- You feel ashamed of your body. You might not get dressed for days at a time, and then are surprised that your clothes are tight.
- You may feel that you are obsessed with your weight, thinking about it every time you eat anything. At the same time, you haven't done anything about it. This is a typical behavior pattern for those that are low in serotonin. These people think about losing weight all the time, even obsess over it, but ultimately don't have the drive or energy to do anything about it.

ARE YOU A NIGHT EATER?

Night eating is also related to a serotonin deficiency. It is characterized by a lack of appetite in the morning and overeating at night, accompanied by agitation and insomnia. The classic night eater consumes fewer than average calories throughout the day. At night, they raid the refrigerator and pan-

try for high-carb snacks. Albert Stunkard, MD, of the University of Pennsylvania's Weight and Eating Disorders Program,[15] identifies night-eating syndrome as a pattern that has persisted for at least two months with the following signs and symptoms. You may be suffering from night eating syndrome if you:

- Have little or no appetite for breakfast; delay the first meal for several hours after waking up.
- Eat more food after dinner than during that meal.
- Eat more than half of your daily food intake after dinner but before breakfast.
- Leave bed to snack at night.
- Feel guilt and shame, not enjoyment, after eating at night. This night eating seems to be stress related and is often accompanied by depression.
- Have trouble falling asleep or staying asleep; wake frequently and then eat.
- Choose simple carbohydrates in relatively small snacks, but continue to snack frequently throughout the night.
- Continually eat throughout the evening hours.

YOU NEED MORE SEROTONIN DURING MENSTRUAL CYCLES

Sex hormones also play a role in how and why we become addicted to food. Studies have shown that women may be more

Meet Melissa D.: She Found that Living Younger Meant Living Happier

Melissa D was 59 years old, 5' 6", and 205 pounds when she came to see me. This divorced mother of three was extremely unhappy with her life. With nearly 75 pounds to lose, she thought she was locked in a hopeless situation. "I don't understand what's wrong with me," she said. "It's like I have no self-control. I eat constantly. I eat when I'm happy, when I'm sad, when I'm anxious. Afterwards I feel numb."

Melissa also had trouble sleeping, was feeling more depressed each day, and said she cried at the silliest things—including TV commercials. She would plant herself in front of the TV and blindly eat whatever she'd set in front of her: popcorn, potato chips, a pint of ice cream, Chinese takeout. It didn't matter what she ate, Melissa no longer found enjoyment in life. She was unproductive at work, and she avoided her family. Food had become her closest friend.

I tested Melissa for a range of obesity-related symptoms and conditions. I found that she was prediabetic, and suffered from a mild case of obsessive-compulsive disorder (OCD). I immediately recognized her serotonin deficiency and started her on the Younger (Thinner) You Diet, paying attention to her serotonin needs. I also started her on a serotonin-enhancing supplement formula that included thiamine, L-niacinamide, folic acid, Vitamin B_{12}, pantothenic acid, 5-hydroxy tryptophan, and Saint John's wort. I also asked Melissa to keep a food, exercise, and sleep diary so she could see what she was doing—and eating—throughout the day.

These journals proved to be invaluable. Once Melissa realized the quantity and frequency of her binges, she was able to tackle them head-on, as well as confront the emotions that she had been burying under all that food. She is also trying to improve her sleep routine, so that she did not get up at night and eat.

Eight months later, Melissa is 70 pounds lighter, with only five pounds left until she reaches her goal weight. She is much happier at work and spends time with her friends and family, often visiting her son and daughter-in-law. She feels better than she has in years, now that her eating is under control.

vulnerable to cravings for certain foods, like chocolate, or to stimulants like nicotine during the latter part of the menstrual cycle when the hormone progesterone is released.[14] Fiber-rich Younger (Thinner) You superfoods that specifically increase serotonin, such as pears, broccoli, brown rice, and oatmeal, soak up excess estrogen, especially during your period. By making sure that you eat these foods, you'll curb your cravings for more fattening choices that would simply trigger your brain to eat more.[15]

CREATE MORE SEROTONIN BY EATING FOODS HIGH IN TRYPTOPHAN

Tryptophan is an amino acid the brain and body needs, but cannot make on its own. It is vital for those with low serotonin because it induces the creation of this brain chemical. The foods that are key to producing serotonin are those low-calorie foods that are high in tryptophan, such as avocados, eggs, or cottage cheese.

Tryptophan is so effective in creating more serotonin that you might see instant results after eating foods that contain lots of it. For example, if you feel sad, eating foods rich in tryptophan can quickly improve your mood. At the same time, they help to circumvent overeating and serotonin-linked cravings, so you won't fall back into your old bad habits of reaching for salty snacks.

The following is a list of foods that contain significant amounts of tryptophan. If you are low in serotonin, you need to incorporate as many of these foods as possible into your diet each day:

- Avocado
- Chicken
- Chocolate
- Cottage cheese
- Duck
- Egg
- Granola
- Milk (whole)
- Rolled oats
- Pork
- Turkey
- Wheat germ
- Yogurt

Foods to Choose When You're Feeling Blue

Adding more fish to your diet can also change a blue mood. One 2001 study out of Finland found that people who frequently eat fish that have high concentrations of omega-3 fatty acids, such as salmon, are 31% less likely to suffer from depression.[16] Besides salmon, other fish that can improve your mood are trout, herring, sardines, and mackerel. These choices are high in vitamin B_{12}, which can also be found in eggs, sea vegetables, soy products, and kelp.

Aside from fish, other good choices for improving your mood are foods high in the nutrient biotin, including egg yolks, soybeans, and whole grains, or foods high in purine, such as calf's liver and flat mushrooms. However, high-purine foods should be avoided if you have experienced gout.

SPICES INCREASE SEROTONIN

On the Younger (Thinner) You Diet, you'll be incorporating at least three spices into every meal. You'll learn much more about the power of spices in chapter 7. While many spices can make your meals more flavorful, specific spices will act as antidepressants, naturally increasing your serotonin levels.

For example, to improve your mood, choose **saffron**, a Persian herb clinically shown to help depression. Dr. Shahin Akhondzadeh, at Ruzbeh Psychiatric Hospital in Tehran University of Medical Sciences has done several studies proving that saffron is especially useful as an antidepressant that doesn't have the side effects often associated with medications like Prozac. Other good choices include seasoning your favorite dishes with **marjoram**, **peppermint**, **spearmint** or **dill**.

Nutmeg, licorice (anise), and **turmeric** have scientifically proven potent antidepressant activity. In a 2006 experiment using mice, nutmeg extract was shown to be comparable to Prozac in several standard tests. The same year, similar results were shown with licorice in a study from India. Specifically, nutmeg was shown to markedly affect levels of adrenaline, dopamine, and serotonin. One theory is that the active compounds in nutmeg have pharmacological properties similar to amphetamines and the recreational drug, ecstasy. A 2002 turmeric study out of Nanjing University also showed a correlation between MAO inhibition and turmeric.

Cinnamon and **fennel** are known to reduce carbohydrate cravings. By adding these to other nutrient groups like proteins or fats, you'll eat less carbs throughout the day. I sprinkle cinnamon into my morning tea, and add fennel to my eggs to start my day off right.

SUPPLEMENTS BOOST SEROTONIN WITHOUT ADDING CALORIES

Many foods that are high in tryptophan do not provide significant levels in diet-size portions. For example, if you look at the tryptophan chart, you would need to eat a whole cup of granola to get the levels you need. Another way to increase your tryptophan and other serotonin-boosting nutrients without adding calories is through vitamin and mineral supplements. Tryptophan supplements can naturally raise blood sugar and decrease appetite for carbohydrates. Many others improve mood and relieve depression. Follow the directions as noted: Some are best taken from the late evening until bedtime because they will help put you to sleep. Now that's a side effect I can live with!

Consult your healthcare provider to see which of the following supplements may be appropriate for you. It is very important to make sure supplements do not interfere with your medications, especially if you are taking antidepressants.

Serotonin Boosters

TREATMENT	SUGGESTED DAILY DOSAGE	WHAT IT DOES
Vitamin D	5000 IU	Take this supplement in the morning for more energy; vitamin D is known to elevate your mood and causes weight loss as it contributes to the ability to burn fat[17]
Melatonin	0.3–10 mg	Take this supplement in the evening; known to suppress body weight and visceral fat accumulation the next day
5-HTP (5-hydroxytrypto-phan)	50–500 mg	Take this supplement in the evening; reduces appetite and promotes weight loss
Vitamin B6	10–500 mg	Take this supplement in the morning for more energy; may reduce fatigue
Fish oils (EPA/ DHA)	500–3000 mg	Take this supplement in the evening; supplements high in omega-3s facilitate loss of adipose tissue, decrease appetite
Magnesium	300–1000 mg	Take this supplement in the morning for more energy
Sceletium tortuosum	50–100 mg	This supplement elevates mood, decreases anxiety, stress, and tension; also works as an appetite suppressant
Fucoxanthin	200 mg	Take this supplement in the evening; an antioxidant that can prevent inflammation and help burn body fat[18]
Acetyl-l-carnitine (ALC)	500–5,000 mg	Take this supplement in the evening; a special form of L-carnitine, which is necessary to create more acetyl-choline; shown to be most effective fighting depression in elderly people as it helps to restore memory and attention
DHEA	Males: 10–100 mg Females: 5–50 mg	This is a steroid hormone that can be converted to other hormones, including estrogen and testosterone; can be taken at night or in the morning
Phenylalanine	500–5000 mg	Taken in the morning, you can balance a low-serotonin brain with more dopamine; this nutrient can be converted to tyrosine, which in turn is converted to dopamine to provide energy
SAMe	400–1600 mg	Taken in the morning, SAMe is the first metabolite of the essential amino acid, L-methionine
Tryptophan	500–2000 mg	Taken in the evening, tryptophan can increase the effectiveness of prescription antidepressants, and provides additional serotonin
Saint John's wort	500–1000 mg std. to hypericin or hyperforin	Taken in the evening, Saint John's wort can be as effective for depression as most prescription medications

SEROTONIN-ENHANCING HORMONES

These bioidentical hormones can help kick-start your serotonin. Using them may give you increased weight loss while following the Younger (Thinner) You Diet. Discuss each with your doctor:

- Progesterone
- Human growth hormone (HGH)
- Pregnenolone
- Leptin
- Aldosterone

THE LAST RESORT: SEROTONIN-ENHANCING MEDICATIONS

Antidepressants, when properly administered by medical professionals, can improve your mood and may also help with weight loss. They work by altering your brain chemistry to restore a chemical balance, making serotonin and other brain chemicals more available.

Antidepressants, like many things, are often misinterpreted. Just like many believe aspirin is a drug that prevents heart disease, some people think that antidepressants cure depression. The fact is, antidepressants treat

Rescue Remedy: Oxytocin

Oxytocin is often called the happy hormone because it is naturally released when you feel loved. Oxytocin raises your emotional capacity for empathy and interpersonal generosity. It also raises your serotonin levels so you feel emotionally satisfied. For some people, its release will curb appetite.

If you found that you are low in serotonin from the quiz in Chapter 2, you can discuss oxytocin supplementation via a prescription nasal spray with your doctor.

brain chemical imbalances, regardless of whether or not you're depressed. They assist the amino acids by filling in the gaps in your brain and preventing the neurons from leaking.[19] As we age, our brain gets "leaky," loses its core chemicals, and gets dehydrated. Antidepressants help us grow new brain cells.[20]

Antidepressants may be effective, but don't turn to them as a cure-all. If you and your doctor choose to follow this route, keep in mind there are many different kinds of antidepressants, and some will be more effective for you than others. The core antidepressants that are used are primarily Wellbutrin, Paxil, and occasionally Zoloft, Prozac, and Effexor.

Meridia is not an antidepressant, but works by changing the levels of serotonin

Antidepressants Often Affect Other Medications

If you're going to take an antidepressant, tell your doctor about any other medicines you take, including over-the-counter medicines and supplements. For example, taking antidepressants with certain over-the-counter medicines for colds and flu can cause a dangerous reaction.

in the brain. It is thought to influence feelings of hunger and fullness. It works by making you feel full sooner. However, this or any other weight loss medication should be considered a last resort. Stick with the Younger (Thinner) You Diet for at least three months before considering this option, especially if you have other existing medical conditions.

PERSONALIZING THE YOUNGER (THINNER) YOU DIET

You've now explored the four distinct brain chemical pathways that can lead to obesity. The quiz in Chapter 2 pointed to your specific issue, and you now have the information you need to identify the foods that you have been abusing as you've learned to self-medicate your imbalance. Each person's path to gaining weight is different, so the weight lose cure needs to be equally personalized:

- If you can now recognize that you eat tons of sugar and coffee to get your energy going, you need to create more dopamine by focusing on lean proteins.
- If you can now recognize that you eat too much high-fat food, you need to focus on

improving your acetylcholine by eating foods containing healthier fat options.

- If you have been binging mindlessly, you're eating to support your imbalanced GABA. Instead, you need to get your portions under control, and focus on high-fiber, complex carbs.
- If you can now recognize that your answer to a bad day is a bag of salty snacks, your serotonin is out of whack. You'll find success when you choose better carbs and other foods that promote an increase in serotonin.

The next section will cover the details of the Younger (Thinner) You Diet so that you can get started. No matter what your deficiency is, there are many constants on the diet that apply to everyone. You'll learn how to best balance your proteins, carbs, and fats effortlessly. You'll learn new ways to incorporate thermogenic teas and spices that will help you add nutrients and raise your metabolic rate to burn calories at the same time. And, you'll learn my ten secrets for weight loss success. By combining this information with your specific needs, you'll finally be able to lose weight, because you will be approaching dieting headfirst.

PART II

How to Make the Diet Work for You

CHAPTER 7

The Basics of the
Younger (Thinner) You Diet

THE YOUNGER (Thinner) You Diet allows you to choose from a wide variety of fresh foods, herbs, spices, and teas that will help you to lose weight and keep those pounds from coming back. These foods have been specially chosen to create long-lasting satiety so you won't feel hungry. They also promote excellent brain chemistry, so you will have an increased sense of well-being and high energy. Many have dopamine-boosting properties, so they increase your metabolism and curb your cravings. High-acetylcholine foods reduce your need for "bad" fats. High-GABA foods alleviate stress and enable you to have better portion control. High-serotonin foods allow you to get the rest you need to recharge your brain and body.

At this point you should understand your particular brain chemical deficiencies, and can recognize the foods you will focus on to remedy your specific issues. If you have multiple deficiencies and have read all the earlier chapters, you may have noticed that some foods will benefit the production of more than one brain chemical. I consider these to be Younger (Thinner) You superfoods: They are nutrient-dense and support overall brain health.

Eating foods that are nutrient dense, rather than calorie dense, is the key to maintaining weight loss and a balanced brain chemistry. You want every square inch of your food to be packed with nutrients, not calories. Low-volume, high-caloric foods can delay the brain's and stomach's activation of the feeling of fullness, so you end up eating more of these poor food choices.

The Younger (Thinner) You Diet offers hundreds of good choices: complex carbohydrates, which include lots of fruits and vegetables; lean meats; healthy fats; wonderful herbs and spices that are chock-full of thermogenic nutrients including antioxidants; and soothing, healing teas. Younger (Thinner) You foods are also rich in fiber to aid in digestion. These choices are considered "high volume": You can eat lots of them and feel full because they take up

Your Eyes Can Fool Your Brain

Using a smaller plate (rather than a large dinner plate) can trick your body into thinking you're eating more food than you actually are.[1]

space in your stomach, yet they are still low in calories. Best of all, you can eat healthy-sized portions of these foods and still lose weight, because the nutrient-to-calorie ratio is the highest of any diet around. You won't feel hungry all day, and at night, you'll sleep well. This way of eating has been proven to improve the way you use and burn your food, which means that not only will you lose weight, but these foods support an antiaging strategy to get you feeling healthier and younger.

WHY I DON'T WORRY ABOUT CALORIE RESTRICTION

A satisfying meal comes from the amount of food you eat, and not the number of calories or the grams of fat, protein, or carbs it contains. Remember, I'm not focusing on those numbers and neither should you. Instead, the trick of the Younger (Thinner) You Diet is to fill up on foods that aren't full of calories.

Yet in order for you to experience weight loss, you need to create a calorie deficit: You need to teach your body to burn more calories than you take in. My superfoods, herbs, spices, and teas do this job so well that you don't have to count calories. And because you will be exercising regularly, you will

need lots of calories to support your energy needs. Your metabolism will be working better due to the foods you choose and the exercise program you follow, so you can eat more and still lose weight.

In fact, I don't believe restricting calories is the way to achieve weight loss at all. It certainly is not the way to become younger or achieve better health. Intense calorie restriction will lead to weight loss over a very short period of time, but I guarantee that as soon as you start increasing your calories, your weight will come right back on. What's worse, you run the risk of becoming frail and experiencing premature aging if you don't get adequate nutrients over a long period of time. Without proper nutrients, your brain will not have the vital raw materials to create enough dopamine, acetylcholine, GABA, and serotonin, and the rest of your body will begin to cascade into a downward spiral of illness, disease, and completely preventable conditions. That's why I say that depriving yourself of vital nutrition like complex carbohydrates, healthy fats, and lean protein is an undeserved punishment, and one that has been proven—time and time again—to not work.

Remember, you are rebalancing your brain by eating the right quantities of the right nutrients, which will then lead to weight loss. At first, balancing your brain and losing weight may be diametrically opposed: You may need more calories than you are used to eating just to get your brain back to full functioning. But once your brain chemistry is on track, you'll see the pounds melt off. What's more, you'll experience greater energy, which will make you look and feel younger and healthier.

NUTRIENT DENSITY: THE KEY TO THE YOUNGER (THINNER) YOU DIET

In the summer of 2007 a new food rating system was unveiled in supermarkets. The overall nutritional quality index (ONQI) was developed by the Yale Griffin Prevention Center to help consumers make more conscientious food choices. This team has developed a scale for ranking foods, assigning each a score from 1 to 100 (100 being the healthiest) based on their overall nutritional quality. The scale is based on each food's nutrient content and nutritional properties. This overall nutritional quality index is an attempt to illustrate what I am suggesting: It's not just calories that matter for weight loss; it's the total nutrient value or nutrient density that will support both weight loss and improved brain health.[3]

Nutrient density is a measure of the nutrients provided per calorie of food, or the ratio of nutrients to calories. Simply stated, nutri-ent density means quantifying how many nutrients you get from a given food, based on the number of calories it contains. Foods that supply generous amounts of one or more nutrients compared to the number of calories they supply are called nutrient dense. What's important for us is the fact that the greater the nutrient density, the greater the weight loss. That's because healthy foods can offer a 1000:1 ratio of nutrients compared to junk, and you need the nutrients to increase your metabolic power. Without nutrients, you simply can't burn your food efficiently. Bad foods offer just a fraction of the nutrients that good foods contain, even if they are calorically equivalent! That's why you shouldn't be fooled by "100 calorie snack packs": They are still just empty calories compared to 100 calories of any nutrient-packed fruit or vegetable that will feed the fire of your metabolism: Fruits and vegetables are "thermogenic."

> ### Quick Fix: Soup's On
>
> A warm bowl of vegetable soup or low-sodium chicken broth makes a great snack. And if you have one about twenty minutes before lunch or dinner, it can help curb your hunger for the next meal by as much as 20%.[2]

Nutrients Matter Most

What did you have for breakfast this morning? Say you ate a small fruit Danish and drank a cup of coffee. Do you know what you got with your food? Nothing of value: empty calories, sugar, and refined carbs. What you did get was a calorie-dense, sugary, fat-laden meal.

A better choice would have been eating an apple and drinking a cup of green tea. Both the apple and the green tea contain phytonutrients, as well as a variety of phytochemicals—including quercetin, catechin, phloridizin, and chlorogenic acid: powerful, healthful antioxidants.

Junk food is just that: garbage. Like the old computer programming adage: garbage in, garbage out. If you feed your body junk food, you'll feel junky and gain weight. But if you feed your brain and body great, healthy, nutrient-dense foods, you'll have increased energy, better thinking, more overall calmness, and more restful sleep. And I haven't even gotten to better sex or better health yet! (That's my teaser for reading Part III!)

Another example: What do you think is the better choice, a medium orange or a plain mini bagel (2½" in diameter)? They both contain around the same number of calories (approximately 80). But the orange provides dozens of nutrients, including vitamin C (crucial for cancer prevention and healthy circulation), B vitamin folate (essen-tial for preventing birth defects and fighting heart disease), potassium (needed for proper fluid balance), water-soluble fiber (which helps reduce blood cholesterol levels, critical for lowering risk for heart disease), antioxi-dants (to help protect from free-radical dam-age), and phytochemicals (such as flavonoids, which act as antioxidants and may protect against heart disease). Additionally, a single orange contains amino acids (such as trypto-phan, threonine, lysine, and alanine), 20+ vitamins (including vitamin A, vitamin B_{12}, beta-carotene, and choline), minerals (such as calcium, magnesium, and phosphorus), omega-3 fatty acids, and omega-6 fatty acids. The orange contains 4.3 grams of fiber. In order to consume an equal amount of fiber, you'd have to eat two bagels, and that would double your calories.

Go Organic

In order to make sure that you are eating the cleanest, most nutrient-dense foods available, all your foods from dairy products, meats, poultry, and fish to produce, teas, herbs, and spices, should be from fresh, natural food sources, and organic whenever possible. A recent four-year European Union (EU) study showed that organic fruit and vegetables contain as much as 40% more antioxidants than nonorganically-grown produce; and organic milk contains between 50 and 80% more antioxidants and more vitamin E than conventionally pro-duced milk. These results suggested that eating organic food would be equivalent to eating an extra portion of fruit and vegetables a day.[4] That's important, because most of us aren't getting the daily recommendation of five servings of fruits and vegetables anyway. By choosing organic, you are packing more nutrients into each serving.

For foods to be certified organic by the USDA, they must meet certain criteria. For example, organic produce is not sprayed with harmful pesticides, and the soil is free of chemicals like mercury and lead. These chemicals can destroy your metabolism and may be linked to certain illnesses, including cancer. Organically raised ani-mals are not treated with artificial growth hormones.

I also find that locally grown fruits and vegetables that are "in season" are often more flavorful than those flown from across the country or from across the world, leaving you more satisfied with your healthier food choices.

The bagel provides very little nutrition. It's made of nutrient devoid ingredients: flour, water, and sugar (high-fructose corn syrup). It's got 650 mg of sodium (more than 25% of your recommended daily intake, but 100% more than the amount of salt I think you should eat!); almost no dietary fiber (2 grams) or protein (2 grams). By comparison, the orange contains 86 calories, no saturated fat or sodium, and double the fiber.

So while a bagel will give you a small amount of fiber and protein, the orange is the much better choice. The bagel provides empty calories; the orange is loaded with nutrient-rich calories. You could eat bagels until the cows come home and never equal the nutrition you get from eating a single orange. The orange will spike your metabolism, but all the bagel will do is slow it down. Remember: Nutrient density trumps calories. A calorie is not a calorie is not a calorie. This program is about counting nutrients, not calories. You may be used to counting calories, but now you'll learn to live a normal-calorie life but change your weight by improving your nutrients.

THE YOUNGER (THINNER) YOU DIET RULES

There are ten simple things you need to remember on this diet:

1. Upgrade every meal with spices.

2. Drink tea with every meal.

3. Eat yogurt.

4. Choose proteins carefully.

Don't Skip Meals

You should never skip meals in order to reduce your caloric intake. This is especially true for breakfast, which is still the most important meal of the day. Without breakfast, you'll find yourself hungry way before lunch. Worse, you will start your day off with a deficit: Your brain needs the nutrients derived from a healthy breakfast to keep functioning throughout the day.

5. Choose expanding and balanced foods.

6. Eat fiber-filled foods.

7. Drink water throughout the day.

8. Add color to every meal.

9. Eat fruits and vegetables both raw and cooked.

10. Have three foods for each meal.

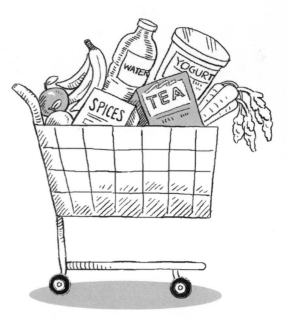

It's easy to follow the 10 Younger (Thinner) You Diet Rules: just consistently choose the right nutrient-dense foods that will balance your unique brain chemistry.

Think of these as the Younger (Thinner) You Ten Commandments. Each rule provides you with an opportunity to boost your weight loss efforts in different and unique ways, ranging from creating a stronger, hotter metabolism to enhancing your digestion. Many of these rules will also help enhance your brain chemistry. The end result is not only the ability to lose weight faster for permanent results, but equally important, to feel younger and healthier in every aspect of your life.

RULE #1: UPGRADE EVERY MEAL WITH SPICES

Herbs and spices add many benefits to your food without adding a single calorie: They are an integral part of the Younger (Thinner) You Diet. Every time you flavor your meals with herbs or spices, you are literally "upgrading" your food to the status of a Younger (Thinner) You superfood. You are taking something ordinary and turning it into something extraordinary by adding color, flavor, vitamins, and often medicinal properties to your blandest dishes. Here's why:

- **Spices and herbs maximize nutrient density.** Herbs and spices contain antioxidants, minerals, and multivitamins, so every time you add spice, you're adding nutrients and upgrading your meal without adding a single calorie. For example, if you slice an apple and sprinkle it with a couple of teaspoons of cinnamon, which contains dozens of nutrients, you now get the benefit from the apple as well as from the cinnamon. You can take even mediocre foods, like plain whole wheat toast, and upgrade it into a quality food by sprinkling the same cinnamon on top.

- **Spices and herbs create a more thermogenic diet.** Because spices are nutrient dense, they are thermogenic, which means they naturally increase your metabolism. As your metabolism revs higher, you will burn more of your food as fuel, and store less as body fat.

- **Spices and herbs make you younger through their medicinal properties.** Study after study shows the benefits of distinct herbs and spices. Many of these are listed in the table below, and can be used to treat your specific illnesses and conditions. For example, specific spices and herbs have tremendous blood sugar benefits. A study at Malma University Hospital in Sweden showed that up to two hours after eating, people who ate cinnamon-spiced rice pudding measured significantly lower blood glucose levels than those who had eaten the unspiced version. It was shown that their blood sugar was moving more efficiently into cells, as well as appearing to have moved more slowly from the stomach into the small intestine. When food enters the intestine more slowly, carbohydrates are broken down slower, which lead to a lower blood glucose concentration. Other studies suggest that cinnamon may improve blood glucose levels by increasing a person's insulin sensitivity. One

2003 trial of sixty people with type 2 diabetes reported that consuming as little as 2 teaspoons of cinnamon daily for six weeks reduced blood glucose levels significantly. It also improved blood cholesterol and triglyceride levels, perhaps because insulin plays a key role in regulating fats in the body.

- **Some spices and herbs increase your overall feeling of fullness and satiety, so you'll eat less.** One study conducted at Maanstricht University in the Netherlands showed that when healthy subjects consumed an appetizer with half a teaspoon of red pepper flakes before each meal, it decreased their calorie intake by 10 to 16%.
- **Spicy foods force you to drink more water.** This is another Younger (Thinner) You rule for weight loss (see Rule #7).
- **You can eliminate salt by replacing it with spices and herbs.** When you flavor your foods with spices instead of salt, you'll immediately see health and physical benefits. Without salt intake, you will no longer have excessive bloating and water retention caused by salty foods, so you will lose water weight immediately. Without salt in your diet, your overall health improves, especially if you have high blood pressure. Excessive salt intake keeps water inside your body, which then increases the circulatory volume, creating excess fluid pressure on blood vessel walls. These walls react by thickening and narrowing, leaving less space for the fluid already cramped in the blood, which then requires higher pressure to move the blood throughout the body. Because of this, the heart has to pump against this high-pressure system at a higher rate, causing the heart to enlarge dramatically. Meanwhile, the kidneys contain a million blood vessels that work as filters. The increased pressure transmitted to the kidneys damages its vascular system leading to a second disorder known as hypertensive nephrosclerosis, which is a major cause of kidney disease.

When you take salt out of your diet, you'll also lose the salty snack cravings associated with low serotonin. That's because using salt begets using more salt: After a while it's impossible to use just a pinch because you've trained your brain to require a salty taste for everything you eat. By following the diet, in just a few days you'll lose your cravings for salt. Over time, spices will also lessen your cravings for simple, nutrient-poor carbohydrate snacks, because you will not be yearning for a savory, salty taste.

- **You will be able to exchange your cravings.** Instead of blindly following your cravings when your brain chemistry is low, spices will change your flavor palate and expand the possibilities for enhancing brain chemistry without the added pounds. Instead of craving something sweet when you are low in dopamine, you'll retrain your brain to feed your need with the flavor of a dopamine-enhancing spice, like black pepper or ginger. This alone can completely change your eating habits, and end your addictive relationship with food. You will no longer rely on the wrong, fattening food choices to boost your brain chemistry.

HOW TO USE SPICES ON THIS DIET

On Younger (Thinner) You Diet, you will be adding at least three different spices to every meal. Appendix A lists the spices and their nutrient properties, as well as their relationship to the specific brain chemicals. One good place to start is to determine which spices will enhance your primary deficiency.

If you use the recipes and meal plans in Chapters 9 and 10, the spices have been added in for you. Most cookbooks suggest using spices sparingly because of their strong flavor. But you'll need more than a pinch or sprinkle in order to get the most benefit. On this diet I want you to use spices liberally to get the most benefits. For example, you'll use as much as a tablespoon of cinnamon sprinkled over a baked sweet potato.

Exotic Spices

There are thousands of spices and spice blends out there, and each offer unique health benefits. Some varieties may be new to you. If you can't find them in your local supermarket, check out Penzeys Spices (www.penzeys.com), which is famous for their quality and have garnered quite a following from chefs and home cooks.

However, your stomach and taste buds need to be able to tolerate higher amounts of spices, especially those that are hot, so experiment to see what works best for you. Don't start adding a tablespoon of cayenne or chili or paprika to all of your meals if you know that you're sensitive to hot foods. Instead, increase your personal tolerance to spice and heat by building it up in small increments. Start by adding a quarter teaspoon of each spice to the recipes in Chapter 10 until you're sure what you can handle. Then, increase the amount of spices incrementally until you get to the full serving suggestion. Because you will be eating spices every day, you'll build your tolerance quickly. So don't get discouraged, and keep experimenting until you reach a comfort level. In the end, you might find that there are some spices that you just can't tolerate, and that's okay, too. Stick with the ones you enjoy so that you can get the most nutritional and metabolism-boosting benefit. In the end, one spice is not much more effective than another, but any spice is better to use than none at all.

Once you get rid of the junk foods that you were relying on for flavor and taste, you'll still want foods that are full of flavor. Traditionally, diet foods are bland and boring. You'll find that when you cook with spices, your meals will be more interesting and more flavorful. This is another reason why spices are so important to the Younger (Thinner) You Diet.

Add any of these spice combinations to a plain skinless, boneless chicken breast and you'll see how easily you can have an entirely different meal:

- Traditional savory combination: rosemary, thyme, and sage
- Middle Eastern exotic: cinnamon, nutmeg, and paprika
- Mediterranean flair: oregano, fennel, and garlic
- Asian feast: ginger, garlic, and lemongrass
- Bollywood fantasy: allspice, turmeric, and saffron
- Mexican fiesta: cilantro, cumin, and cayenne
- French escape: fennel, mustard seed, and bay leaves

THE DIFFERENCE BETWEEN HERBS AND SPICES

The way to distinguish an herb from a spice is to note from where on the plant the item is taken. Herbs, such as basil, peppermint, rosemary, and sage, usually come from the leafy part of a plant, and can be bought either fresh or dried. Spices, such as coriander seed, cinnamon, pepper, turmeric, and cumin, on the other hand, are always dried, and can be obtained from the seeds, roots, bark, or other part of the plant. Spices are often ground into a fine powder, but can also be sold as dried seeds, pods, or sticks.

Cayenne Caution

Consult with your doctor about increasing your cayenne intake if you are on blood-thinning drugs or taking an asthma drug containing theophylline.

Some argue that there is no distinction between herbs and spices, considering both have similar uses and benefits. To make matters more confusing, in certain areas of the United States, a dried herb is considered a spice. So for the purposes of this book, I'll refer to all herbs and spices and "spices" unless otherwise noted.

Fresh herbs will always have the most intense flavor and nutrient density, but they don't store well. Fresh herbs can last as long as a week in the refrigerator if you keep them wrapped in paper towel inside a plastic zip-top bag. Or you can start your own kitchen garden with a few clippings and a small pot to plant them in. Snip the leaves off and use as needed. A potted planting will last from spring until fall. Some of the most successful kitchen gardeners experiment with different varieties

Fresh Herb Facts

- 1 teaspoon dried herbs = 3 teaspoons fresh herbs
- Add fresh herbs near the end of your cooking time for the most flavor and benefits.
- Refrigerate herbs at 35°F to 50°F, except basil, which is best stored at 55°F to 60°F.

Uncommon Sense

As Dostoevsky said, "I admit that two times two makes four is an excellent thing, but if we are to give everything its due, two times two makes five is sometimes a very charming thing too." So it is that adding three spices to each meal will be better than just adding one. If you can do this, you will be adding literally hundreds of nutrients to your diet every day. This is the best way to keep your metabolism strong and burning all day long, so that you can lose the weight and keep it off.

of basil, rosemary, sage, and peppermint, among others.

Dried spices and herbs are an entirely different option. It's best to buy spices in the smallest quantities available and whole seeds or pods whenever possible. This way you'll be able to grind the spices as you need them, and their essential oils and vitamins will stay intact. Store all dried herbs and spices in airtight containers in cool, dark, dry places: heat, light, and moisture drain spices of their flavor. Once opened, most whole spices will keep for a year. Ground spices are best used within three to six months. Mark the labels of all spices with the date of purchase so you know when you are ready to toss them. If the fragrance or flavor of a spice fades, throw it out.

Are You a Cinnamon Girl?

If you love the taste of cinnamon, and want more of its fat-busting properties, add ¼ teaspoon to your cup of coffee each morning. For the most thermogenic effects, add the cinnamon directly to your coffee filter with the coffee grounds before brewing. Or sprinkle a medium-sized banana or any other fruit with cinnamon.

RULE #2: DRINK TEA WITH EVERY MEAL

Just like spices, tea is now thought to be beneficial as a weight loss and antiaging tool. This is due mainly to the nutrients—namely the polyphenols—it contains, which have powerful antioxidant properties. The darker teas have much higher concentrations, which offer higher antioxidant values.

Tea has absolutely no calories (if you don't drink it with milk or sugar) and can stimulate digestion, cleanse the body, reduce inflammation, lower cholesterol, and give you lots of energy. These are all necessary for losing weight and reversing the aging of every part of your body.

The health benefits of drinking tea add up fast. Not only does it get you in the habit of drinking more beverages, you are simultaneously flushing out of your system the toxic foods you've been eating. The nutrients in tea speed up your metabolism. Best of all, tea benefits your overall health and makes you younger. Tea drinkers have:

- A lower risk of cancer
- Healthier intestinal flora, which inhibit bacteria

- A lower risk of heart disease
- Improved their glucose tolerance, preventing diabetes
- Continuously detoxified their liver

ACCEPTABLE TYPES OF TEA

The main types of tea (white, black, green, and oolong) all come from the same plant (*Camellia sinensis*), so any type of tea is acceptable to drink on this diet. The differences in color and taste result from the degree of fermentation the tea leaves undergo after harvesting. The fermentation, in turn, determines the type and amounts of healthful polyphenols that are present.

The most research has been recorded for green teas. The high caffeine content in green tea can increase metabolism, decrease appetite, and provide more energy for exercise. Green tea may also reduce the absorption of dietary fats by approximately 40% by blocking the production of digestive enzymes that facilitate the absorption of dietary fats. It can also help reduce fat by inhibiting the effects of insulin so that sugars are sent directly to the muscles for instant use, instead of being stored as body fat.[5,6]

However, one 2003 study from Japan's University of Tokushima School of Medicine reports than oolong tea has greater metabolism-boosting properties that green tea. Oolong tea may increase the number of calories burned by 10%, while green tea was only shown to have a metabolic increase

of 4%. Another Japanese study showed that oolong tea is able to reduce the absorption of fats, so that more dietary fat is passed through the body as waste instead of being digested. Another positive benefit is that oolong tea has about half the caffeine of green tea, so if you are caffeine sensitive or like to drink tea in the evening, it might be a better option.[7]

Herbal teas are not officially teas at all, but are acceptable options on this diet. These herbal varieties should really be called "herbal infusions" or "tisanes." They are not made from the same plant as regular teas: Instead they are brewed from the roots, stems, bark, leaves, and flowers of other plants. Herbal teas are naturally decaffeinated and each have their own unique taste as well as their own set of reported health benefits. Herbal teas count as servings of tea on the diet, not servings of fruits or vegetables, even if they are derived from a fruit or vegetable.

However, "designer" bottles of tea aren't all that they appear to be. Bottled tea's antioxidant levels are ten to one hundred times lower than those in brewed tea, and many brands are filled with sugar. Instead of drinking any bottled tea, I brew it myself

Rooibos Herbal Tea Is Pure Nutrients

This South African herbal tea is packed with vitamin C, and has 50% more antioxidants than its caffeinated rival, green tea. For an added nutrient bonus, look for a rooibos tea brewed with cinnamon.

and often combine two or three teas to get the most color, and therefore the most benefit. For example, I brew a pot that makes 3 to 4 cups, and I combine red rooibos, blueberry, and green tea.

There are many other great combinations. These include:

- Green tea, peach, and black cherry
- Green tea, orange spice, and cinnamon apple
- Green tea, orange spice
- Lemon green tea with rooibos
- Green tea, mint, chamomile

DAILY TEA STRATEGY

Whichever type of tea you prefer, you need to drink 1 cup of tea or more *after* each meal to achieve the greatest affect. By doing so, I believe that you can lose 5% more weight. Follow these suggestions for best results.

- Breakfast: Within two hours of waking, drink green tea after breakfast.
- Mid-morning: Keep energy going with a cup of flavored black tea.
- Lunch: Follow this meal with a strong cup of oolong tea.

- Midday: Improve digestion with a cup of peppermint tea.
- Dinner: No later than three hours before bedtime, drink a weaker cup of oolong or chamomile tea.
- Before bed: Drink a cup of white tea to help you relax before bedtime.

RULE #3: EAT YOGURT EVERY DAY

On the Younger (Thinner) You Diet you will be eating a single 8-ounce cup of low-fat yogurt every day. You can have this for breakfast, lunch, or a snack, no matter what your brain chemistry deficiency is. Yogurt is high in both calcium and protein, which together are known to raise metabolic rate and improve digestion and bowel health, so you will not be constipated during the diet. It also supports your immune system, reduces overall inflammation, and lowers your LDL, or "bad" cholesterol. Best of all, yogurt may help burn fat and promote weight loss. A University of Tennessee study in 2005 shows that dieters who ate three servings of yogurt a day lost 22% more weight and 61% more body fat than those who simply cut calories and didn't add cal-

Upgrade Your Tea

Taking your tea with a slice of fresh lemon upgrades your tea, because you are adding more nutrients to your beverage. The same is true if you take your tea with low-fat milk. But don't add sugar! If you need a sweetened taste, make a wise choice with a flavored herbal tea, like apple or berry.

Calcium Reduces Belly Fat!

Another reason I love yogurt is that it is a low-fat food packed with calcium—and calcium reduces belly fat. A recent study presented at the Obesity Society Meeting of 2007 showed significant abdominal fat reduction following calcium supplementation.[8] During the course of the seven-week study, participants ate three to four servings of dairy foods each day. The data showed that an exercise program combined with a reduced-calorie, nutrient-rich diet, like the Younger (Thinner) You Diet, and an increase in dairy consumption changed metabolism significantly enough to affect the amount of body fat burned.

cium to their eating plan. Those that lost the most weight were also able to protect their lean muscle mass, which is critical when dieting, because the muscle mass is essential to maintaining high metabolism.[9]

While other dairy products also contain calcium and protein, to my mind, yogurt is the best bet for many reasons. Full-fat dairy options, like milk or cheese, add tons of unnecessary calories even as they promote weight loss, leaving you with a net loss of zero pounds. These dairy products can also promote the production of cellulite on the body. Low-fat yogurt provides all the benefits of dairy without the added fat or calories, and actually contains more calcium and protein per serving than other choices because of the way it is made. Last, many people have problems digesting lactose, a carbohydrate that is found in milk and milk products, because their bodies do not produce enough of the enzyme lactase. Yogurt naturally contains lactase, making it a healthy alternative for the people who cannot tolerate other milk products to get the calcium they need. That's why I want you to eat some every day.

Yogurt has become such a staple to the American diet that there are literally hundreds of options to choose from. I suggest that you choose plain, low-fat yogurts. Plain yogurts have fewer calories and little sugar. Full-fat yogurts are too high in calories, and fat-free yogurts do not have the essential fat you need to lose weight. Strained (Greek-style) yogurt is currently the rage and is thicker than traditional yogurt, if you like that type of consistency. Yogurts with probiotics, like Dannon's Activia, are good for those who have digestive ailments, but are not necessary for people who do not have them. Probiotics can help regulate your digestive system by helping reduce bloating and difficult and painful defecation. For those who can't tolerate traditional yogurts, you can also try goat's milk or soy varieties.

Upgrade Your Yogurt

Sprinkle 1 teaspoon of cinnamon on top of a cup of plain yogurt to create a delicious and fat-burning Younger (Thinner) You superfood.

Fresh Fish Is Just a Click Away

I tell my patients to eat fish until they start sprouting gills. We live in a world where fresh fish is available all year long. Purveyors like Vital Choice can send your order in the mail: You don't even have to leave your home to shop! There is fabulous variety, and literally hundreds of different ways to prepare each type.

If you find plain low-fat yogurt unappealing and you really need to sweeten it, add a teaspoon of sugar-free all-fruit preserves, or a teaspoon of honey. You can also add more yogurt to your diet by substituting it for mayonnaise in your favorite recipes, like tuna salad or egg salad, or use as a base for salad dressings. In the recipe section you'll find great ideas for yogurt smoothies and dessert options, too.

RULE #4: CHOOSE PROTEINS CAREFULLY

Too much red meat may thwart your best weight loss efforts, which is why the emphasis on this diet is on fish and poultry for

Where to Find Omega-3s

Aside from natural sources of protein, many food manufacturers are fortifying their products with additional omega-3s. Look for the varieties listed below to boost your consumption. Remember to stick to the suggested portion size recommended in the Younger (Thinner) You Diet.

- Energy bars: KeriBars
- Eggs: Christopher Eggs, Eggland's Best
- Cereals: Nature's Path Organic Flax Plus Pumpkin Raisin Crunch
- Soymilk: Silk Soymilk Plus Omega-3 DHA

protein choices. Red meat may also contribute to a higher risk of cancer and heart disease. I suggest that you choose red meat options like steak only in moderation, which on this diet will mean that you can eat them weekly, not daily.

Chicken can be eaten every day. However, I often find that my patients get bored looking at the same boneless, skinless chicken breast every night. The spice combinations and recipes included in the next chapter will make chicken meals more appealing, flavorful, and less redundant.

Fish, on the other hand, offers a low-fat, healthy variety of choices that can be consumed every single day for breakfast, lunch, or dinner. Eating fish on a regular basis can significantly reduce your risk of heart disease, especially if you have been diagnosed with diabetes. Cold-water fish, such as salmon, are high in the good omega-3 fats and are well documented for their blood-thinning properties. That's why the American Heart Association recommends two fish meals per week. But I recommend more. On this diet, you can choose to have one fish meal every day. Refer to the recipes and meal plans for great ideas for cooking fish. Or you can simply bake, broil, or steam plain fish with a touch of olive oil and three of your favorite spices to create your own Younger (Thinner) You recipes.

RULE #5: CHOOSE EXPANDING AND BALANCED FOODS FOR WEIGHT LOSS AND LONGEVITY

I've given up on the United States government's food pyramid and its heavy emphasis of carbohydrates. In my opinion it is a medical disaster. Instead, I classify foods in a few distinct categories: expanding foods and balanced foods. Expanding foods are those that have extreme effects on the body and cause a seemingly positive short-term effect (an energy boost) while creating a nutritional disaster over time. Once we start to eat expanding foods, we find ourselves craving more of them to restore our energy. Simple carbohydrates, refined foods, or "white foods" are all expanding foods because they boost our energy in the short term but often create food cravings, dopamine deficiencies, and worse, food addictions. These are foods that can zap energy and attention, and make us feel "flighty."

Foods in this category include:

- Processed foods (fast food, "just add water" mixes)
- Foods high in sugar (candy, "health" bars, sweetened breakfast cereals, fruit juices, sweetened tea beverages)
- White bread (French bread, sourdough, bagels, English muffins)
- Foods made from white flour (cookies, cakes, muffins, pancakes, waffles)
- White rice
- Pastas
- Fried foods (French fries, potato pancakes, fried chicken, fried fish)
- Foods filled with saturated fats (donuts, pizza, cheeseburgers)
- Foods high in salt

How Much Sugar Can I Have?

According to the World Health Organization, no more than 10% of calories should come from sugars. That translates to a daily maximum of 12 teaspoons of sugar (48 grams) in a 2,200-calorie diet. However, the Younger (Thinner) You Diet is based on roughly 1,800 calories a day, which means that you should have no more than 9 teaspoons or 36 grams of sugar on any given day. Remember, each teaspoon of sugar is 4 grams,[10] and fruits and vegetables are packed with natural sugars. And although sugar is not considered a balanced food, many balanced foods, like fruits, do contain natural sugars that need to be accounted for while you are following this diet.

Read nutrition labels on packaged foods, even if they are considered balanced or expanding, because sugar adds up fast. A single bowl of Frosted Mini Wheats contains 3 teaspoons (12 grams) of sugar; some raisin bran cereals contain 20 grams; and a 20-ounce fruit drink can pack nearly 18 teaspoons (71 grams) of sugar. And be sure to count the "hidden" sources of sugar, too—soups, pasta sauce, and even salad dressings may

Younger (Thinner) You foods are balanced foods. Our bodies still need carbohydrates and proteins in order to stay healthy. But instead of making bad food choices in the extreme range of these categories, you can choose a middle option. Moderate portions of lean meats, fish, and poultry are all in the range of balanced foods. So are whole grains like millet, brown rice, barley, corn, oats, quinoa, and buckwheat. These foods are absorbed slowly by the body, thus keeping glucose and insulin low and providing long-lasting energy. They provide the unique ability to prevent the steep declines in blood sugar levels that give rise to fatigue, mood swings, and food cravings.

The best way to stave off cravings is by eating complex carbohydrates, such as whole grains and vegetables, with small amounts of animal products. You'll find your energy levels will stay up between meals. Each of your three meals, plus one snack, should be at least 70% plant based and no more than 30% animal based. The portion sizes are set in the recipes and meal plan chapter. Use those suggestions as a guideline if you plan to create your own meals instead of following the Younger (Thinner) You Diet as directed.

Where the Sugar Is

Fruits are packed with natural sugars, some more than others. Take these numbers into consideration as you are planning your day's worth of sugar.

FRUIT	GRAMS OF SUGAR PER CUP
Date	73.0
Banana	20.4
Fig	19.0
Pomegranate	17.0
Grapes	15.5
Mango	15.0
Cherry	13.0
Pineapple	12.0
Apple	11.8
Pear	11.5
Blueberry	11.0
Orange	10.6
Plum	9.6
Kiwi fruit	8.8
Apricot	8.0
Papaya	8.0
Watermelon	8.0
Blackberry	8.0
Peach	7.9
Grapefruit, red	6.6
Melon, cantaloupe	6.3
Strawberry	5.1

RULE #6: EAT FIBER-FILLED FOODS EVERY DAY

Diets that are low in fat and high in fiber may be the most effective combination that promotes weight loss. Fiber is like a scrub brush for your digestion, scouring your system until it is sparkling clean. It cleans out your colon, controls your blood sugar, pulls fat from you arteries, raises your "good" (HDL) cholesterol, and detoxifies your body. What's more, it's bulky: Fiber fills you up so that you aren't hungry, and you will eat less and feel full faster.

Check labels for fiber content in baked goods, and choose breads, cereals, and pastas made from whole grains. Leafy greens, root vegetables, beans, and lentils are all

Choose from Balanced Proteins

On the Younger (Thinner) You Diet, you'll enjoy a wide range of proteins in tailored portions for maximum weight loss. These include lean cuts of meat such as beef, lamb, pork, and veal; poultry such as chicken, turkey, or Cornish hen; all types of fish, particularly salmon and mackerel; beef liver; soy proteins; eggs and egg whites; and low-fat dairy products, such as skim or low-fat milk, and of course, yogurt.

good sources. Other recommended fiber-abundant foods are quinoa, millet, bulgur, buckwheat, seeds, and nuts. They are absorbed slowly by the body, thus keeping glucose and insulin low and providing long-lasting energy. They provide the unique ability to prevent the steep declines in blood sugar levels that give rise to fatigue, mood swings, and low-dopamine food cravings.

The following chart shows some great sources of fiber. The recommended dosage of daily fiber for weight loss is 40 to 45 grams every day. I tell my patients to gradually increase their fiber intake over several weeks. The goal for the first week of the Younger (Thinner) You Diet should be 15 grams of fiber daily; the second week should be 20 grams; the third week 30 grams, and so on until you can reach the final goal. Read packaged food labels carefully to determine fiber contents of whole wheat breads and other grains.

FOOD	TOTAL GRAMS OF FIBER
½ cup pinto beans	11
1 cup peas	9
½ cup kidney beans	8
½ cup blueberries	8
½ cup blackberries	8
½ cup cranberries	4
5 prunes	4
1 pear	4
1 sweet potato	4
¼ cup almonds	4
½ cup Brussels sprouts	4
½ cup corn	4
½ cup lentils	4
1 cup oatmeal	4
1 orange	3
1 cup strawberries	3

Psyllium

Forty grams of fiber daily will keep your metabolism running and your bowels moving like clockwork. However, we can't always get all the fiber we need from the foods we eat. So fiber supplementation is a good option. One popular fiber supplement is made from psyllium. When added to water, this fiber swells, adding bulk to the stool. In the stomach, this slows gastric emptying, which helps to regulate blood sugar levels and reduce the appetite.

Fiber and PMS

High-fiber foods, such as oatmeal, brown rice, and broccoli, absorb excess estrogen compounds, which are produced during menstruation. Fiber can be used as a powerful appetite suppressant, especially when you are experiencing PMS cravings.

RULE #7: DRINK WATER THROUGHOUT THE DAY

Patients ask me all the time: Can drinking water give me weight loss? The answer is definitively yes. Water continuously flushes your digestive system, moving food particles along at a rapid rate, which leads to weight loss. And, if you're busy drinking your 3 to 4 liters of water all day, you won't have the time or the desire to drink higher-calorie beverages like sodas or juices. Drinking coffee and teas counts, especially those with deep colors for a greater nutritional punch.

Drinking plenty of water will make your metabolism more thermogenic because water raises your dopamine levels. Another benefit is that if you drink water thirty minutes prior to a meal, it will actually fill you up so you will eat less. This is especially true for older individuals.

SKIP ALL OTHER "NO CALORIE" BEVERAGES

Don't run to diet sodas to quench your thirst. It's true they have no calories, but diet sodas contain phosphates that rot your teeth and bones as they deplete your calcium, raise your blood pressure, and damage your brain chemistry. They can increase your chance of developing osteoporosis, especially if you are older than 40. Dr. Earl Mindell notes in his book *Earl Mindell's New Vitamin Bible* that diet soft drinks are especially hazardous to people older than 40 because older kidneys are less able to process phosphorus, which can lead to the depletion of calcium. Without calcium, bones will weaken.[11]

And what about vitamin waters? While many are low in calories, these new beverages don't pack nutrients in the same quantities as whole food sources. You're better off sticking with regular water, and focusing your diet on fresh fruits and vegetables, and supplements if necessary.

Quick Fix: Keep Chugging

Don't wait until you feel thirsty to go for another glass of water. Although most healthy people meet their daily needs judging by thirst alone, this is not always the case. If you live in hot environments, are chronically ill, exercise regularly, or are entering your senior years, make sure that you are constantly drinking water throughout your day until you hit 3 liters (twelve 8-ounce glasses) for women, and 4 liters (sixteen 8-ounce glasses) for men.

OTHER GOOD WATER SOURCES

Just by following the Younger (Thinner) You Diet you will be increasing your water intake. Fresh fruits and veggies are mostly composed of water. The following Younger (Thinner) You choices are comprised of between 80 to 90% water:

- Apples
- Broccoli
- Cantaloupe
- Grapes
- Lettuce
- Milk
- Oranges
- Peaches
- Pears
- Strawberries
- Tomatoes
- Watermelon

RULE #8: EAT COLOR IN EVERY MEAL

On the Younger (Thinner) You Diet, each meal will reflect a variety of the colors of the rainbow. Remember, there is no "white" in the rainbow, because white foods are usually simple carbs that don't contain essential nutrients to support a fast-burning metabolism. So, on the Younger (Thinner) You Diet you'll be avoiding white foods like white bread, white rice, white pasta, white potatoes, and white flour.

A diet that is diverse, with a whole range of colorful fruits and vegetables, has been shown to provide many benefits to your overall health. Colorful foods are mainly fruits and vegetables, and you'll be striving to get nine servings of these every day.

NUTRIENTS COME IN EVERY COLOR

Colorful fruits and vegetables are high in powerful antioxidants, which are integral to becoming younger. I'm sure that you've heard that antioxidants are the nutrients that prevent "free radicals." But you need to know exactly what free radicals are and how they work to understand their effect on aging. Free radicals are very unstable atoms that react with other compounds. In order to gain stability, free radicals will attack the nearest stable molecule, beginning a chain reaction. Once the process is started, it can cascade, breaking down your body on the cellular level, leading to accelerated aging and illnesses like cancer and heart disease.

Eat Plenty of Pomegranates

Pomegranates are a Younger (Thinner) You superfood because they are packed with nutrients. Each of those tiny seeds contains important amino acids, lipids, and minerals such as zinc, and copper. They also contain vitamin C, B_2, B_5, B_1, B_3, B_6, K, and E, as well as folic acid. One hundred percent pomegranate juice is the best way to get a red fix, but make sure it is unsweetened. My favorite is POM Wonderful.

It's thought that this fruit:

- prevents and reverses atherosclerosis
- lowers blood pressure
- helps prevent skin cancer
- slows the progression of prostate cancer
- lowers cholesterol

Dr. Braverman's Top Twenty Rainbow Fruits and Vegetables

Red: cranberries, raspberries, cherries, red beans, pomegranates

Orange: sweet potatoes, oranges, peppers

Yellow: squash, artichokes, peppers

Green: kale, spinach, broccoli, peppers

Blue: blueberries, grapes

Indigo: eggplant

Violet: prunes, plums

Some free radicals arise normally during metabolism. We also create more free radicals naturally as we age. Sometimes the body's immune system cells purposefully create them to neutralize viruses and bacteria. Environmental factors such as pollution, radiation, cigarette smoke, and herbicides, can also spawn free radicals.

So here's where antioxidants come in. These vitamins, including vitamins C and E, protect the body against the destructive effects of free radicals because they neutralize free radicals. In short, increasing your antioxidants counteracts the damage of aging and the environment, so that you can look and feel younger longer. Each time you eat one of these colorful fruits, vegetables, teas, or spices that contain these and other antioxidants, you are helping to make your body younger. By constantly rotating through all of the colors and the choices within the colors, you are creating the best environment for eating the most antioxidants. The lists of colorful fruits and vege-tables below provide their individual nutrient properties.

THE NUTRIENTS IN COLORFUL FOODS

A complete list of all the colored fruits and vegetables is in Appendix B. The following breaks down the different properties of each color group.

Red: Red pigments contain antioxidants that support heart health, improve memory function, protect blood vessels, cartilage, tendons, and ligaments from damage, and may reduce the likelihood of cancer by preventing tissue degeneration that sometimes follows chronic irritation. They may also improve urinary tract health.

Orange: Orange fruits and vegetables are high in carotenoids, which have anti-cancer and antioxidant properties. They can also improve your vision and heart health. Try to eat at least two to three different orange foods daily.

A research study from Arizona State University presents a clear link between low levels of vitamin C and obesity.[12] Vitamin C is needed for the breakdown of the amino acid carnitine. If you don't have enough carnitine, you will increase the accumulation of fat in your muscles.[13] Boosting your vitamin C will help reduce body mass index, lower body fat percentage, shrink your waist circumference, and create lean, strong muscles. Vitamin C is found in many citrus fruits and fresh vegetables, like oranges.

I suggest you stay away from fruit juices, which have lots of unnecessary calories. For example, an 8-ounce glass of orange juice has more than 100 calories. The calorie count may not be tremendously higher than eating whole fruit, but you're missing the health benefits of eating the whole fruit, such as the fiber that is found surrounding the orange segments.[14] By juicing and removing the pulp from citrus fruits, you're removing the flavonoids, which have diverse beneficial biochemical and antioxidant effects. And don't be fooled by containers that say "added pulp." It may not be the pulp originally found in the whole fruit, and it's highly doubtful the amount added back will equal the amount you'd find in a whole piece of fruit. Vitamin C is also concentrated in the inedible parts of fruits, such as the leaves and peel.

Yellow: Yellow fruits and vegetables contain large amounts of phytochemicals as well as carotenoids and bioflavonoids (bonus vitamins and minerals found in many foods that naturally reduce inflammation), which have anticancer and antioxidant properties. They can also improve your vision and heart health. Try to eat at least two to three different yellow foods daily.

Yellow and red grapefruit are high in naringin, the compound that provides its characteristic bitter flavor. It can also enhance the effects of caffeine and could increase its fat-burning action. So it's not the grapefruit alone that makes it a great diet breakfast: It's the combination of grapefruit and coffee that packs the most punch.

Potassium, found in yellow fruits like bananas, is a key nutrient. It gives your heart cells a needed lift. Some soy drink manufacturers (like Bolthouse Farms) make protein soy drinks that contain seven times more potassium than sodium. This is a powerful weight loss agent. The higher the potassium-to-sodium ratio in any food, the better the reduction of water retention. Water retention slows metabolism.

Green: Chlorophyll, present in all green plants, has anticancer and detoxifying properties. Green fruits and vegetables are high in lutein, which is currently being studied for its antioxidant properties. In addition, green leafy veggies are high in carotenoids, vitamins, and minerals that naturally reduce inflammation. Many green foods contain calcium, which helps build strong bones and teeth and improves vision. It is recommended you eat at least one serving daily of leafy green vegetables.

Blue: Many of these foods contain anthocyanins and phenolics, two powerful phytochemicals currently being studied for their antiaging benefits. Blue fruits and vegetables are extremely high in antioxidants. Blue foods can protect your blood vessels, cartilage, tendons, and ligaments from damage, and may reduce the likelihood of cancer by preventing tissue degeneration that follows chronic irritation. They can improve memory function and urinary tract health.

Some nuts, like brazil nuts, macadamia nuts, and black walnuts fall into the category of blue foods because of their particular

The Power of Prunes

Prunes and other dried fruits are great sources of fiber, especially if you cannot tolerate fiber supplements. They are also handy to eat if you are craving something sweet: They are an excellent substitute for sugary snacks.

nutrient content. Macadamia nuts are a particularly good source of fiber and have antioxidant properties. They may also be beneficial for helping to lower cholesterol and preventing heart disease.

Indigo/violet: Indigo- and violet-colored foods also contain an abundance of antioxidant compounds. Dark blue and indigo foods reduce "oxidative stress," one of the main factors that cause aging. They also contain high levels of resveratrol, which is believed to reduce the risk of heart disease and cancer, and other important vitamins and minerals that can improve memory function and urinary tract health.

RULE #9: EAT YOUR FRUITS AND VEGETABLES BOTH RAW AND COOKED

Raw fruits and vegetables contain higher amounts of fiber than cooked ones. And many of the important nutrients, vitamins, and enzymes (which may help with digestion) are destroyed or inactivated during cooking: They are thrown out with the boiling water. For example, steaming broccoli on a stovetop can deplete its vitamin C content by as much as 34%, reports the *Journal of Food Science*. Microwaving is a better alternative: The broccoli retains as much as 90% of its nutrients.[15]

Raw fruits and vegetables also provide the wonderful sense of chewing, which is important not to lose while dieting. Chewing raw food provides a greater sense of satiety with your meal. And you will feel fuller when you have to chew your food vigorously. If you're not chewing your food, you're going to fall into the trap of eating too much too quickly, and filling your mouth with excess calories. A non-chewing mouth is an overeating mouth.

Yet cooked vegetables do have merit. They are usually more easily digested, and any pathogens (a microbe or organism that can cause disease) will be destroyed when food is cooked, which is important as you get older and if you have autoimmune issues. Nutrients like carotenoids (found in red, orange, and yellow veggies) are more available to the body when processed by heat. Cruciferous vegetables including cauliflower, Brussels sprouts, broccoli, cabbage, kale, kohlrabi, mustard greens, rutabagas, and turnips, as well as soybeans, peaches, strawberries, peanuts, radishes, spinach, and millet grain are considered goitrogens (they negatively affect the thyroid) when presented raw, but are inactivated when cooked.

To create a balance and get the most out of your colorful foods, I recommend that you create a mix throughout the day of raw and cooked fruits and veggies. When you cook vegetables, choose a method that keeps the nutrients intact: microwaved, stir-fried, or broiled. On this diet you will be rotating your fruits and vegetables to get a full range of nutrients. You can also rotate your cooking methods so you can experience each one in many different ways.

RULE #10: CHOOSE THREE FOODS FOR EACH MEAL

At every Younger (Thinner) You meal, you'll eat at least three foods. Each should come from a different food group: one must be a protein, and the other two should be different colors of either complex carbohydrates or healthy fats. At the same time, make each meal at least 70% plant based and no more than 30% animal based.

Three foods per meal will make it much easier for you to stick to the pre-scribed serving sizes. It will teach you how to create meals so that you don't eat too much of any one nutrient group. As you learn to cut down your portions of protein and increase your portions of fruits and vegetables, you'll look forward to the addition of different types of food to each meal. For example, if you were used to eating half a chicken for dinner, the Younger (Thinner) You Diet will have you eating much less: 4 to 6 ounces of chicken in total. To compensate, you'll be able to choose two different vegetables, or one vegetable and one healthy grain, to fill your plate. This way, you can look forward to variety instead of dwelling on the fact that you aren't eating as much chicken as before.

Stuck in a Rut?

I've often broken stubborn weight loss plateaus by following a modified green tea fast. I spend one day drinking green tea and eating as many servings of vegetables as possible. On that day, I do not eat any proteins or fats. The next day I go back and eat as on a regular Younger (Thinner) You Diet day.

Tomato Products Are Good Cooked Fruits

Lycopene is a powerful member of the carotenoid family, which forms the red pigment found in tomatoes, watermelon, papayas, and pink grapefruit. Lycopene seems to have the strongest antioxidant properties of all the carotenoids studied to date. Cooked tomato products (such as tomato sauce, paste, powder, ketchup) are the best food sources, since cooking makes lycopene more available for the body to use. Remember, when choosing a condiment, look for the low-sodium, low-sugar version for the best weight loss results.

Pace Yourself

The foods on the Younger (Thinner) You Diet are so delicious and satisfying that you will want to savor every bite. So slow down. Chew your food thoroughly for better digestion and absorption of the greatest amount of nutrients. Put down your utensils between bites to prevent gobbling food, and make each meal last longer.

Include one complete serving of one of the following appetite-suppressing foods each day:

- Apples
- Broccoli
- Carrots
- Eggs
- Pomegranate juice
- Salmon
- Spinach
- Almonds (unsalted)

DON'T GIVE UP ON THE YOUNGER (THINNER) YOU DIET

The latest research in dieting science is showing that the ninety-day rehabilitation model first developed by Alcoholics Anonymous (AA) is just about how long it takes for the brain to reset itself and shake off the influences of your deficiency. So give yourself three months of following the Younger (Thinner) You Diet before you decide it's not right for you. If you follow these ten steps, use the recipes and meal plans, and incorporate exercise into your daily life, you will see results.

These ten steps not only set up the building blocks for the diet, they ensure that you stay focused on changing your brain chemistry, even if you make a few bad choices along the way. Your new brain chemistry will be able to support your lapses, so that the results won't be as drastic. We all mess up from time to time, even with our best intentions. However, the trick is to get right back to making those good choices, so that you can continue with the diet. If you have retrained your brain to rev your metabolism, small transgressions won't matter as much, and you'll be able to get back on track quickly.

My favorite aspect of this diet is that it is one that your whole family can benefit from, whether or not they are trying to lose weight. Just as you are learning to eat better, you will be doing your family an enormous favor by getting them to eat healthier, even at an early age. You'll see in the following chapter the enormous variety in the meal plans. Use these to introduce new fruits and vegetables to your children, and help them make better food choices and break their own rut of eating that same few beige favorites (macaroni and cheese, chicken nuggets, pasta, and so forth).

I also appreciate the newfound energy I feel when I'm following the diet, which I carry into every aspect of my life. As your brain chemistry improves and true neurogenesis begins, you'll find that not only are you losing weight, you're literally feeling younger every day.

CHAPTER 8

Younger (Thinner) You Exercise Strategies

EXERCISE IS an important component of the Younger (Thinner) You Diet. An exercise routine that you enjoy and can maintain will help to keep your internal systems in great shape, as well as improving your outward appearance. Exercise burns calories and stored body fat. It improves your cardiovascular health, keeping your heart pumping strongly. Consistent exercise is important specifically for building muscle. I also find that it helps to relieve stress, especially while you are dieting.

This chapter will help you tailor an exercise program based on your individual needs. You will need to take your brain chemistry into account when choosing which types of exercise are best for you. On the Younger (Thinner) You Diet, you need to be exercising not only to shape and tone your body and raise your metabolic rate, but to improve and enhance your brain functionality. A healthier brain leads to more aggressive weight loss and a younger you. Exercise is one of the greatest brain-balancing choices you can make. And as I've said before, good choices foster more good choices. So the more you exercise, the more you'll want to continue.

There are basically two types of exercise: anaerobic exercise that strengthens and builds muscle, and aerobic exercise that conditions your heart and your stamina. As in all aspects of life, balance is the key. You will need to incorporate both types of exercise into your program in order to increase your metabolism, which will help you achieve weight loss now, and keep the weight off afterward. It is your most effective weapon against storing body fat.

When Should I Work Out?

To get the most out of any workout, exercise in the morning so you can get the benefits of increased metabolism all day. If you just can't get yourself out of bed early enough, though, don't write off your workout. The best time to exercise is whenever you will do it.

STRONG MUSCLES SUPPORT SUPER METABOLISM

If you want to look and feel younger, it's not good enough just to be thin: You need to be thin with great muscle mass that will literally support you and your metabolism well into your later years. Not only will stronger muscles keep your body looking toned, the more musculature you have, the more vibrant and youthful you will feel. Bigger, stronger muscles also protect your body from injury as you become stronger. And you'll find that you have more energy than ever before.

Increasing your muscle mass is an important part of the weight loss equation because lean muscles consume a large percentage of your body's total energy requirement. By creating more muscle, you will burn more of the calories that you consume, and store less as body fat. Muscles burn energy continuously, not just while you are moving around or working out. Even as you sleep, your muscles continue to burn calories simply to maintain their existence, growing new cells and repairing muscle tissue. Anaerobic exercise, more commonly known today as resistance or weight training, is the only way to develop more muscle.

You can easily lose 100 pounds of fat by following this diet, but that might not be enough to make you truly healthy or younger. In fact, with weight loss at that level, it would be a real challenge not to lose muscle or bone density while dieting.

The key, then, is to lose weight without losing your strength or bone mass. By combining anaerobic exercise with aerobic exercise supported by good nutrition, you'll end up losing the weight without sacrificing muscle and bone.

Last year I met a new patient named Carla. She was 5' 4½", and weighed 225 pounds. Based on her BMI, Carla needed to drop down to 125 pounds, losing approximately 100 pounds. But once I took her DEXA scan into consideration, we realized that she had a dangerous level of body fat as well. With a careful assessment of 45% body fat, Carla needed to lose 120 pounds, while adding 20 pounds of muscle. By following the Younger (Thinner) You Diet and incorporating exercise into her life every single day, Carla was able to reach her goal within a year.

THE SECRET OF RESISTANCE TRAINING: WEIGHT-BEARING EXERCISE

Resistance training includes the use of free weights, weight machines, resistance bands, or water exercises to strengthen the muscles and bones in your arms and upper spine. Strength training works directly on your bones to slow mineral loss, so it is especially important if you know that you have osteoporosis. Resistance training involves regularly working your muscle groups against weights to a point where they fatigue, or become tired. Over time, the constant fatiguing of the muscle and increasing of the weight amount signals your body to repair and grow new stronger and thicker muscle tissue to adapt to their new workload. These bigger, stronger muscle fibers require more energy just to exist, and will use up your energy stores in order to properly function. This constant requirement of energy is what gives you the maximum boost in metabolism. Resistance training exercises also increase bone density, which can help ward off osteoporosis. Now, I'm not asking you to look like a bodybuilder. You only need to create a small increase in your overall muscle mass to see weight loss results.

Many of my patients do their resistance training with a variety of sizes of weights or weight machines, in a home gym or workout center. These activities are effective, but need to be closely monitored by a professional. If you choose to work out at a gym, make sure that you take a few classes with a personal trainer who can teach you how to use free weights effectively and safely. If you choose to purchase free weights for home, there are many books and DVDs available that teach you the basics of weight training. Use weights that are heavy enough so you feel a level of exertion as you complete 10 to 15 repetitions for each exercise, and then increase the weight when the repetitions become easy.

If you have access to a personal trainer, either at your local gym or someone who can come to your home, I highly recom-

> ### A Recipe for Successful Exercise
>
> The typical exercise routine for the Younger (Thinner) You Diet is rigorous, but it is important. I strongly believe that you have to prioritize your health: Your health drives everything else in your life, so taking care of yourself has to come first. I recommend:
>
> - 1 hour of dumbbells on Tuesday and Thursday
> - 30 minutes on the treadmill or an incline run of 8 minutes at 4.5 mph speed, Monday, Wednesday, and Friday
> - A swim on Saturday
> - A rest day on Sunday

mend it. A trainer can create a muscle-building workout that is tailored to your current health and weight loss goals. What's more, trainers get you to do what you don't want to do: extra push-ups, curls, and other exercises in which the benefits really add up.

Another type of resistance exercise falls under the category of weight-bearing exercise. These have both aerobic and resistance components to them because they require your muscles to work against gravity. They are one of the best ways to incorporate both aerobic and anaerobic activity into one workout. You are your own set of free weights. Walking briskly with a slight pounding to the ground is considered a weight-bearing exercise, which will help increase your dopamine and your metabolism. At the same time, you're getting an aerobic workout and increasing your GABA. You should be moving at a pace in which it is difficult but not impossible to talk and walk at the same time.

Swimming and simply walking, although good for cardiovascular fitness, are not the best exercises for building bone. Thirty minutes of weight-bearing exercise daily benefits not only your bones, but improves heart health, muscle strength, coordination, and balance. Those 30 minutes don't need to be done all at once: 10 minutes at a time is all it takes to start to see a significant change.

These activities include:

- Weight lifting
- Jogging
- Hiking
- Stair climbing
- Step aerobics
- Dancing
- Racquet sports

AEROBIC EXERCISE

Aerobic activity increases your heart rate for extended periods of time, and improves the way that the body uses the oxygen we breathe. You need to sustain a high level of aerobic activity for at least 20 minutes to get the best results. Additionally, you need to incorporate a warmup and a cooldown period into your routine.

You can create a simple aerobics routine right in your own home using DVDs created by professional trainers to guide you. Or you can start a fast-paced walking program. To get started, you'll need a pair of comfortable walking shoes, a watch, and a pair of hand-held weights of no more than 1 to 2 pounds. The goal of this routine is to get you moving at a variety of paces. If you can, walk outdoors, no matter what the weather is!

Start walking slowly with a 5-minute warm-up. Carry the light weights with you and pump your arms as you walk. Your pace should be one in which you can easily carry a conversation.

Then, for the next 20 minutes, pick up the pace. You want to reach a momentum in which you are panting but can carry on a quick conversation at the same time. Vary your terrain: Walk up and down a staircase, or walk up and down a hill. Pump your arms faster as you go, deliberately alternating your left and right sides. Bring the weights to the level of your heart.

For the last 5 minutes, progressively slow down your pace. Take long strides, and stretch your legs as you bring your walk to an end. Stop pumping your arms and carry the weights at your sides. Don't stop moving until you have walked a total of 30 minutes.

30 Minutes a Day or 1½ Hours Twice a Week?

A longer session of exercise is great, especially if you can let off some steam in a tennis match or during a good, long run. But these stretches of exercise do not make up for your daily 30 minutes. A combination of the two will yield the best results.

Cardio vs. Resistance

You need to tailor your specific exercise programs to your health issues and your brain chemistry. However, I recommend that you include both aerobic and anaerobic exercises for a complete workout program. Cardio work burns calories in the moment that the exercise is being performed. Your metabolism quickly returns to its normal level not long after the exercise is stopped. However, increasing muscle mass boosts metabolism permanently, so you are burning more fuel all day long.

Make sure to select aerobic activities in which you have the least chance of being injured. Swimming is an excellent option, especially if you have not exercised regularly in a long time. Walking is a low-impact exercise with numerous health benefits, including improved heart health (lowering risk of heart attacks). Walking can help you lower bad cholesterol levels and raise good cholesterol levels. It can help manage your blood pressure; reduce your risk of developing type 2 diabetes or help control existing diabetes; burn calories; and reduce stress levels and feelings of depression and anxiety. Running and sprinting, either indoors on a treadmill or outdoors, are excellent choices for aerobic activity that also risk few injuries.

EXERCISE AND BRAIN HEALTH

Different types of exercise can stimulate the production of the four primary brain chemicals. This may be another reason why exercise programs have not helped you in the past: You may have been focusing on one type of exercise while your brain chemistry

required another. By creating a diet that's just right for you, and an exercise program that's equally personalized, you are in the best situation to lose weight and feel younger.

Dopamine: Exercise has been linked to stimulating the dopamine pleasure and satisfaction circuits. This may explain why some people are actually addicted to exercise. You may have experienced that satisfied feeling when you are exercising. Some describe it as a "runner's high" or have heard it linked to the release of pleasure-producing hormones, such as endorphins. These are the same hormones that are released during sex.

A dopamine-enhancing workout should feature aerobic activity followed by weight training every day, if possible. This combination will give you the energy you may be lacking.

Acetylcholine: Although you may have the best intentions about exercise, it's quite possible you spend more time thinking about when you'll do it than actually getting around to working out. Studies have shown aerobic exercise can restore acetylcholine. You'll need at least half an hour of aerobic exercise every day to increase your acetylcholine levels.

You do not need to do your 30 minutes of aerobic exercise all in one session. Three power walks for ten minutes each can be substituted for a 30-minute workout, but they are never really as effective. Figure out which is better for your schedule, and mix it up whenever necessary. Just be sure to get your thirty minutes in every day, for a total of three hours of aerobic exercise a week.

GABA: If you are GABA deficient, one of your daily goals should be to use aerobic exercise as a form of relaxation. Some of my favorite forms of exercise for increasing GABA are power yoga and Pilates. It may sound counterintuitive, but physical exercise works as a tranquilizer and it actually helps to restore your GABA imbalance. Many low-GABA individuals have trouble getting involved with exercise. But once you experience the high of exercise and the relaxation state that it produces, you'll realize what you've been missing.

Serotonin: Just as getting good sleep provides the opportunity for your brain to reset, the same can be said for exercise: Physical movement—whether aerobic or anaerobic—helps to reset the brain and release serotonin. I always tell my patients to balance an aggressive workout with some brain exercise. In the case of low serotonin, you won't need to work on crossword puzzles or Sudoku. Instead, you might consider incorporating prayer, yoga, meditation, and/or chanting into your weekly routine. All of these activities boost serotonin and an overall feeling of serenity.

For example, a chanting exercise is ideal for improving serotonin levels: It shuts off your thinking pattern, blocks negative thoughts, and slows the mind and body down in order to resynchronize. Best of all, you can access this serotonin-enhancing exercise whenever you want, wherever you want.

DR. B'S BEST EXERCISE TIPS

- Warm up before starting and cool down at the end of each exercise session.
- Don't pick one type of exercise and stick to it. Just like you are rotating your foods to get the most nutrients, rotate your exercise routine for the best workout.
- As you begin to feel stronger, increase resistance or weight, rather than the number of repetitions.
- Drink plenty of water whenever exercising.
- Add more physical activity to every part of your day: take the stairs whenever you can; park at the back of the parking lot instead of right in front of the store; and get out of your house and talk to your friends and family, instead of e-mailing or using the phone.

CHAPTER 9

The Younger (Thinner) You
Daily Meal Plans

THIS CHAPTER provides a thirty-day meal plan for the Younger (Thinner) You Diet. It features loads of easy-to-prepare meals for breakfast, lunch, dinner, and daily snacks, many of which follow recipes found in Chapter 10. You'll find these suggestions incredibly satisfying: You will never walk away from the table hungry if you follow this plan.

You can use this meal plan in many different ways. First, you can follow it exactly as written for thirty days, and repeat until you've lost all the weight you want. In fact, you can continue using this meal plan forever, even after you've reached your goal. That's because I'm promoting a wide variety of foods that are healthy, satisfying, and natural. These choices are also dopamine enhancing, which will not only boost your brain chemistry but will increase your metabolism: tools you'll need for a lifetime of good health.

Meal suggestions followed by an asterisk (★) indicate the recipe for that meal is in the next chapter. Many of the other meal suggestions are simple to prepare, or can be store-bought. Make sure that whenever you purchase pre-made meals, you choose low-sodium and low-sugar varieties. Read labels carefully and watch out for these hidden sugars:

- Cane juice
- Corn syrup
- Dextrose
- Fructose
- Glucose
- Lactose
- Maltodextrin
- Rice syrup
- Sucrose
- High-fructose corn syrup

You can also use these meal plan suggestions for any of your brain chemical deficiencies, and substitute similar items when necessary. For example, if you are low in acetylcholine, you might want to eat more fish than chicken. In this case you can swap the protein choices. Your specific deficiency will guide you to pick foods high in the nutrients that will support your

Don't Be Fooled: Sugar Is Sugar

High-fructose corn syrup is not food, it's a science experiment! High-fructose corn syrup is produced by processing corn starch to yield glucose, and then processing the glucose to produce a high percentage of fructose. Two of the enzymes used in production, alpha-amylase and glucose isomerase, are genetically modified to make them more stable. Animal studies have shown a link between increased consumption of high-fructose corn syrup and adverse health effects, such as diabetes and high cholesterol.

Here are some ways to eliminate high-fructose corn syrup from your diet.

- Buy 100% fruit juice instead of fruit-flavored drinks. Or better yet, eat fruit rather than drink it. You'll get an extra boost of fiber and fewer calories than you do by drinking juice. Even 100% fruit juice has a high concentration of sugar.
- If you opt for canned fruit, make sure it's packed in its own juices, rather than in heavy or light syrup. These syrups are just sugar.
- Eliminate soda, even the diet version.

needs. Appendix C gives you an index of recipes to help you boost a particular brain chemical. If you have specific health issues, read through the chapters in Part III to further modify your personal Younger (Thinner) You Diet.

USING THE MEAL PLANS EVERY DAY

The Younger (Thinner) You Diet allows for three full meals plus one snack. You can choose when you want to have your snack during the day. Just make sure your last meal is no fewer than 2 to 3 hours before bedtime so that breakfast can be a "break fast." Many individuals who have hypoglycemia have to have a snack or meal before bed. The best snack can be dried fruit, which is filled with powerful nutrients and ensures that your bowels don't fall asleep when you do.

If you are hungry at any point during the day, help yourself to a full 8-ounce glass of room-temperature water with lemon or a cup of tea. Wait twenty minutes. If you are still hungry, have a large apple (start with half, wait again, then eat the other half). These tricks should curb your appetite until the next full meal or snack.

I always tell my patients that they need to plan their meals like they plan the rest of their day. Just as you look over your calendar in the morning to see what's in store for the day, look over the meal plans for each day every morning. Make sure you have all the ingredients you need, or have access to prepared meals that closely resemble the meal plan. At the end of the day, write down exactly what you ate in the log in Chapter 11, so you can keep track of your success.

YOUNGER (THINNER) YOU DAILY EATING PLANNER

BREAKFAST	LUNCH	DINNER	SNACK
DAY 1			
2 poached eggs over steamed spinach and garlic sprinkled with fresh rosemary and thyme; small orange	Green salad with ½ avocado, 4 ounces roasted turkey, 1 tomato, 5 black olives drizzled with olive oil, sesame seeds, black pepper, and garlic	Curried Shrimp★ served with ½ cup brown rice and steamed asparagus	Apple slices and 2 tablespoons natural low-sodium peanut butter
DAY 2			
Italian Omelet★	Navy Bean and Kale Soup★ served with 1 slice of whole wheat bread	Baked Chicken with Yogurt★ served with 8 ounces of roasted beet and onion salad	½ cup red grapes with ½ cup low-fat cottage cheese
DAY 3			
Rainbow Fruit Salad★	4 ounces turkey slices with mustard, served with ½ cup cooked quinoa seasoned with rosemary and garlic powder, and broccoli	Salmon with Dill Crust and Tomato Fennel Sauce★, steamed spinach, and raw carrot slices with dill	1 slice whole wheat bread dipped in 2 tablespoons olive oil seasoned with a touch of balsamic vinegar and cayenne pepper
DAY 4			
¾ cup bran cereal with ¾ cup low-fat milk and ½ cup sliced strawberries, sprinkled with 1 teaspoon each cinnamon, nutmeg, and allspice	Tuna Pita Pocket★ served with an 8-ounce glass of no-sugar-added pomegranate juice	Flank Steak Fajitas★ with Mango Salsa★ served with ½ cup of black beans and brown rice	1 cup plain low-fat yogurt with ½ cup fresh fruit and 2 teaspoons cinnamon

Breakfast Supports Metabolism

I know I've said it already, but make sure you eat breakfast every day. Skipping out on this essential meal slows your metabolism and triggers the body to go into "hoard mode," in which it thinks it's starving because you've gone for a long period of time, usually 8 to 10 hours, without food. By doing this, the body believes it needs to store new calories. The result is a slowdown of digestion, and you'll end up storing excess fuel as fat. People who eat breakfast every day reduce the number of total calories they consume, which may prevent overeating during the day and lowers the risk of weight gain.[2]

BREAKFAST	LUNCH	DINNER	SNACK
DAY 5			
Apple Walnut Cinnamon Oatmeal★	Tuna Stuffed Tomatoes★ served with 2 slices rye toast	Tandoori Chicken★ served with steamed snow peas and medley of red beans and corn	1 cup plain low-fat yogurt mixed with fresh berries and 2 teaspoons cinnamon
DAY 6			
1 cup plain low-fat plain yogurt mixed with ¼ cup whole grain granola, 2 tablespoons raisins, 1 teaspoon cinnamon, and ½ teaspoon nutmeg or allspice	Black Bean Soup★ served with tossed salad greens and tomato drizzled with 1 tablespoon of olive oil, balsamic vinegar, herbs, and 10 walnuts	Lamb Chops with Herbs and Tabouli★ served with steamed or roasted broccoli	4 whole-grain crispbread crackers served with ¼ cup cottage cheese
DAY 7			
2 scrambled eggs with ½ teaspoon each turmeric, cumin, and tarragon; 1 medium-sized banana sprinkled with a pinch of allspice or cinnamon	Soy veggie burger seasoned with mustard, cayenne, and black pepper on a whole wheat bun served with a mixed salad of 2 ounces blue cheese, red and orange peppers, and tomato slices	Broiled Halibut with Yogurt Dill Sauce★ served with ½ cup brown rice and 1 cup sautéed broccoli rabe; ¼ of a small cantaloupe	¼ cup hummus dip and red pepper sticks
DAY 8			
1 cup plain low-fat Greek yogurt sprinkled with ½ cup fresh berries, ¼ cup granola, and cinnamon, nutmeg, and allspice	Sprouted Pea Soup★ sprinkled with 1 tablespoon toasted sesame seeds served with a slice of whole wheat toast; 1 pear	6 ounces roasted pork with ½ baked eggplant sprinkled with rosemary, thyme, and black pepper, and cooked carrots seasoned with dill and garlic and a sprinkle of olive oil	¼ cup unsalted nuts
DAY 9			
Egg Bruschetta★ served with ½ grapefruit	Rainbow Fruit Salad★	Jasmine Tea–Infused Brown Rice Salad with Sweet Peas and Duck★	2 ounces lean roast beef slices served with a Granny Smith apple sprinkled with 1 teaspoon allspice

BREAKFAST	LUNCH	DINNER	SNACK
DAY 10			
1 whole wheat English muffin spread with 2 tablespoons hummus and tomato slices	Tofu Curry with Green Beans★ with ½ cup brown rice	Herb-Rubbed Mackerel with Snow Peas & Lemon★	1 cup plain low-fat yogurt mixed with ¼ cup walnuts and 1 teaspoon cinnamon
DAY 11			
1 slice whole wheat bread topped with 1 ounce baked salmon and tomato slices sprinkled with black pepper, rosemary, and garlic	Asian Chicken Lettuce Wrap★ served with 1 cup tomato soup and 1 apple	Baked Sweet Potato Casserole with Pecans★ served with steamed spinach	1 cup plain low-fat Greek yogurt with 1 tablespoon all-fruit strawberry preserve

My Favorite Spice Combinations

Take a plain chicken breast or salmon fillet and literally change your life by adding any of these no-calorie, high-nutrient spice combinations. These recipes are enough for at least two portions. Don't forget to use your spices liberally!

1. Chili powder (¼ teaspoon) + oregano (½ teaspoon) + basil (½ teaspoon)
2. Cayenne (½ teaspoon) + cumin (1 teaspoon) + coriander (1 teaspoon)
3. Black pepper (½ teaspoon) + garlic (1 teaspoon) + ginger (1 teaspoon)
4. Turmeric (½ teaspoon) + cumin (1 teaspoon) + curry (½ teaspoon)
5. Oregano + thyme + rosemary + cayenne (combine to your taste: Use more cayenne if you like spicy foods and your digestive system can tolerate it)
6. Basil + rosemary + thyme + garlic (combine to your taste)
7. Bay leaves (2) + cinnamon (½ teaspoon) + cloves (½ teaspoon) + cardamom (½ teaspoon) + black pepper (½ teaspoon) + cumin (1 teaspoon) + coriander (1 teaspoon)
8. Nutmeg + cinnamon + cardamom (combine to your taste)
9. Fennel (½ teaspoon) + mustard (½ teaspoon) + fenugreek (½ teaspoon) + cumin (½ teaspoon)
10. Saffron (a few strands) + cumin (½ teaspoon) + cardamom (½ teaspoon) + clove (¼ teaspoon) + cinnamon (½ teaspoon)
11. Marjoram (½ teaspoon) + thyme (1 teaspoon) + basil (½ teaspoon) + oregano (½ teaspoon) + savory (½ teaspoon)

BREAKFAST	LUNCH	DINNER	SNACK
DAY 12			
Baked Bananas★ served with 1 cup plain yogurt sprinkled with 2 teaspoons cinnamon and a pinch of allspice	Egg Salad Tomato Cup★ served with 1 slice whole wheat bread	Lemon Garlic Rooibos Chicken★ served with tabouli and tomato salad	¼ cup dried cherries, apricots, pears, apples, or prunes mixed with ¼ cup almonds
DAY 13			
2 hard-boiled eggs sprinkled with rosemary, oregano, and parsley flakes; 8 ounces no-sugar-added pomegranate juice	Spicy Kale and Yams★ served with ½ cup whole wheat couscous	Sautéed Liver with Caramelized Onions★ served with ½ cup mashed sweet potatoes and 1 baked apple	1 cup plain low-fat yogurt sprinkled with 1 tablespoon ginger
DAY 14			
1 cup high-fiber cereal (I like to rotate, and sometimes even mix these together: Kashi, Fiber One, All-Bran, Shredded Wheat, Grape Nuts, Cheerios, Bran Flakes, or Quaker Oat Bran) with ¾ cup 1% milk and 1 medium banana	Sweet Potato and Chickpea Curry★ served with ½ cup barley	Rosemary Chicken with Broccoli★ served with steamed pea pods	½ cup frozen blueberries mixed into 1 cup of low-fat vanilla yogurt
DAY 15			
Herb Frittata★ served with ½ grapefruit	Super Salad★ served with 1 cup potato-leek soup	Herb Crusted Halibut★ served with ½ cup wild rice pilaf and pinto beans	1 cup plain low-fat yogurt sprinkled with ¼ cup low-fat granola and 1 teaspoon cinnamon

Delicious and Meatless Do Go Together

If you happen to be a vegetarian or are just looking for meat alternatives, there are some amazing soy- and vegetable-based products on the market. Give these a try: Boca Burgers, Morningstar Farms, Dr. Praeger's Veggie Burgers, Trader Joe's Meatless Meatballs, Amy's Veggie Burgers, Gardenburger, and Tofurky products.

BREAKFAST	LUNCH	DINNER	SNACK
DAY 16			
½ small cantaloupe served with 1 cup low-fat yogurt sprinkled with cinnamon, nutmeg, and allspice	Salade Niçoise with Olives, Oranges, and Bell Pepper★	Shrimp Fajitas★	1 cup popcorn, such as Smart Balance Low-Fat or Bearitos No Oil Added
DAY 17			
1 cup low-fat yogurt parfait: layer with 1 cup mixed strawberries and raspberries and sprinkle with cinnamon and nutmeg	Spicy Seared Tofu with Mandarin Orange Sauce★ served with ½ cup quinoa	Herb Frittata★ served with 1 baked sweet potato sprinkled with cinnamon	10 low-sodium olives sprinkled with fennel seeds, rosemary, and red pepper flakes
DAY 18			
1 cup oatmeal seasoned with cinnamon, ginger, and nutmeg; ¼ fresh whole pineapple	Mediterranean Turkey Leg★ served with salad greens and sliced pear	Baked Tilapia★ served with ½ baked whole winter squash	1 cup low-fat chocolate yogurt and ½ cup strawberries
DAY 19			
2 soft-boiled eggs with garlic, rosemary, thyme, and fresh radishes	Spinach and Strawberry Salad★ served with 1 cup plain low-fat yogurt	6 ounces lean steak seasoned with garlic, paprika, black pepper, and oregano, served with steamed green beans, toasted almonds, and dried cranberries	1 cup low-sodium chicken broth served with 5 whole wheat crackers

Choose from the Best

McCormick is famous for their herbs and spices, and for good reason. They use high quality raw materials and deliver a terrific product. Give these a try: allspice, ancho chile, anise, basil, bay leaves, black pepper, caraway seed, cardamom, celery seed, chervil, chipotle chile, chives, cilantro, cinnamon, cloves, coriander, cumin, dill, fennel, ginger, mace, marjoram, mint, mustard, nutmeg, oregano, paprika, parsley, poppy seed, red pepper, rosemary, saffron, sage, savory, sesame seed, tarragon, thyme, turmeric, vanilla, white pepper.

BREAKFAST	LUNCH	DINNER	SNACK
		DAY 20	
1 cup apple and watermelon cubes mixed with ½ cup assorted nuts (walnuts, almonds, etc.) and sprinkled with wheat germ, cinnamon, and nutmeg	Baigan Ka Bharta (Mashed Eggplant)★ served with ½ cup brown rice and steamed broccoli	Grilled salmon with fennel, oregano, and garlic, served with roasted corn and steamed edamame	1 cup plain low-fat Greek yogurt drizzled with 1 teaspoon honey
		DAY 21	
Cinnamon Fruit Smoothie★	Garden salad with beets, mandarin oranges, and grapes, mixed with a touch of olive oil and 2 tablespoons balsamic vinegar, seasoned with fresh mint, basil, and black pepper	Chicken with Prunes and Olives★ served with English Breakfast Tea Green Beans★ and 1 small baked sweet potato sprinkled with cinnamon	2 tablespoons peanut butter on apple slices

Dress Your Salad Tasty

When it comes to salad dressings, low-fat doesn't always mean healthy. Low-fat dressings are often loaded with extra sugar or salt to make up for the missing fat. Read the labels: Carefully check the sugar, salt, and fat content of dressings, and look for brands that use only natural ingredients. Be aware that most dressings are loaded with calories, so use sparingly. Even healthy can be fattening!

Look for special spiced olive oils, or oils infused with herbs and spices like rosemary, garlic, and cayenne. Or try making your own. Add fresh rosemary sprigs or fresh whole garlic cloves to extra-virgin olive oil, and let marinate for a day or two for more nutritious, flavor-infused oils.

There are many healthy, flavorful salad dressings on the market, including brands like Annie's Naturals Balsamic Vinaigrette, Annie's Naturals Goddess, Fresh Direct dressings, Newman's Own, Harriet's Original dressings, and Simply Delicious. Also consider trying one of the salad sprays that are new to the market, including Wish-Bone Salad Spritzers, which contain about 1 to 2 calories per spray and allow you to carefully control the amount of dressing you're using. Or buy a spray bottle or mister and fill it with olive oil, balsamic vinegar, and your favorite spices, like garlic, oregano, basil, and thyme. You can always add additional spices to bottled dressing for extra flavor and nutrients.

BREAKFAST	LUNCH	DINNER	SNACK
DAY 22			
Pineapple Upside-down French Toast★ served with ½ grapefruit	Sprouted Pea Soup★ served with 1 whole wheat English muffin and 8 ounces no-sugar-added pomegranate juice	Salmon and Tomato Stew★ served with oven-roasted fennel and carrots	1 cup plain low-fat yogurt and 1 small red apple
DAY 23			
2 hard-boiled eggs sprinkled with garlic, rosemary, and red pepper flakes	Tuna salad sandwich made with garlic, dill, and oregano served on whole wheat bread with lettuce and tomato slices	Middle Eastern Turkey Kebabs★ served with ½ cup whole wheat couscous	1 cup low-fat yogurt mixed with ½ cup frozen blackberries
DAY 24			
1 slice whole wheat toast with 1 tablespoon peanut butter, served with 1 cup banana and strawberry slices sprinkled with cinnamon, nutmeg, and allspice	1 skinless chicken breast baked with Plain Yogurt Cumin Marinade★ served with 1 cup diced tomatoes and cucumbers sprinkled with rosemary, thyme, and dill	Moroccan Lamb Tagine with Cinnamon, Apricots, and Almonds★ served with roasted eggplant	¼ cup hummus and celery sticks
DAY 25			
2 hard-boiled eggs sprinkled with paprika, rosemary, and sage served with ½ cup melon	1 cup of steamed mixed vegetables served over ½ cup whole wheat couscous seasoned with turmeric, basil, and rosemary	½ Cornish hen with Garlic Lover's Rub★ served with a small green salad	1 cup low-fat yogurt sprinkled with cinnamon; 1 plum (or 4 prunes if not in season)

Take Your Spices with You

Restaurants come up short when it comes to herbs and spices. Look at the table in a typical restaurant—what are your options? Salt and years-old ground pepper. Always ask if you can have the right spices served with your meal "on the side" so you can add them yourself. And don't be afraid to carry along your own small bottles of spices and herbs to supplement your meals with powerhouse nutrients and mega-boosts of flavor.

BREAKFAST	LUNCH	DINNER	SNACK
DAY 26			
1 banana yogurt smoothie sprinkled with wheat germ and 1 teaspoon cinnamon	Egg salad seasoned with dill, black pepper, and garlic powder, served over tomatoes, green peppers, and romaine lettuce.	Citrus Tuna★ served with ½ cup whole wheat couscous and steamed spinach and orange sections	¼ cup mixed unsalted nuts and ¼ cup raisins
DAY 27			
Rainbow Yogurt Parfait with Fresh Fruit★	Black Bean, Jicama, Corn, and Mango Salad★	Blood Orange Salmon★ served with Mint and Cranberry Tea Basmati★	1 cup plain popcorn seasoned with rosemary and garlic
DAY 28			
Scrambled Eggs with Broccoli★	1 cup low-fat vanilla yogurt with strawberry slices, wheat germ, ginger, cinnamon, and nutmeg	Veal medallions with Garlic Lover's Rub★ served with wild rice and steamed artichokes; 1 apple	1 cup organic butternut squash soup

Eating and Your Health Issues

If you have certain illnesses that involve inflammation—any of the "itises"—cut back on nightshade fruits like tomatoes, eggplant, bell peppers, potatoes, and cayenne. Instead, choose from the anti-inflammatory spices like rosemary and basil. A person suffering with GERD should drink green tea, and eat smaller, more frequent meals. Break up each of the three big meals in these meal plans and spread the same foods over six small meals.

Younger (Thinner) You Treats for Kids

Healthier Chicken Nuggets: Cut one chicken breast into 1-inch chunks and brush with no-sugar-added fresh fruit jam or jelly (try Smucker's Simply Fruit or Sugar-Free, Sorrell Ridge 100% Fruit, or Trader Joe's Organic Fruit Spreads); roll in seasoned nut meal, and bake for 30 minutes at 350°F.

Younger (Thinner) You Pops: Combine 1 cup fresh fruit puree (no added sugar) with 2 tablespoons of plain, low-fat yogurt and 1 teaspoon cinnamon. Fill an ice cube tray with mixture. Cover trays with plastic wrap and poke the sticks through so that they stand up. Freeze overnight.

BREAKFAST	LUNCH	DINNER	SNACK
DAY 29			
Oatmeal with bananas and raisins sprinkled with cinnamon, nutmeg, and allspice	Super Salad★	Tandoori Chicken★ served with sautéed spinach and corn on the cob	1 cup plain low-fat yogurt poured over a diced peach (or other fruit in season)
DAY 30			
Baked Bananas★ served with 1 cup plain low-fat yogurt	Hearty tomato vegetable soup seasoned with cayenne, oregano, and basil served with 1 slice whole wheat toast	Mahimahi with Ginger Glaze★ served with baked fruit compote and ½ cup cooked buckwheat (kasha)	1 slice whole wheat bread dipped in 2 tablespoons of olive oil seasoned with a touch of balsamic vinegar and cayenne pepper

THE YOUNGER (THINNER) YOU DIET ON THE GO

Our fast-paced lives are such that most of us don't eat three meals a day at home anymore. I've tried to vary these menus so that there will always be something on a menu at a restaurant that resembles one of my meals.

Before you leave your home, stock up on Younger (Thinner) You foods that you can take with you. Go to a local grocery store like Whole Foods or Wild Oats and load up with small packages of unsalted sunflower seeds, apples, oranges, celery sticks, different kinds of unsalted nuts, and of course, tea bags. Parcel out single servings in small plastic bags so that you don't fall back on repetitive or "hand to mouth" eating.

If you find that you are stuck at a business meeting, a hotel, or even a restaurant that can't accommodate this diet, just remember to "think fruit." You can always substitute a platter of fresh fruit, with or without a small low-fat yogurt, for any meal. Otherwise, you'll fall back on old habits and order a hamburger with French fries and ketchup. This meal has so much sodium that you'll blow up like a balloon. Worse, it'll take you two to five days just to get rid of the grease from a burger.

Great Grilling Tips

Grilled foods taste great. Grilling vegetables concentrates their flavor and seals in their nutrients. For a great veggie side dish, sprinkle carrots and parsnips with cumin, coriander, and turmeric. Wrap them loosely in tin foil that has been sprayed lightly with olive oil. Cook directly over high heat until tender. Carefully open the packet away from your face to avoid steam burns.

CHAPTER 10

The Younger (Thinner) You Recipes

I NEVER FEEL LIKE I'm dieting when I prepare these foods. Each one is packed with metabolism-boosting spices and is made with fresh ingredients you can find in any supermarket. Best of all, they are family-friendly: Make sure to prepare enough for your whole crew so they can also benefit from the Younger (Thinner) You Diet.

You'll find special occasion breakfasts that we serve whenever we entertain for brunch, or for special treats on the weekend. I've made sure the lunches are very easy to prepare for busy people like us, and that they are as tasty as they are filling. I often double the lunch recipes and cook in batches to ensure I have enough for a couple of days each week. The dinner recipes are slightly more complicated, but worth the extra work. There are also special sauces and marinades to help you jazz up your favorite chicken, fish, or meat.

You can use these recipes as they have been laid out in the Younger (Thinner) You meal plans in Chapter 9, or you can create your own meal plans based on your brain chemistry. Review the chapters in Part I that highlight your specific deficit(s). Then choose foods that will boost your brain chemistry for each meal. Pair the recipes with the right vegetables, fresh fruits, or side dishes that will boost your brain chemicals.

By following this diet, you will be able to see positive results in just a matter of

Younger (Thinner) You Shopping Tips

- Make lots of room in the refrigerator and pantry for Younger (Thinner) You foods.
- Shop for food on a full stomach.
- Stock the refrigerator with healthy foods from the outside perimeter of the supermarket, where the fresh foods are stationed.
- Buy fruits and veggies in season, and local whenever possible.
- Check for the green USDA "organic" label on all food products: Everything you need for the Younger (Thinner) You Diet comes in an organic version.

weeks. Aside from losing weight, you will have renewed energy during the day, and experience better, more restful sleep at night. In short, you'll look and feel younger than you have in years, just by eating appropriately to support your health.

SHOPPING LIST

Every diet starts with you emptying your cupboards of the foods that you will not eat. So go ahead: Throw away all the pasta, leftover Chinese takeout, white rice, canned vegetables, chips, cookies, salty snacks, pickles, and hidden chocolates (yes, even those tiny ones), and let's start over.

Here are the items you will need to have on hand to prepare the dishes specified in the following recipes. Personalize this shopping list with the foods you'll need to balance your brain chemistry that were listed in the chapters that match your

deficits. Then, look over the tea recipes in Chapter 7 to see which appeal to you, and add those to your list.

Remember, fresh is best, so you may want to buy the vegetables on an "as needed" basis instead of having them go bad at the bottom of your refrigerator. Fresh herbs like basil and parsley have more nutrients than their dried counterparts. When

Buying Salad Blends

There are so many salad mixes, it's hard to choose the right one. To get the most from salads, pick the darkest green leaves. Stay away from iceberg lettuce; it contains almost no nutrients. Look for mixes with these leaves that are high in nutrients:

Arugula: packed with folate and calcium
Spinach: high in lutein and zeaxanthin
Red leaf: bone-building vitamin K
Curly endive: tons of beta-carotene
Romaine: an old standby that provides almost 100% of your vitamin A requirements

On the Road

It's happened to all of us: You're starving and the only place in town has a giant "M" on the door. Typical fast food options are harmful to your weight loss. Fast food means indigestion, poor metabolism, extra fat, extra salt, and extra sugar. The good news is that the fast-food industry has finally woken up to what Americans really need. There are new choices available, so that if you end up at a fast-food joint, you can stay on the Younger (Thinner) You Diet.

Order the salad, and throw away the dressing. Get the chicken grilled instead of fried. Remember, eating slowly and enjoying your food is a GABA brain exercise.

Keep some healthy snacks like granola or unsalted nuts in the car so you won't be tempted by the latest super fabulous Half-Pounder.

One More Reason to Lay off the Booze

A 2007 Swedish research study demonstrated what we all have seen around the party circuit: High alcohol intake is associated with abdominal obesity.[1] While the study monitored elderly men, you can guess that anyone could develop the proverbial beer belly. So lay off the wine, vodka, and beer as you learn to eat and drink for a younger, thinner, and flatter body the Younger (Thinner) You way.

If you must, indulge in a single alcoholic drink a week. Think low calorie with distilled alcohol (vodka, gin, tequila) without the juices or mixers. You can add club soda or fresh citrus juice (lemon or lime). Or try vodka with a splash of flavored tea (like berry, apple, or peach). A hot toddy is comparatively low in calories (skip the sugar—use Splenda instead). Cheers!

you are choosing fruits and vegetables, pick the firmest, most colorful ones. A deep color is a sign that it is fresh and packed with vitamins and nutrients; firmness shows that it won't spoil immediately, and hasn't over-ripened during shipping. Frozen is a fine alternative if the fruits or veggies needed are out of season. Canned fruit is okay only if no sugar or salt is added. And always buy organic—and local, in season—whenever possible; this goes for produce as well as prepared foods, like whole wheat couscous, tomato sauces, condiments, and so forth.

Now that we're talking about the grocery aisles, it's a great habit to check labels on your staples and other dry goods, and choose varieties that have the lowest amounts of sugars, salt, and preservatives.

Ingredients are listed on labels in the order of quantity or volume: If sugar is the first ingredient, the item contains mostly sugar. So, make sure to choose wisely, where sugar or salt is not one of the first five ingredients in any item. This goes for breads as well: Look for breads that are high in protein (4 grams or more a slice), high in fiber, whole wheat, or whole grain.

I also suggest to my patients that they shop for their nonperishables through the Internet. You can set up an account with PeaPod or Fresh Direct that allows you to place a consistent order every week. That way, you won't be tempted to buy the foods you know are bad for you when you go to the store.

YOUNGER (THINNER) YOU DIET SHOPPING LIST

SPICES AND HERBS

Allspice
Basil
Bay leaf
Black pepper
Cardamom
Cayenne pepper
Red pepper flakes
Chili powder
Chives

Cinnamon, ground
Cinnamon stick
Cloves
Coriander
Cumin
Curry powder
Dill
Fennel seeds

Ginger
Green chilies
Lemongrass
Marjoram
Mint
Mustard seed
Nutmeg
Oregano
Paprika

Parsley
Red pepper
Rosemary
Sea salt
Serrano chili pepper
Thyme
Turmeric

FRUIT

Apples, green
Apples, red
Apple juice
Apricots, dried
Bananas
Blueberries

Cantaloupe
Cherries, dried
Figs, dried
Grapefruit
Grapes, red
Lemons

Limes
Mangoes
Oranges
Pears
Pineapple
Pomegranate juice

Prunes, pitted
Raspberries
Raisins
Strawberries
Watermelon

VEGETABLES

Artichoke
Avocados
Belgian endive
Bell peppers: red, yellow, orange, and green
Black beans
Broccoli florets
Broccoli rabe
Cabbage: red and purple
Carrots
Cauliflower
Celery

Corn
Cranberries, dried
Cucumbers
Edamame (soybean pods, found in the freezer section)
Eggplant
Fennel bulb
Garlic
Green beans
Hot chili peppers, such as Scotch bonnet

Jalapeño chili pepper
Kale
Leeks
Mixed salad greens
Mushrooms (choose your favorites)
Onions, white (small to medium)
Onions, red (large)

Radicchio
Romaine lettuce
Scallions
Snow peas
Spinach
Sweet potatoes
Swiss chard
Tomatoes, cherry
Tomatoes, whole
Watercress
Winter squash

PROTEINS

Almond butter
Beef liver
Chicken breasts
Flank steak
Flounder
Halibut

Lamb chops
Mahimahi fillets
Peanut butter
Red snapper fillets
Soy burgers
  (frozen)

Shrimp
Tilapia fillets
Tuna, white,
  packed in water
Tuna steaks
Turkey bacon

Turkey breast,
  roasted
Unsalted nuts:
  almonds,
  walnuts,
  macadamias,
  cashews

EGGS & DAIRY

Butter
Eggs: omega-3
  enriched

Milk, low-fat or
  fat-free

Sour cream,
  fat-free or
  reduced-fat

Yogurt, low-fat,
  plain, or Greek-
  style

BREAD

Croutons, whole
  wheat
Pita pockets, whole
  wheat, small

Whole wheat
  bread, sliced

Whole wheat
  flour tortillas

Whole wheat
  hamburger buns/
  rolls

GROCERY

Almonds
Barbecue sauce, low
  sodium
Barley
Black beans
Black olives
Bread crumbs, whole
  wheat
Brown rice
Brown sugar
Buckwheat
Capers
Chickpeas, canned
Coconut milk
Couscous, whole wheat

Green olives, low sodium
Honey
Mayonnaise, reduced fat
Mustard
Navy beans, dried
Olive oil spray
Olive oil, extra virgin
Orange juice concentrate
Pecans
Pie crust, 9-inch prepared
Pine nuts
Quinoa
Safflower oil
Sesame oil

Soy sauce, reduced sodium
Tamarind paste
Tomato purée
Tomato sauce, no sugar
  added
Tomatoes, canned whole
Vegetable broth, low
  sodium
Vinegar, red wine
Vinegar, white balsamic
Walnuts
White wine, dry
Worcestershire sauce, low
  sodium

BEVERAGES

Green tea bags or loose leaves

Rooibos tea bags or loose leaves

Your favorite herbal teas (recipes, Chapter 7)

Your favorite caffeinated teas

Coffee

Low-sodium seltzer or club soda

HEALTHY BRANDS

I've culled the aisles looking for the healthiest products. Here are my best recommendations.

MICROWAVE POPCORN

Smart Balance Low-Fat

Bearitos No Oil Added

BREAD

Natural Oven's Multi-Grain Stay Trim, 100% Whole Grain, Multigrain or Mild Rye

Oroweat 100% Whole Wheat, Whole Grain or any Light variety

Healthy Choice 100% Whole Grain

Brownberry 100% Whole Grain

Alvarado Street Bakery Sprouted Breads

Trader Joe's Sprouted Breads

Arnold Bakery Carb Counting Wheat

Sara Lee 100% Whole Wheat or Multi-Grain

Baker's Inn 100% Whole Wheat

Earth Grain's 100% Whole Wheat

Bohemian Hearth 100% Whole Wheat

Healthy Life, All Varieties

BAGELS

Natural Oven's Brainy Bagel or Whole

Brownberry Health Nut

Oroweat 100% Whole Wheat or Health

Thomas' Carb Counting Wheat

Thomas' 100% Whole Wheat

BUNS/ROLLS

Natural Oven	The Baker 9-Grain Whole	Healthy Life	Oroweat Health Nut

PITA BREAD

Sahara Whole Wheat Pita	Trader Joe's Whole Wheat Pita	Sara Lee 100% Whole Wheat

ENGLISH MUFFINS

Thomas' Honey Wheat	Thomas' Light	Oroweat Whole Wheat or Multi-Grain

TORTILLAS

La Tortilla Factory Original Low Whole Wheat	Trader Joe's Low Carb Flour or Whole Wheat Tortillas	Alvarado Street Bakery Ezekiel Sprouted Tortillas

WAFFLES

Kashi	Van's	Optimum

COUSCOUS

Trader Joe's Whole Wheat	Near East	Casbah

PASTA

Eddie's Whole Wheat Spaghetti / Trader Joe's Whole Wheat Pasta	Westbrae Natural Whole Wheat or Spinach Spaghetti	Hodgson Mill Whole Wheat Spaghetti	Prince Healthy Harvest Whole Wheat Blend Pasta

QUINOA

Trader Joe's
Organic Quinoa

Ancient Harvest
Quinoa

RICE

Success Boil-in-the-Bag
Brown Rice

Trader Joe's California
Aromatic Brown Rice

Trader Joe's California
Rice Trilogy

Trader Joe's Brown Rice
Medley

Lundberg Brown Rice

Trader Joe's Brown
Basmati

COLD CEREAL

Kashi
Nature's Path
Health Valley
Fiber One or All-Bran
Shredded Wheat

Wheat Chex
Grape Nuts (limit to ½
cup portion)
Grape Nut Flakes
Cheerios

Bran Flakes
Barbara's Bakery
Uncle Sam Cereal
Quaker Oat Bran or
Crunchy Corn Bran

HOT INSTANT CEREAL

Quaker Instant Oatmeal,
regular

Erewhon Instant Oatmeal
with Oat Bran

Erewhon Instant Oatmeal,
flavored

Arrowhead Mills Instant
Multigrain

Roman Meal Instant
Cream of Rye

Nature's Path Instant
Oatmeal

HOT NON-INSTANT CEREAL

Kashi Breakfast Pilaf

Nature's Path
Multi-Grain or Oat
Bran Cereal

Roman Meal Cream of
Rye or Multi-Grain

Arrowhead Mills Oat Bran,
Cracked Wheat, 4-Grain
with Flax or 7-Grain

Wheatena

Quaker Oat Bran or
Multi-Grain

Erewhon Oat Bran with
Wheat Germ

Mother's Oat Bran or
Whole Wheat Hot
Natural

CHEESE

Heavenly Light Swiss
Jarlsberg Lite Sliced
 Reduced Fat Swiss
Alpine Lace Reduced Fat
Cabot Reduced Fat
 Cheddar

Sargento Reduced Fat,
 shredded or Deli Style,
 sliced
Laughing Cow Light
 Creamy Swiss, Garlic
 Herb or French Onion
 Cheese Wedge

Laughing Cow Mini
 Babybel Light Original
Kraft 2% sliced, shredded
 or block

SOUR CREAM

Knudsen Fat-Free or Light
Naturally Yours Fat-Free

Lucerne Low-Fat
Deans Low-Fat

Breakstone Low-Fat

SMOOTHIES

Nouriche Light

Dannon Light
 and Fit

YOGURT

Axelrod
Dannon Light and Fit
Fage Greek-style 2%
Yoplait Light, Nonfat

Horizon Organic Fat-Free
Stonyfield Farm Low-Fat
 or Nonfat

Cascadian Farms Nonfat
 or Low-Fat

SOY CHEESE

Yves Good Slices and
 Good Shreds

TofuRella

Soya Kaas

SOY MEAT ALTERNATIVES

Boca—all varieties
Morningstar—all varieties
Yves—all varieties
Gimmie Lean

Dr. Praeger's Veggie
 Burgers
Trader Joe's Meatless
 Meatballs
Amy's Veggie Burgers

Lightlife—all varieties
Gardenburger—all
 varieties
Tofurky—all varieties

SOY MILK

Silk Soy Milk
8th Continent Plain &
  Vanilla

8th Continent Light
  Chocolate, Light Vanilla
Trader Joe's

Westsoy Low-Fat or Fat
Free

SOY YOGURT

Whole Soy

Silk Soy Yogurt

Stonyfield Farm

JAMS/JELLIES

Smucker's Simply Fruit or
  Sugar-Free

Sorrell Ridge 100% Fruit
Knott's Light

Trader Joe's Organic Fruit
  Spreads

PEANUT/NUT BUTTERS

Laura Scudder's Natural
Peter Pan Natural

Adam's Natural
Trader Joe's Natural

Maranatha Natural
  Almond Butter

CRACKERS

Health Valley Low-Fat
  Whole Wheat
Ry-Krisp
Ryvita
Wasa Fibre Rye
Ak-Mak

Reduced Fat Triscuit
Kashi TLC 7-Grain
Hain Wheatettes
Whole Foods 365 Baked
  Woven Wheats

Trader Joe's Woven
  Wheat Wafers
Barbara's Bakery
  Wheatines

SHAKES

Kashi GoLean
Balance
Myoplex

Glucerna Weight
  Management or Regular

Boost
Zone Perfect

THE RECIPES

In the following Younger (Thinner) You recipes "active ingredients"—the herbs and spices—are marked in bold. The recipes are also marked to indicate the brain chemicals they most affect. And there is a box to show how to swap out an ingredient or add another to make it more beneficial for other brain chemicals. The calories are listed in case you are curious, and the diet is set up for an average of 1,800 calories a day, including three meals and one snack.

Dark Chocolate May Keep the Doctor Away

Dark chocolate is a potent antioxidant that can help lower blood pressure. Dark chocolate bars (milk chocolate may interfere with the absorption of antioxidants from chocolate, so only dark qualifies here) with high cocoa content contain epicatechin, which is a member of a group of compounds called plant flavonoids, which help keep cholesterol from gathering in blood vessels, reduce the risk of blood clots, and slow down the immune responses that lead to clogged arteries. Additionally, dark chocolate contains compounds called cocoa phenols, which are also known to lower blood pressure.[1]

If you have to succumb on occasion, better to indulge in something heart healthy at the same time. Keep your chocolate treats to an absolute minimum, but know you're lessening the damage to your health when you indulge in dark chocolate.

SPECIAL BREAKFASTS

Ⓐ ACETYLCHOLINE BOOSTING RECIPE

Herb Frittata

Eggs are a perfect protein and support all of your brain chemicals. Both the eggs and the sour cream are great sources of choline, making this a super acetylcholine-boosting meal.

1 tablespoon safflower oil

8 egg whites

¼ cup fat-free sour cream

❀ **2 teaspoons Dijon mustard**

❀ **¼ teaspoon freshly ground black pepper**

❀ **1 teaspoon basil**

❀ **½ cup fresh parsley, chopped**

Serves 4
190 calories per serving
Swap Box
● For a dopamine boost, add ½ cup sautéed mushrooms, spinach, or broccoli.
● For a GABA boost, add ½ cup sautéed carrots.
● For a serotonin boost, add 2 teaspoons sage

1. Preheat broiler.

2. Warm safflower oil in a large ovenproof frying pan over medium heat.

3. In a large bowl, whisk together egg whites, sour cream, mustard, pepper, and basil; stir in parsley.

4. Add to skillet and cook 5 to 6 minutes. Frequently lift the mixture from the sides of the pan to allow any uncooked eggs to run to the bottom. Place frittata under broiler and cook until golden on top, 1 to 2 minutes. Cut into 4 slices and serve.

NUTRITION INFORMATION: Per serving: 190 calories; 13 g fat (3.5 g sat); 375 mg cholesterol; 190 mg sodium; 5 g carbohydrate; 0 g fiber; 2 g sugars; 12 g protein

More Flavorful and Healthier Coffee

Flavored coffees are simply regular coffee beans that have been coated with flavored oils. You can create the same, less fattening option right at home. Add a few drops of hazelnut, vanilla, or almond extract, cinnamon sticks, or nutmeg to your morning coffee. This way you're adding flavor and nutrients.

D DOPAMINE BOOSTING RECIPE

Scrambled Eggs with Broccoli

Eggs and broccoli increase dopamine and boost metabolism.

4 large eggs

2 teaspoons safflower oil

❋ **1 teaspoon rosemary**

❋ **1 teaspoon fresh minced dill**

❋ **1 teaspoon chopped chives**

❋ **1 teaspoon paprika**

❋ **Freshly ground black pepper to taste**

1 cup broccoli florets

1. Whisk eggs in a metal bowl.

2. Heat oil in a nonstick skillet over low to medium heat. Pour the eggs in. Add spices; stir the eggs gently with a soft spatula to keep from sticking and burning. Add the broccoli and continue to stir until the eggs are fully cooked. Divide eggs between two plates and serve.

Serves 2
290 calories per serving

Swap Box

- For an acetylcholine boost, serve with a 6-ounce glass of unsweetened orange or grapefruit juice.
- For a GABA boost, add ½ cup of cooked corn kernels.
- For a serotonin boost, fold ½ cup low-fat cottage cheese into the eggs before cooking.

NUTRITION INFORMATION: Per serving: 290 calories; 24 g fat (5 g sat); 375 mg cholesterol; 350 mg sodium; 6 g carbohydrate; 1 g fiber; 2 g sugars; 12 g protein

Try Not to Say Cheese

Fat cravings indulged with hunks of cheese will not lead to weight loss! There isn't much benefit to cheese, and the cons outweigh the pros (saturated fat and high concentration of calories versus small amounts of calcium). Thank goodness there are plenty of healthier good-for-you fat alternatives, like nuts, nut butters, and even eggs. But if you can't live without your cheese, sample some of these lower-fat options: Alpine Lace Reduced Fat, Jarlsberg Lite, Cabot Reduced Fat Cheddar, Sargento Reduced Fat, Laughing Cow Mini Babybel Light Original, or Laughing Cow Light Creamy Swiss, Garlic Herb, or French Onion cheese wedges.

D **S** DOPAMINE AND SEROTONIN BOOSTING RECIPE

Italian Omelet

Eggs and spinach both increase your brainpower, making this a super *dopamine-boosting* meal, while the basil boosts serotonin.

4 large eggs

1 cup spinach, chopped

❉ **1 teaspoon dried basil or thinly sliced fresh**

¼ cup chopped scallions

❉ **1 teaspoon oregano**

❉ **Freshly ground black pepper to taste**

1 tablespoon safflower oil

❉ **1 garlic clove, minced**

2 large tomatoes, chopped

4 slices whole wheat or oat bran toast

> **Serves 4**
> **220 calories per serving**
>
> ## Swap Box
>
> Eggs are a perfect protein and support all of your brain chemicals. For an extra brain enhancement try the following:
>
> ● For an acetylcholine boost, serve with ½ cup blueberries.
>
> ● For a GABA boost, add 1 teaspoon fresh cilantro.

1. Combine eggs, spinach, basil, scallions, oregano, and pepper in a bowl and beat until blended. Set aside.

2. Coat a small nonstick skillet with the oil and heat over medium heat. Add garlic and stir until lightly browned.

3. Add the egg mixture to pan. Cook until bottom is lightly browned and firm, 5 to 6 minutes. Sprinkle tomatoes over half the eggs and fold omelet in half. Once set, flip the entire omelet. Cook until center is set, about 3 minutes more.

4. Allow to stand 1 minute. Divide into four portions and serve with toast.

NUTRITION INFORMATION: Per serving: 220 calories; 11 g fat (3 g sat); 215 mg cholesterol; 250 mg sodium; 17 g carbohydrate; 3 g fiber; 4 g sugars; 12 g protein

G GABA BOOSTING RECIPE

Egg Bruschetta

Eggs and whole wheat bread both increase your ability to calm the brain, making this a super *GABA-boosting* meal. The capers featured in this recipe are an excellent food for those living with heart disease.

❋ **2 garlic cloves, halved**

4 slices whole wheat bread, toasted

3 large ripe tomatoes, diced

❋ **¼ cup finely chopped fresh basil**

2 tablespoons capers, chopped

½ teaspoon extra virgin olive oil

❋ **1 teaspoon oregano**

½ cup finely chopped black olives

Safflower oil spray

4 large eggs

❋ **Freshly ground black pepper to taste**

> **Serves 4**
> **200 calories per serving**
>
> **Swap Box**
>
> - For a dopamine boost, sprinkle with 2 teaspoons wheat germ.
> - For an acetylcholine boost, serve with a 6-ounce glass of unsweetened orange or grapefruit juice.
> - For a serotonin boost, increase pepper to ½ teaspoon.

1. Rub the garlic onto the toast, infusing into the bread. Set aside.

2. To make the bruschetta mixture, combine the tomatoes, basil, capers, olive oil, oregano, and olives in small bowl and mix. Set aside.

3. Spray a skillet with safflower oil and warm over medium heat. Break the eggs into the skillet and cook as you prefer: scrambled or fried.

4. To assemble, cover each slice of garlic toast with bruschetta mixture. Season with salt and pepper if desired. Top with the eggs and serve immediately.

NUTRITION INFORMATION: Per serving: 200 calories; 12 g fat (4 g sat); 220 mg cholesterol; 480 mg sodium; 16 g carbohydrate; 3 g fiber; 2 g sugars; 9 g protein

D A G S TOTAL BRAIN CHEMICAL BOOSTING RECIPE

Rainbow Fruit Salad

This colorful, highly spiced meal supports all of your brain chemicals.

2 large green apples, chopped

2 large red apples, chopped

2 cups cubed cantaloupe

2 cups sliced pears

1 cup grapes

1 cup strawberries, halved

1 large banana, sliced

½ teaspoon fresh lemon juice

1 cup low-fat vanilla or plain yogurt

1 tablespoon orange juice concentrate

❋ **2 tablespoons chopped fresh mint**

❋ **2 teaspoons cinnamon**

❋ **1 teaspoon nutmeg**

❋ **1 teaspoon cumin**

½ teaspoon vanilla

½ teaspoon lemon zest

> **Serves 6**
> **210 calories per serving**

1. Toss the fruit together with the lemon juice.

2. In a small bowl, mix the yogurt with the orange juice concentrate, spices, vanilla, and lemon zest. Drizzle over fruit mixture, and serve.

NUTRITION INFORMATION: Per serving: 210 calories; 2 g fat (.5 g sat); 0 mg cholesterol; 35 mg sodium; 48 g carbohydrate; 7 g fiber; 39 g sugars; 4 g protein

A Rainbow of Apples

Apples are high in fiber and packed with nutrients. Don't forget you have many colorful options when it comes to apples. Rotate from all that are seasonally available: Golden Delicious, Red Delicious, Granny Smith, Winesap, Gala, Rome, McIntosh, Pink Lady, or Fuji. Sprinkle some cinnamon or allspice for a boost of flavor and nutrients. Try dipping your apple slices in plain fat-free yogurt flavored with cinnamon, honey, and allspice. However you eat them, leave the skins on. That's where the vitamins and fiber are.

D **A** **G** **S** TOTAL BRAIN CHEMICAL BOOSTING RECIPE

Cinnamon Fruit Smoothie

Yogurt and cinnamon both boost metabolism, making this a super *dopamine-boosting* meal. The fruit and spices also increase the other biochemicals.

2 bananas

1 cup raspberries, fresh or frozen

1 cup blueberries, fresh or frozen

1 cup orange juice

1 teaspoon vanilla

❋ **2 teaspoons cinnamon**

❋ **1 teaspoon nutmeg**

❋ **1 teaspoon allspice**

1 tablespoon honey

2 to 3 ice cubes

> **Serves 2**
> **280 calories per serving**

Put all ingredients in a blender, blend until smooth, and serve immediately.

NUTRITION INFORMATION: Per serving: 280 calories; 1.5 g fat (0 g sat); 0 mg cholesterol; 10 mg sodium; 69 g carbohydrate; 10 g fiber; 54 g sugars; 3 g protein

D DOPAMINE BOOSTING RECIPE

Pineapple Upside-Down French Toast

Eggs and pineapple both increase your brain power, making this a super *dopamine-boosting* meal.

4 large eggs

⅔ cup low-fat milk

❋ **1 teaspoon cinnamon**

1 teaspoon vanilla extract

½ teaspoon orange zest

❋ **½ teaspoon nutmeg**

❋ **½ teaspoon cumin**

4 slices whole wheat or oat bran bread

1 teaspoon safflower oil

2 teaspoons brown sugar

4 round slices fresh pineapple, ½" thick

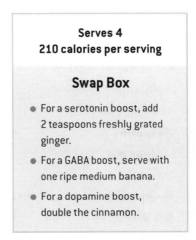

> **Serves 4**
> **210 calories per serving**
>
> ## Swap Box
>
> ● For a serotonin boost, add 2 teaspoons freshly grated ginger.
>
> ● For a GABA boost, serve with one ripe medium banana.
>
> ● For a dopamine boost, double the cinnamon.

1. Combine eggs, milk, cinnamon, vanilla, orange zest, nutmeg, and cumin in a large bowl. Soak bread in egg mixture for about 1 minute.

2. Heat oil in a nonstick skillet over medium heat and place two slices of bread in a single layer in skillet. Sprinkle ½ teaspoon sugar over each slice and cook bread until well-browned, 4 to 5 minutes. Flip bread and place a pineapple ring on top of each slice. Flip bread again; cook until sugar is melted and pineapple is warm, about 3 minutes. Serve immediately.

NUTRITION INFORMATION: Per serving: 210 calories; 8 g fat (2.5 g sat); 215 mg cholesterol; 230 mg sodium; 23 g carbohydrate; 3 g fiber; 10 g sugars; 11 g protein

Your Daily Bread

I know that many people love their bread. But most of us are choosing varieties that add little value because they are so deficient in nutrients. Today there are some terrific nutrient-rich breads to choose from, but you have to read the labels carefully. Choose organic whenever possible. Always choose whole wheat or oat grain breads that are high in fiber and protein (at least 4 grams of each per slice) and low in sugar (watch carefully for all the various forms of sugar in the ingredients list). I personally rotate the following favorites: Trader Joe's sprouted breads, Sara Lee Multi-Grain, Baker's Inn 100% Whole Wheat, and Bohemian Hearth 100% Whole Wheat.

EASY LUNCHES

D **A** **G** **S** TOTAL BRAIN CHEMICAL BOOSTING RECIPE

Sprouted Pea Soup

A hearty, highly seasoned vegetable soup is a satisfying lunch that boosts all of your brain chemicals. That's because it's a total-nutrient meal.

1 large onion, chopped

3 celery stalks, chopped

2 tablespoons safflower oil

8 cups water

2 cups sprouted peas

1 bay leaf

½ teaspoon reduced-sodium soy sauce

❋ **½ teaspoon marjoram**

❋ **½ teaspoon oregano**

❋ **¼ teaspoon basil**

❋ **2 garlic cloves, minced**

❋ **Freshly ground black pepper to taste**

> **Serves 4**
> **160 calories per serving**
>
> ### Swap Box
>
> - For an extra dopamine boost, serve with a tablespoon of low-fat sour cream.
> - For more acetylcholine, season with an additional teaspoon of sage.
> - For more GABA, serve with a slice of whole wheat bread.
> - For more serotonin, serve with a slice of fresh roasted turkey.

1. In a large stockpot, sauté onion and celery in the oil over medium heat until the onion is translucent, about 5 minutes.

2. Add water, peas, bay leaf, soy sauce, marjoram, oregano, basil, garlic, and pepper. Bring to a boil, cover, and simmer for 1 hour, until peas are soft.

3. In a blender or food processor, puree soup in batches. Return soup to stockpot. Add additional water to create desired consistency, and serve.

NUTRITION INFORMATION: Per serving: 160 calories; 8 g fat (1 g sat); 0 mg cholesterol; 95 mg sodium; 22 g carbohydrate; 4 g fiber; 3 g sugars; 6 g protein

D A G S TOTAL BRAIN CHEMICAL BOOSTING RECIPE

Navy Bean and Kale Soup

A hearty, highly seasoned vegetable soup is a satisfying lunch that boosts all of your brain chemistry. That's because it's a total-nutrient meal. The beans in this soup support both *GABA* and *acetylcholine*.

½ pound dried navy beans

¼ cup safflower oil

1 small onion, chopped

2 small carrots, diced

1 stalk celery, diced

4 cups shredded kale

1 large potato, diced

2 cups chopped Swiss chard

1 large tomato, diced

❋ **2 garlic cloves, minced**

❋ **2 teaspoon minced fresh rosemary**

❋ **1 tablespoon minced fresh parsley**

❋ **1 teaspoon fresh thyme leaves**

❋ **Freshly ground black pepper to taste**

> ### Serves 6
> ### 310 calories per serving
>
> ## Swap Box
>
> ● For an extra dopamine boost, serve with a tablespoon of low-fat sour cream.
>
> ● For more serotonin, serve with a slice of roasted turkey.

1. Place beans in large saucepan with enough cold water to cover. Let stand at room temperature overnight. In the morning, drain the beans and return to saucepan. Add enough water to cover and bring to a boil over high heat. Reduce heat and simmer until tender, 1 hour 30 minutes. Drain, reserving the liquid. Transfer half of beans to a blender and puree.

2. Heat oil in large pot over medium-high heat. Add onion, carrots, and celery and sauté 5 minutes. Stir in kale, potato, pureed beans, and reserved bean cooking liquid. Add water to make 6 cups. Simmer over medium heat for about 30 minutes, just until vegetables are tender.

3. Add chard, tomato, garlic, rosemary, parsley, thyme, and pepper to taste. Simmer for at least 1 hour. Add additional water if the soup becomes too pasty, but it should be quite thick.

4. Stir in reserved whole beans and simmer until heated through, 5 to 10 minutes, before serving.

NUTRITION INFORMATION: Per serving: 310 calories; 10 g fat (1.5 g sat); 0 mg cholesterol; 70 mg sodium; 45 g carbohydrate; 13 g fiber; 7 g sugars; 12 g protein

D **A** **G** **S** TOTAL BRAIN CHEMICAL BOOSTING RECIPE

Spicy Black Bean Soup

A hearty, highly seasoned vegetable soup is a satisfying lunch that boosts all of your brain chemistry. That's because it's a total-nutrient meal. The beans in this soup support both *GABA* and *acetylcholine*.

1 tablespoon safflower oil

1 small onion, chopped

½ carrot, grated

❀ **2 garlic cloves, chopped**

❀ **1 teaspoon cumin**

2 teaspoons chopped jalapeño chili pepper with seeds, divided

1 (16-ounce) can black beans (do not drain)

1 medium tomato, diced

¾ cup low-salt chicken broth

❀ **Freshly ground black pepper to taste**

❀ **Chopped fresh cilantro**

> **Serves 2**
> **320 calories per serving**
>
> **Swap Box**
>
> - For an extra dopamine boost, serve with a tablespoon of low-fat sour cream.
> - For more serotonin, top each serving of the soup with ¼ sliced avocado.

1. Heat oil in large pot over medium-high heat. Add onion, carrot, and garlic; sauté until vegetables begin to soften, about 5 minutes. Mix in cumin and 1 teaspoon jalapeño pepper.

2. Add beans (including liquid), tomatoes, and broth. Bring to a boil. Reduce heat to medium, cover, and cook until carrots are tender, about 15 more minutes.

3. Transfer 1½ cups of soup to blender and puree until smooth. Return puree to pot. Simmer soup until slightly thickened, about 15 more minutes. Season to taste with pepper and remaining teaspoon jalapeño, if desired.

4. Ladle soup into bowls. Top with fresh cilantro and serve.

NUTRITION INFORMATION: Per serving: 320 calories; 9 g fat (1.5 g sat); 0 mg cholesterol; 970 mg sodium; 49 g carbohydrate; 16 g fiber; 7 g sugars; 17 g protein

G GABA BOOSTING RECIPE

Spinach and Strawberry Salad

Spinach is a powerful *GABA enhancer.*

12 ounces fresh spinach

¼ cup extra virgin olive oil

2 tablespoons red wine vinegar

2 tablespoons sliced scallion

❈ **Freshly ground black pepper to taste**

1 pint strawberries, sliced

❈ **2 tablespoons chopped fresh mint leaves**

❈ **2 tablespoons chopped fresh parsley**

❈ **2 tablespoons fennel seeds**

❈ **2 tablespoons sesame seeds, toasted**

> **Serves 2**
> **390 calories per serving**
>
> ## Swap Box
>
> ● For a dopamine boost, add ½ cup sliced fennel to the salad.
>
> ● For an acetylcholine boost, double the amount of sesame seeds.
>
> ● For a serotonin boost, sprinkle salad with 1 teaspoon cinnamon.

1. Wash spinach thoroughly and discard stems. Dry leaves and tear into bite-sized pieces. Wrap in toweling and refrigerate until ready to use.

2. To make dressing, combine oil, vinegar, scallion, cayenne, and pepper in a small bowl.

3. Combine strawberries, mint, parsley, and fennel in a large salad bowl. Add the spinach and gently toss. Add dressing, toss, and garnish with toasted sesame seeds.

NUTRITION INFORMATION: Per serving: 390 calories; 33 g fat (4.5 g sat); 0 mg cholesterol; 140 mg sodium; 20 g carbohydrate; 9 g fiber; 8 g sugars; 7 g protein

Ⓖ GABA BOOSTING RECIPE

Black Bean, Jicama, Corn, and Mango Salad

Black beans and mango are both considered *GABA-enhancing* foods.

2 teaspoons safflower oil

❋ **1 clove garlic, minced**

2 cups corn kernels

2 cups cooked black beans

2 cups shredded peeled jicama

1 large ripe mango, peeled and diced

½ cup chopped scallions

½ cup diced green pepper

½ cup diced red pepper

¼ cup fresh lime juice

❋ **1 tablespoon cayenne pepper**

❋ **1½ tablespoons chopped fresh parsley**

❋ **1 teaspoon ground cumin**

❋ **Freshly ground black pepper to taste**

Serves 4
280 calories per serving

Swap Box

● For a dopamine boost, add a few dashes of hot sauce to the salad.

● For an acetylcholine boost, sprinkle with ¼ cup sliced almonds.

● For a serotonin boost, exchange half of the black beans for an equal amount of diced avocado (add at the end of recipe).

---

1. Heat oil in a large nonstick skillet over medium heat. Add garlic and cook until lightly browned, about 30 seconds. Add corn, stirring occasionally, until browned, about 8 minutes.

2. Transfer the corn mixture to a large bowl. Stir in remaining ingredients until completely combined.

NUTRITION INFORMATION: Per serving: 280 calories; 5 g fat (.5 g sat); 0 mg cholesterol; 690 mg sodium; 53 g carbohydrate; 15 g fiber; 13 g sugars; 11 g protein

D A G S TOTAL BRAIN CHEMICAL BOOSTING RECIPE

Super Salad

A fresh vegetable salad that is highly seasoned like this one can enhance all of the brain chemicals. This salad is excellent topped with grilled tuna steak.

1 cup spinach, torn into bite-sized pieces

1 cup chopped romaine lettuce

¼ cup shredded red cabbage

½ cup diced red pepper

½ tomato, chopped

½ cup grated carrot

¼ cup dried cranberries

¼ avocado, peeled and cubed

❋ **1 teaspoon minced fresh rosemary**

❋ **1 teaspoon thyme**

❋ **¼ cup chopped fresh basil leaves**

2 tablespoons extra virgin olive oil

1 tablespoon balsamic vinegar

> **Serves 4**
> **160 calories per serving**

1. Combine spinach, romaine, cabbage, red pepper, tomato, carrot, cranberries, and avocado in a large bowl. Sprinkle with rosemary, thyme, and basil leaves.

2. For the dressing, whisk together the olive oil and vinegar.

3. Toss the dressing with the salad.

NUTRITION INFORMATION: Per serving: 160 calories; 13 g fat (2 g sat); 0 mg cholesterol; 15 mg sodium; 11 g carbohydrate; 3 g fiber; 7 g sugars; 1 g protein

D A G DOPAMINE, ACETYLCHOLINE, AND GABA BOOSTING RECIPE

Salade Niçoise with Olives, Oranges, and Bell Pepper

Both tuna and oranges are *acetylcholine- and GABA-boosting* foods. They are also excellent *dopamine* precursors.

¼ cup extra virgin olive oil

¼ cup white balsamic vinegar

❋ **1 tablespoon minced garlic**

3 seedless oranges, peeled and segmented

1 small red onion, thinly sliced

1 red pepper, thinly sliced

1 (9-ounce) can white tuna packed in water, drained and flaked

¼ cup low-sodium black olives

❋ **¼ cup chopped fresh parsley**

4 cups mixed salad greens

❋ **1 tablespoon fennel seeds**

❋ **1 tablespoon dill**

⅓ cup walnuts, toasted

> **Serves 4**
> **360 calories per serving**
>
> ## Swap Box
>
> For an extra brain enhance-ment try the following:
>
> ● For a GABA boost, add ½ cup sliced beets.
>
> ● For a serotonin boost, ex-change walnuts for a sliced hard-boiled egg.

1. Whisk oil, vinegar, and garlic in large bowl. Add orange sections, onion, red pepper, tuna, olives, and parsley; toss.

2. Divide salad greens among plates. Divide tuna mixture over greens and sprinkle with fennel and dill. Garnish with walnuts.

NUTRITION INFORMATION: Per serving: 360 calories; 23 g fat (3 g sat); 25 mg cholesterol; 340 mg sodium; 22 g carbohydrate; 5 g fiber; 14 g sugars; 19 g protein

Experiment with Color

Change your favorite recipe by experimenting with the colors of the rainbow. Try using red, yellow, or orange peppers instead of green, or yellow tomatoes instead of red, or even purple broccoli. This way you'll sample different flavors and different nutrients.

ⓖ GABA BOOSTING RECIPE

Asian Chicken Lettuce Wrap

Poultry, as well as spices such as lemongrass, can increase your ability to calm the brain, making this a super *GABA-boosting* meal.

Olive oil spray

4 scallions, chopped

1 red pepper, chopped

1 cup fresh mushrooms (any variety), chopped

2 tablespoons pine nuts, chopped

❋ **1 teaspoon basil**

❋ **2 teaspoons curry powder**

❋ **1 teaspoon oregano**

❋ **2 tablespoons chopped fresh lemongrass**

1 pound grilled chicken breast, chopped

Low-sodium soy sauce

4 large romaine lettuce leaves

> **Serves 4**
> **210 calories per serving**
>
> **Swap Box**
>
> - For a dopamine boost, sprinkle with 2 teaspoons wheat germ.
> - For an acetylcholine boost, double the amount of pine nuts, or substitute an equal amount of peanuts.
> - For a serotonin boost, add 1/2 teaspoon of freshly ground black pepper.

1. Spray a large sauté pan with olive oil spray. Over medium heat, sauté the scallions, pepper, and mushrooms until tender, about 3 minutes. Add the pine nuts, spices, and lemongrass. Add chicken and cook about a minute to heat it through.

2. Remove from heat. Sprinkle the mixture with soy sauce to taste.

3. Place a large lettuce leaf on each of 4 plates, and spoon one-fourth of the mixture into each. Fold and serve, using toothpicks to hold the wraps if necessary.

NUTRITION INFORMATION: Per serving: 210 calories; 6 g fat (1 g sat); 65 mg cholesterol; 125 mg sodium; 10 g carbohydrate; 2 g fiber; 1 g sugars; 29 g protein

Ⓐ ACETYLCHOLINE BOOSTING RECIPE

Tuna Salad Pita Pocket

Fish, such as tuna, is an excellent source of choline, making this recipe an *acetylcholine-boosting* meal.

1 (6-ounce) can white tuna packed in water, drained

2 teaspoons low-fat mayonnaise

¼ cup diced onion

¼ cup diced celery

¼ cup diced green peppers

❈ **Freshly ground black pepper**

❈ **1 teaspoon oregano**

❈ **1 teaspoon celery seeds**

2 small whole wheat pita pockets

1 large tomato, sliced into 4 rounds

2 large romaine lettuce leaves

Makes 2 servings
210 calories per serving

Swap Box

- For a dopamine boost, add 1 tablespoon fresh lemon juice to the tuna salad.

- For a GABA boost, serve with a cup of diced cantaloupe.

- For a serotonin boost, substitute an equal amount of cooked chicken breast for the tuna.

---

1. Place tuna in a bowl and add the mayonnaise. Mix in the diced vegetables and the spices.

2. Open each pita pocket and carefully place 2 slices of tomato and a lettuce leaf into each. Spoon in the tuna salad, and serve.

NUTRITION INFORMATION: Per serving: 210 calories; 2 g fat (0 g sat); 25 mg cholesterol; 490 mg sodium; 23 g carbohydrate; 4 g fiber; 6 g sugars; 26 g protein

D **A** DOPAMINE AND ACETYLCHOLINE BOOSTING RECIPE

Tuna-Stuffed Tomatoes

Fish, like tuna, is an effective *acetylcholine enhancer.* Fish is also an excellent source of protein, which boosts *dopamine* as well.

2 (6-ounce) cans white tuna packed in water, drained and flaked

1 scallion, chopped

❋ **1 clove garlic, minced**

1 tablespoon reduced-sodium soy sauce

1 orange pepper, chopped

❋ **1 tablespoon oregano**

❋ **1 tablespoon marjoram**

❋ **1 tablespoon thyme**

❋ **Freshly ground black pepper to taste**

4 large tomatoes, tops sliced off, cored, and seeded

2 teaspoons sesame oil

> **Serves 4**
> **190 calories per serving**
>
> ## Swap Box
>
> - For a GABA boost, serve over brown rice, $1/2$ cup per serving.
> - For a serotonin boost, swap the tuna for a light egg salad made with 2 eggs, low-fat mayonnaise, and the rest of the ingredients, omitting the soy sauce and sesame oil.

1. Preheat oven to 350°F.

2. In a mixing bowl, combine all ingredients except the tomatoes and sesame oil.

3. Spoon the mixture into the tomatoes until they are full. Brush the outsides of the tomatoes with sesame oil. Place stuffed tomatoes on a baking sheet.

4. Bake tomatoes for 12 to 15 minutes and serve.

NUTRITION INFORMATION: Per serving: 190 calories; 10 g fat (1.5 g sat); 0 mg cholesterol; 300 mg sodium; 19 g carbohydrate; 4 g fiber; 9 g sugars; 11 g protein

Alternate Seasonings

Bottled condiments are easy to use. When you can't get fresh seasonings together, try San.J's (www.san-j.com) tamari peanut and tamari sesame sauces; Annie's (www.annies.com) shiitake sesame vinaigrette; any bottled hot sauce, or Organicville (www.organicvillefoods.com) sesame tamari vinaigrette. These are all healthy, delicious alternatives to replace soy sauce or salt.

D A G S TOTAL BRAIN CHEMICAL BOOSTING RECIPE

Baigan Ka Bharta (Mashed Eggplant)

Indian dishes are loaded with spices. Here is one of my favorites. There are so many spices in this dish that it enhances all of your brain chemicals, and really revs your metabolism. You'll need to make a large batch of spice mix, garam masala. Keep the rest in the refrigerator in a container with a tight-fitting lid and use to spice up any poultry, fish, or meat dish.

Olive oil spray

2 eggplants, halved

1 tablespoon safflower oil

1 onion, diced

❋ **2 teaspoons garlic**

❋ **⅓ teaspoon mustard seed**

❋ **2 bay leaves**

❋ **2 green chili peppers, minced**

❋ **1 tablespoon minced fresh ginger**

❋ **1 teaspoon turmeric**

❋ **½ teaspoon chili powder**

2 tomatoes, chopped

½ cup plain yogurt

❋ **2 teaspoons garam masala** (opposite)

½ teaspoon lemon juice

❋ **Fresh chopped cilantro leaves for garnish**

Lime slices for garnish

> Serves 4
> 190 calories per serving

1. Preheat the oven to 400°F.

2. Spray the eggplant lightly with olive oil, place on a baking sheet, and bake for 20 minutes, or until soft. Cool and remove the peel. Mash until smooth.

3. Meanwhile, in a large nonstick skillet, heat the safflower oil and sauté the onion, garlic, mustard seed, bay leaves, green chilies, ginger, turmeric, and chili powder until onions are translucent, about 3 minutes. Remove the bay leaves.

4. Add the eggplant, tomatoes, yogurt, garam masala, and lemon juice to the skillet. Continue to cook for up to 10 minutes, stirring continuously. Garnish with fresh chopped cilantro and lime slices and serve.

NUTRITION INFORMATION: Per serving: 190 calories; 8 g fat (1.5 g sat); 0 mg cholesterol; 40 mg sodium; 28 g carbohydrate; 8 g fiber; 15 g sugars; 6 g protein

GARAM MASALA

❋ **1 tablespoon minced fresh ginger**

❋ **1 teaspoon paprika**

❋ **½ teaspoon cinnamon**

❋ **½ teaspoon ground coriander**

❋ **½ teaspoon garlic powder**

❋ **½ teaspoon cayenne pepper or red pepper flakes**

❋ **½ teaspoon cardamom seeds**

❋ **½ teaspoon cumin**

❋ **½ teaspoon ground cloves**

❋ **½ teaspoon nutmeg**

❋ **½ teaspoon sesame seeds**

❋ **½ teaspoon mustard seeds**

❋ **½ teaspoon turmeric**

❋ **½ teaspoon fennel**

Combine all the ingredients in a small bowl and stir until mixed.

(S) SEROTONIN BOOSTING RECIPE

Spicy Seared Tofu with Mandarin Orange Sauce

Tofu and other soy-based products are used to create terrific *serotonin-boosting* meals.

1 block firm tofu, drained

❋ **1½ teaspoons dried basil**

❋ **¼ teaspoon cayenne pepper**

1 tablespoon safflower oil

❋ **1 teaspoon minced fresh ginger**

❋ **1 teaspoon red pepper flakes**

½ cup finely chopped onion

½ cup low-sodium chicken broth

1 (11-ounce) can mandarin orange segments, drained and rinsed, reserving 2 tablespoons liquid

1 teaspoon cornstarch

> **Serves 4**
> **260 calories per serving**
>
> ### Swap Box
>
> - For a dopamine boost, add ½ cup steamed snow peas to each serving.
> - For an acetylcholine boost, sprinkle 2 tablespoons crushed peanuts over each serving.
> - For a GABA boost, serve with quinoa or another whole grain.

1. Rinse tofu and pat dry. Cut into 4 slices of equal size. Season the tofu with the basil and cayenne pepper.

2. Heat the safflower oil in large nonstick skillet. Add the ginger, garlic, and red pepper flakes. Stir over medium heat for 2 to 3 minutes. Add tofu and pan sear until lightly browned, about 3 minutes per side. Remove tofu from pan and keep warm.

3. Add the onion to the skillet and cook 4 to 6 minutes.

4. In a small bowl, combine the chicken broth, reserved orange liquid, and cornstarch; blend well. Pour mixture into the skillet and cook, stirring, until thick and bubbly.

5. Gently stir in orange segments; cook until heated through. Pour over the tofu slices and serve.

NUTRITION INFORMATION: Per serving: 260 calories; 14 g fat (2 g sat); 0 mg cholesterol; 40 mg sodium; 19 g carbohydrate; 3 g fiber; 12 g sugars; 18 g protein

G **S** GABA AND SEROTONIN BOOSTING RECIPE

Tofu Curry with Green Beans

Tofu and other soy products are *serotonin enhancers*. The green beans are also great *GABA* precursors and are high in nutrients.

1½ cups skim milk

❋ **1 tablespoon curry paste**

1 tablespoon low-sodium soy sauce

❋ **3 red chilies, seeded and diced**

2 teaspoons brown sugar or 3 packets of Stevia

8 shiitake mushrooms, sliced

1 block firm tofu

1 cup green beans

2 scallions, sliced

❋ **1 teaspoon Asian seven spice seasoning***

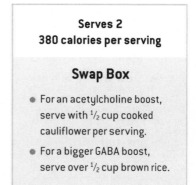

Serves 2
380 calories per serving

Swap Box

- For an acetylcholine boost, serve with ½ cup cooked cauliflower per serving.
- For a bigger GABA boost, serve over ½ cup brown rice.

1. Warm the milk in a pot until it starts to boil. Quickly add the curry paste, soy sauce, chilies, and sugar.

2. Add in the mushrooms and tofu and bring to a boil.

3. Add the green beans and let it simmer until the beans are cooked through. Add the scallions and cook for a minute or so more. Sprinkle with the seven spice seasoning and serve.

* Seven spice seasoning, also called shichimi (or hichimi) togarashi is a peppery Japanese condiment made of seven seasonings: red pepper flakes, sansho, white sesame seeds, nori (seaweed) flakes, dried mandarin orange peel, black hemp seeds, and white poppy seeds. It is available in hot, medium, and mild strengths in most Asian markets.

NUTRITION INFORMATION: Per serving: 380 calories; 15 g fat (2.5 g sat); 5 mg cholesterol; 760 mg sodium; 37 g carbohydrate; 6 g fiber; 16 g sugars; 33 g protein

DELICIOUS DINNERS

Ⓓ Ⓐ Ⓖ Ⓢ TOTAL BRAIN CHEMICAL BOOSTING RECIPE

Tandoori Chicken

The vibrant mix of spices in this dish will not only boost all of your brain chemistry, it will also effectively boost your metabolism. Chicken is an excellent source of protein, and is listed to enhance all of your brain chemicals as well. That's why I consider this dish to be a Younger (Thinner) You superfood.

❋ **¼ cup garam masala** (page 177)

1 cup plain low-fat yogurt

1 teaspoon lemon juice

1 pound boneless, skinless chicken breasts

> **Serves 4**
> **180 calories per serving**

1. Combine the garam masala with the yogurt and lemon juice.

2. Place the chicken in a container and spread the yogurt marinade over the chicken. Cover and refrigerate for at least 2 hours to marinate.

3. Preheat oven to 350°F.

4. Place the chicken in a baking dish and bake until the juices run clear when pierced or internal temperature reaches 160°F, 25 to 30 minutes, depending on thickness of chicken breasts.

NUTRITION INFORMATION: Per serving: 180 calories; 3 g fat (1 g sat); 70 mg cholesterol; 120 mg sodium; 7 g carbohydrate; 1 g fiber; 4 g sugars; 30 g protein

D A G S TOTAL BRAIN CHEMICAL BOOSTING RECIPE

Chicken with Prunes and Olives

Chicken is an excellent source of protein that can enhance all of your brain chemicals.

1 tablespoon safflower oil

❋ **2 teaspoons rosemary**

❋ **1 teaspoon minced garlic**

❋ **1 teaspoon basil**

❋ **1 bay leaf**

2 pounds boneless, skinless chicken breasts

2 cups low-sodium chicken broth

½ cup red wine vinegar

½ cup chopped pitted low-sodium green olives

½ cup chopped pitted prunes

❋ **Freshly ground black pepper to taste**

> **Serves 8**
> **190 calories per serving**
>
> ## Swap Box
>
> - For more dopamine, serve with English Breakfast Tea Green Beans (see page 207).
> - For more acetylcholine, serve with roasted cauliflower or broccoli.
> - For more GABA, serve with cooked peas and lentils.
> - For more serotonin, serve with pan-seared tofu.

1. Heat oil in a large nonstick skillet over medium heat; add rosemary, garlic, basil, and bay leaf, gently cooking for one minute. Add the chicken and sauté until browned, about 2 minutes per side.

2. Add broth and vinegar and bring to a simmer. Stir in olives and prunes. Reduce heat to low.

3. Cover and cook until juices run clear when chicken is pierced and internal temperature reaches 160°F, about 30 minutes. Season with pepper. Transfer the chicken to a plate. Discard the bay leaf and spoon sauce over the chicken.

NUTRITION INFORMATION: Per serving: 190 calories; 4.5 g fat (1 g sat); 65 mg cholesterol; 180 mg sodium; 8 g carbohydrate; 1 g fiber; 5 g sugars; 27 g protein

D A G S TOTAL BRAIN CHEMICAL BOOSTING RECIPE
Lemon-Garlic Rooibos Chicken

This chicken dish is infused with rooibos tea, which is packed with vital nutrients. Chicken is a lean protein that supports all of your brain chemistry.

1 cup brewed rooibos tea

½ cup sliced carrots

2 tablespoons lemon juice

❋ **3 to 6 cloves garlic, chopped**

❋ **1 tablespoon rosemary**

❋ **1 tablespoon oregano**

❋ **1 teaspoon cumin**

❋ **Freshly ground black pepper to taste**

4 skinless, boneless chicken breasts, sliced

½ teaspoon olive oil

½ cup sliced green beans

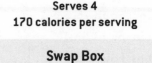

Serves 4
170 calories per serving

Swap Box

- For a dopamine or acetylcholine boost, use this same preparation with salmon.
- For a GABA or serotonin boost, use this same preparation with turkey.

1. Combine tea, carrots, lemon juice, garlic, and spices in a large pot. Add about 2 cups water. Bring to a boil, reduce heat, and simmer for 30 minutes.

2. Sauté chicken breasts in medium skillet in olive oil until browned, 3 to 5 minutes. Add chicken to pot and simmer for 1 hour. Stir in the green beans, cook another 15 minutes, and serve.

NUTRITION INFORMATION: Per serving: 170 calories; 2.5 g fat (0 g sat); 70 mg cholesterol; 90 mg sodium; 8 g carbohydrate; 1 g fiber; 2 g sugars; 28 g protein

Did You Know... about Oregano

There are three distinct varieties of oregano. The most familiar one, found in kitchens across the country, is Greek or Mediterranean oregano. Mexican oregano has a more "earthy" flavor. Cuban oregano is not well known outside the Caribbean, but its distinct taste makes it worth looking for.

D A G S TOTAL BRAIN CHEMICAL BOOSTING RECIPE

Baked Chicken with Yogurt

I love this dish because it hits all of the brain's chemicals. The chicken and spices each support your brain function as well.

3 ounces plain yogurt

¼ cup orange juice

❋ **2 cloves garlic, finely chopped**

❋ **2 teaspoons minced fresh ginger**

❋ **1 teaspoon rosemary**

❋ **½ teaspoon cumin**

❋ **½ teaspoon paprika**

❋ **½ teaspoon cayenne pepper**

❋ **2 teaspoons dried parsley**

❋ **Freshly ground black pepper to taste**

6 boneless skinless chicken breasts

> **Serves 6**
> **240 calories per serving**

1. In medium bowl, combine yogurt, orange juice, garlic, ginger, rosemary, cumin, paprika, cayenne, parsley, pepper, and a pinch of salt and mix well.

2. Dip chicken breasts in yogurt-spice mixture until well coated. Arrange in baking pan. Cover and marinate in the refrigerator for at least 1 hour.

3. Preheat oven to 350°F.

4. Bake chicken until thermometer registers 170°F, 30 to 40 minutes depending on thickness of breasts. Serve hot.

NUTRITION INFORMATION: Per serving: 240 calories; 4 g fat (2 g sat); 80 mg cholesterol; 190 mg sodium; 13 g carbohydrate; 0 g fiber; 13 g sugars; 36 g protein

D A G S TOTAL BRAIN CHEMICAL BOOSTING RECIPE

Rosemary Chicken with Broccoli

This dish is one of my favorites because it is a complete Younger (Thinner) You superfood. Broccoli is one of the most nutrient-dense vegetables, and both a *GABA* and *dopamine* precursor. Chicken supports both *dopamine* and *serotonin*, making this dish a super dopamine food. The spices provide lots of nutrients as well: The sage is particularly good for increasing *acetylcholine*.

❈ **2 tablespoons rosemary**

❈ **1 tablespoon sage**

❈ **2 tablespoons marjoram**

⅓ cup dry white wine

3 pounds chicken, cut into pieces

❈ **Freshly ground black pepper to taste**

❈ **1 clove garlic, minced**

1 tablespoon safflower oil

2 cups broccoli florets

> **Serves 4**
> **270 calories per serving**

1. In a small bowl, mix rosemary, sage, and marjoram with wine. Rub chicken pieces with pepper and garlic.

2. Heat oil in a medium to large skillet. Cook chicken pieces over medium heat until browned, about 8 minutes on each side.

3. Add wine mixture to chicken. Lower heat and cover pan; simmer for 20 minutes. Add broccoli, and continue to cook for 10 minutes, or until a thermometer registers 170°F and juices run clear.

NUTRITION INFORMATION: Per serving: 270 calories; 3.5 g fat (1 g sat); 130 mg cholesterol; 150 mg sodium; 2 g carbohydrate; 1 g fiber; 0 g sugars; 53 g protein

D S DOPAMINE AND SEROTONIN BOOSTING RECIPE

Middle Eastern Turkey Kebabs

Turkey is a lean protein that contains tryptophan, a precursor to *serotonin*, as well as *dopamine* precursors tyrosine and phenylalanine.

❋ **2 garlic cloves, minced**

❋ **1 teaspoon cumin**

❋ **1 teaspoon cinnamon**

❋ **½ teaspoon allspice**

❋ **1 teaspoon thyme**

3 tablespoons lemon juice

2 tablespoons extra virgin olive oil

1 pound turkey breast, cut into 1½" cubes

3 green, red, or yellow peppers, seeded and quartered

12 large cherry tomatoes

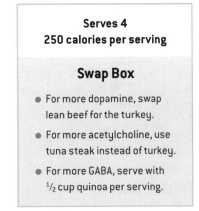

Serves 4
250 calories per serving

Swap Box

- For more dopamine, swap lean beef for the turkey.
- For more acetylcholine, use tuna steak instead of turkey.
- For more GABA, serve with ½ cup quinoa per serving.

1. In a large mixing bowl, mix together the garlic, spices, lemon juice, and oil.

2. Place the turkey in a shallow dish and pour the marinade over the turkey. Cover with plastic wrap and marinate in the refrigerator for at least 1 hour.

3. Preheat oven broiler or outdoor grill. If using wooden skewers, soak in water for at least 30 minutes so they do not burn.

4. Thread a turkey cube onto a skewer, followed by a pepper piece and a tomato. Repeat the process three times, adding a fourth piece of turkey at the end. Repeat with remaining skewers.

5. Grill or broil kebabs for 5 minutes on each side. Reduce the heat to low and continue to cook for 10 to 12 minutes, or until the turkey is cooked through.

NUTRITION INFORMATION: Per serving: 250 calories; 15 g fat (3 g sat); 75 mg cholesterol; 70 mg sodium; 2 g carbohydrate; 1 g fiber; 0 g sugars; 25 g protein

D **S** DOPAMINE AND SEROTONIN BOOSTING RECIPE

Mediterranean Turkey Legs

Turkey is a lean protein that is high in brain chemical precursors. It contains tryptophan, a precursor to *serotonin*, as well as tyrosine and phenylalanine, precursors to *dopamine*.

❋ **2 garlic cloves, finely chopped**

❋ **2 teaspoons cumin**

❋ **2 tablespoons rosemary**

2 tablespoons fresh lime juice

❋ **¼ teaspoon freshly ground black pepper**

2 teaspoons safflower oil

4 turkey legs

Serves 4
480 calories per serving

Swap Box

- For more acetylcholine, swap orange juice for the lime juice in the marinade.

- For more GABA, add 2 teaspoons cinnamon to the marinade.

1. Whisk together garlic, cumin, rosemary, lime juice, pepper, and oil and transfer to a large zip-top bag. Add turkey legs and seal bag, forcing out excess air. Shake until legs are evenly coated. Marinate the legs in the bag for at least 30 minutes in the refrigerator.

2. Meanwhile, preheat oven broiler or outdoor grill. Remove the legs from the marinade and broil or grill 8 to 10 minutes on each side, or until a thermometer registers 170°F and juices run clear.

NUTRITION INFORMATION: Per serving: 480 calories; 20 g fat (4.5 g sat); 2 mg cholesterol; 240 mg sodium; 2 g carbohydrate; 1 g fiber; 0 g sugars; 71 g protein

D A G S TOTAL BRAIN CHEMICAL BOOSTING RECIPE

Jasmine Tea–Infused Brown Rice with Sweet Peas and Duck

This Younger (Thinner) You meal supports all of your brain chemistry. The duck is a precursor to both *dopamine* and *serotonin*. Brown rice and peas are high in glutamine, which is necessary to create *GABA*. *Serotonin* is enhanced with basil. To top it off, this delicious meal is cooked with nutrient-rich tea.

2 quarts low-sodium chicken broth

¼ cup brewed jasmine tea

¼ cup safflower oil

1 large onion, finely chopped

❋ **2 cloves garlic, minced**

1 pound duck breast, cut into thin strips

2 cups brown rice

2 cups sweet peas

❋ **1 teaspoon oregano**

❋ **1 teaspoon coriander**

❋ **2 tablespoons fresh basil, cut into thin strips**

> **Serves 8**
> **400 calories per serving**

1. Combine the chicken broth and tea in a large pot and heat until boiling.

2. In a skillet, heat the oil and sauté the onion and garlic until the onion starts to turn golden. Add duck breast and sauté until firm. Set aside.

3. Add the rice to the chicken-tea broth and reduce heat. Cover and simmer until liquid is completely absorbed, about 45 minutes.

4. Stir in the peas, oregano, coriander, and basil and mix until combined well. Divide into four portions and top with duck breast.

NUTRITION INFORMATION: Per serving: 400 calories; 12 g fat (2 g sat); 50 mg cholesterol; 190 mg sodium; 53 g carbohydrate; 5 g fiber; 3 g sugars; 20 g protein

D A DOPAMINE AND ACETYLCHOLINE BOOSTING RECIPE

Citrus Tuna

Fish, such as tuna, is an effective *acetylcholine enhancer*. Fish is also an excellent source of protein, which boosts *dopamine*.

1 cup orange juice

1 cup pineapple juice

¼ cup lime juice

❁ **1 teaspoon thyme**

❁ **1 teaspoon dill**

❁ **¼ teaspoon cayenne pepper**

Olive oil spray

2 pounds fresh tuna steak

❁ **1 teaspoon paprika**

❁ **Freshly ground black pepper to taste**

> **Serves 4**
> **340 calories per serving**
>
> ## Swap Box
>
> ● For more GABA, serve with a whole grain like quinoa or bulgur wheat.
>
> ● For more serotonin, coat the tuna with 1 tablespoon fennel seeds.

1. To prepare the marinade, combine orange juice, pineapple juice, and lime juice in a shallow baking dish. Add thyme, dill, and cayenne. Add the tuna, turning to coat, and cover. Let fish marinate in the refrigerator for at least 1 hour.

2. Heat a large skillet and spray with olive oil. Remove tuna from marinade, place in skillet, and sprinkle with paprika. Cook 5 minutes and turn. Cook for 5 minutes longer, or until tuna is opaque. Season with salt and pepper and serve.

NUTRITION INFORMATION: Per serving: 340 calories; 6 g fat (1.5 g sat); 0 mg cholesterol; 90 mg sodium; 17 g carbohydrate; 1 g fiber; 15 g sugars; 51 g protein

D A S DOPAMINE, ACETYLCHOLINE, AND SEROTONIN BOOSTING RECIPE

Salmon with Dill Crust and Tomato-Fennel Sauce

Freshwater fish, such as salmon, is a powerful *dopamine* and *acetylcholine enhancer*. Fennel is a precursor to *serotonin*.

1 large tomato, chopped

1 cup finely chopped fennel bulb

2 tablespoons minced red onion

1 tablespoon red wine vinegar

1 pound salmon fillet, skinned

❀ **2 tablespoons minced dill**

❀ **2 tablespoons oregano**

❀ **1 tablespoon parsley**

❀ **Freshly ground black pepper to taste**

2 tablespoons fresh lemon juice

2 tablespoons safflower oil

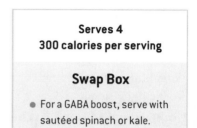

Serves 4
300 calories per serving

Swap Box

● For a GABA boost, serve with sautéed spinach or kale.

1. Combine tomato, fennel, onion, and vinegar in a medium bowl.

2. Cut salmon into 4 equal portions and sprinkle with dill, oregano, parsley, pepper, and lemon juice.

3. Heat oil in a large nonstick pan over high heat and cook the salmon until golden, 3 to 5 minutes. Turn the salmon over and cook 1 to 2 minutes longer, or until opaque. Spoon tomato mixture over salmon and serve immediately.

NUTRITION INFORMATION: Per serving: 300 calories; 18 g fat (2.5 g sat); 80 mg cholesterol; 95 mg sodium; 7 g carbohydrate; 3 g fiber; 2 g sugars; 27 g protein

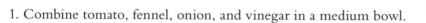

Make Powerful Choices

Whether it's with fresh sage, rosemary, or some paprika, always add two to three spices with every whole grain meal. Forget store-bought sauces unless they are low-sodium and sugar-free. Try Casino di Caprafico pastas, made from 100% farro (whole emmer wheat), or Delallo's line of whole wheat organic pastas like fusilli, shells, penne candeli, gemelli, and fusilli bucati. By combining the right carbs with nutrient-dense spices, you can create a delicious, nutritious, quick, and easy meal.

D **A** DOPAMINE AND ACETYLCHOLINE BOOSTING RECIPE

Blood Orange–Infused Salmon

Salmon is a Younger (Thinner) You superfood because it is versatile and packed with protein and healthy fats that are precursors to both *dopamine* and *acetylcholine*. This recipe combines the health benefits of salmon with the powerful antioxidants of tea.

2 teaspoons sesame oil

2 teaspoons red wine vinegar

1 cup brewed Stash Blood Orange Tea

1 tablespoon honey

❋ **1 tablespoon minced fresh ginger**

½ cup finely chopped shallots

❋ **2 garlic cloves, minced**

❋ **2 teaspoons sesame seeds, toasted**

❋ **1 teaspoon cumin**

❋ **1 teaspoon chili powder**

❋ **1 teaspoon paprika**

2 pounds salmon fillets

> **Serves 4**
> **390 calories per serving**
>
> ## Swap Box
>
> To boost any of the brain chemicals, steep the fish in green tea instead of blood orange tea.

1. Preheat oven to 375°F.

2. Combine all ingredients except salmon in a bowl and stir until mixed. Refrigerate for 1 hour.

3. Place salmon in a baking dish and cover with the sauce. Bake uncovered for 12 to 15 minutes, or until the salmon is opaque. Serve immediately.

NUTRITION INFORMATION: Per serving: 390 calories; 18 g fat (2.5 g sat); 125 mg cholesterol; 110 mg sodium; 10 g carbohydrate; 1 g fiber; 5 g sugars; 46 g protein

D **A** DOPAMINE AND ACETYLCHOLINE BOOSTING RECIPE

Salmon and Tomato Stew

Salmon is a Younger (Thinner) You superfood because it is versatile and packed with protein and healthy fats that are precursors to both *dopamine* and *acetylcholine*.

1½ cups low-sodium chicken broth, divided

1 large onion, diced

1 green pepper, diced

1 red pepper, diced

3 celery stalks, diced

❋ **4 garlic cloves, minced**

1 (32-ounce) can whole tomatoes, coarsely chopped

❋ **1 teaspoon celery seed**

❋ **1 teaspoon paprika**

❋ **½ teaspoon chili powder**

❋ **½ teaspoon cayenne pepper**

❋ **2 bay leaves**

1 pound salmon fillets, cut into 1" cubes

> **Serves 4**
> **260 calories per serving**
>
> ### Swap Box
>
> ● For a GABA boost, serve over ½ cup bulgur wheat.
> ● For a serotonin boost, swap tofu for the salmon.

1. In a large skillet, heat ½ cup of chicken broth over medium heat. Add the onion, peppers, celery, and garlic and cook for 6 to 8 minutes.

2. Add the remaining 1 cup chicken broth, tomatoes, celery seed, paprika, chili powder, cayenne pepper, and bay leaves. Bring to a boil. Lower the heat and simmer uncovered for 30 minutes.

3. Add the salmon and simmer for 8 to 10 minutes, or until opaque. Remove the bay leaves and serve.

NUTRITION INFORMATION: Per serving: 260 calories; 9 g fat (1.5 g sat); 65 mg cholesterol; 480 mg sodium; 21 g carbohydrate; 5 g fiber; 10 g sugars; 27 g protein

Ⓐ Ⓖ ACETYLCHOLINE AND GABA BOOSTING RECIPE

Broiled Halibut with Yogurt-Dill Sauce

Halibut is great for increasing *GABA*. The yogurt in this dish supports *acetylcholine*.

2 tablespoons extra virgin olive oil

❉ **1 clove garlic, minced**

❉ **2 tablespoons finely chopped basil**

❉ **1 tablespoon finely chopped chives**

1 scallion, finely chopped

❉ **Freshly ground black pepper to taste**

1 tablespoon lemon juice

2 pounds halibut fillets

1 cup plain yogurt

❉ **1 tablespoon dill**

1 large lemon, sliced

> **Serves 4**
> **360 calories per serving**

1. In a shallow bowl, combine oil, garlic, basil, chives, scallion, pepper, and lemon juice. Dip fish in spice mixture until coated and place on broiler pan.

2. Mix yogurt and dill in small bowl and set aside.

3. Arrange lemon slices on top of fish. Place under broiler and broil for 5 to 8 minutes, or until fish flakes easily. Serve fish with yogurt–dill sauce.

NUTRITION INFORMATION: Per serving: 360 calories; 13 g fat (2.5 g sat); 75 mg cholesterol; 180 mg sodium; 7 g carbohydrate; 1 g fiber; 5 g sugars; 51 g protein

G GABA BOOSTING RECIPE

Herb-Crusted Halibut

Halibut a nutrient-dense fish that contains high levels of magnesium, niacin, phosphorus, potassium, selenium, and vitamins B_6 and B_{12}. It is also a *GABA* precursor.

1½ pounds halibut fillets

❊ **1 tablespoon rosemary**

❊ **1 tablespoon thyme**

❊ **2 garlic cloves, minced**

❊ **1 teaspoon freshly ground black pepper**

❊ **1½ teaspoons cumin**

❊ **1½ teaspoons cayenne pepper**

¼ cup whole wheat bread crumbs

¼ cup low-sodium Worcestershire sauce

¼ cup water

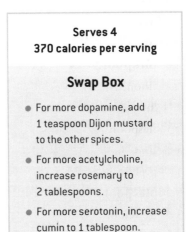

Serves 4
370 calories per serving

Swap Box

- For more dopamine, add 1 teaspoon Dijon mustard to the other spices.

- For more acetylcholine, increase rosemary to 2 tablespoons.

- For more serotonin, increase cumin to 1 tablespoon.

1. Preheat oven to 375°F. Rinse fish fillets and pat dry with a paper towel.

2. In a medium bowl, combine rosemary, thyme, garlic, black pepper, cumin, cayenne pepper, bread crumbs, Worcestershire sauce, and water. Stir to make a thick paste.

3. Using a spatula, spread paste over halibut fillets. Place fish on a roasting rack inside a roasting pan. Bake for 20 minutes, or until just opaque. Serve immediately.

NUTRITION INFORMATION: Per serving: 370 calories; 19 g fat (3 g sat); 55 mg cholesterol; 280 mg sodium; 10 g carbohydrate; 2 g fiber; 1 g sugars; 37 g protein

D A G S TOTAL BRAIN CHEMICAL BOOSTING RECIPE

Baked Tilapia

The spice mixture in this dish creates a Younger (Thinner) You super food. Not only are these spices thermogenic, they help to increase each of your brain chemicals.

Olive oil spray

❋ **1 teaspoon garlic powder**

❋ **1 teaspoon paprika**

❋ **1 teaspoon onion powder**

❋ **1 teaspoon cumin**

❋ **1 teaspoon basil**

❋ **1 teaspoon dry mustard**

❋ **1 teaspoon turmeric**

❋ **¼ teaspoon freshly ground black pepper**

 1 pound tilapia fillets

 ½ cup whole wheat bread crumbs

❋ **2 tablespoons chopped fresh parsley**

 3 tablespoons chopped scallions

 TK extra virgin olive oil

> **Serves 4**
> **200 calories per serving**

1. Preheat the oven to 450°F. Lightly spray a baking sheet with oil.

2. Combine all the spices, except the parsley, in a small bowl. Sprinkle 4 teaspoons of the spice mix over the fish.

3. Combine the bread crumbs, parsley, and scallions. Add the remaining spice mix and blend well. Add the olive oil and blend well with your fingers.

4. Coat the fish with the bread crumbs. Place the fish on the prepared sheet and bake for 5 minutes. Turn the fillets over and bake for 5 minutes longer, or until just opaque. Serve immediately.

NUTRITION INFORMATION: Per serving: 200 calories; 7 g fat (1 g sat); 55 mg cholesterol; 460 mg sodium; 14 g carbohydrate; 1 g fiber; 1 g sugars; 24 g protein

G **S** GABA AND SEROTONIN BOOSTING RECIPE
Mahimahi with Ginger Glaze

Mahimahi is a large, saltwater fish. It is a good source of potassium as well as being an excellent source of selenium, niacin, and vitamin B$_6$, making this fish a perfect *serotonin enhancer.* The ginger in this dish also supports *GABA.*

3 tablespoons honey

3 tablespoons reduced-sodium soy sauce

3 tablespoons balsamic vinegar

❋ **1 teaspoon grated fresh ginger root**

❋ **2 cloves garlic, minced**

2 pounds mahimahi fillets, cut into 4 pieces

❋ **1 teaspoon dried dill**

❋ **Freshly ground black pepper to taste**

2 teaspoons safflower oil

1 teaspoon fresh lemon juice

> **Serves 4**
> **260 calories per serving**
>
> **Swap Box**
>
> - For a dopamine boost, serve with ¹/₂ cup broccoli.
> - For a GABA boost, serve with ¹/₂ cup of whole wheat couscous.

1. In a bowl, stir together the honey, soy sauce, vinegar, ginger, and garlic. Set aside.

2. Season fish fillets with dill and pepper. Heat oil in a large skillet over medium heat. Cook fish for 4 to 6 minutes on each side, or until just opaque. Remove fillets to a serving platter and keep warm.

3. Pour glaze mixture into the skillet and cook over medium heat until thickened and reduced to a glaze. Spoon over fish, sprinkle with lemon juice, and serve immediately.

NUTRITION INFORMATION: Per serving: 260 calories; 7 g fat (1 g sat); 125 mg cholesterol; 560 mg sodium; 17 g carbohydrate; 0 g fiber; 14 g sugars; 32 g protein

D A G S TOTAL BRAIN CHEMICAL BOOSTING RECIPE

Herb-Rubbed Mackerel with Snow Peas and Lemon

This is a complete Younger (Thinner) You powerhouse meal that supports all of your brain chemistry. Mackerel not only increases *acetylcholine* and *serotonin*, it can also help you beat a blue mood. Peas are *dopamine* and *GABA* precursors, and lemon supports *GABA* and *dopamine*.

2 pounds snow peas

❀ **2 tablespoons cayenne pepper**

❀ **2 garlic cloves, minced**

❀ **1 teaspoon thyme**

❀ **1 teaspoon dill**

❀ **3 tablespoons onion powder**

1 pound mackerel fillets

2 tablespoons safflower oil

3 tablespoons lemon juice

| Serves 4 |
| 290 calories per serving |

1. Bring water to boil in a saucepan fitted with a steamer. Add snow peas and cook uncovered until slightly tender, about 5 minutes. Drain; set snow peas aside.

2. Combine cayenne, garlic, thyme, dill, and onion powder on a plate. Coat mackerel in the spice mixture. Heat oil in a large nonstick skillet over medium heat. Add the fish and cook, gently turning once, about 5 minutes, or until fish is just opaque. Transfer fish to a serving plate.

3. Add lemon juice and snow peas to the pan and cook until the snow peas are coated and heated through, about 2 minutes. Serve with the fish.

NUTRITION INFORMATION: Per serving: 290 calories; 10 g fat (1.5 g sat); 55 mg cholesterol; 105 mg sodium; 23 g carbohydrate; 8 g fiber; 9 g sugars; 29 g protein

Ⓓ Ⓐ Ⓖ Ⓢ TOTAL BRAIN CHEMICAL BOOSTING RECIPE

Curried Shrimp

Another Younger (Thinner) You superfood that hits all of the brain's chemicals.

1 pound large shrimp

❋ **2 tablespoons turmeric**

❋ **1 teaspoon cinnamon**

❋ **1 teaspoon basil**

❋ **1 teaspoon cumin**

❋ **1 teaspoon rosemary**

1 to 2 tablespoons safflower oil

❋ **4 cloves garlic, finely chopped**

1 cup finely chopped shallots

1 cup mushrooms (any variety), sliced or chopped

❋ **½ cup chopped fresh parsley**

½ cup water

❋ **Freshly ground black pepper to taste**

½ cup cashews, chopped

1 cup low-fat Greek yogurt

> **Serves 4**
> **380 calories per serving**

1. In a small bowl, combine the shrimp, turmeric, cinnamon, basil, cumin, and rosemary. Set aside.

2. Heat oil in a large skillet over medium-high heat. Add garlic, shallots, mushrooms, and parsley and sauté for 1 to 3 minutes, until tender. Transfer to a plate.

3. Add shrimp to same skillet and cook for about 1 minute, until lightly browned. Turn shrimp and cook other side, about 1 minute longer. Add the water, stirring constantly.

4. Return the mushroom mixture to the pan and add pepper to taste. Stir in the cashews. Cook for another 3 minutes, or until the shrimp are opaque. Remove from heat, slowly stir in the yogurt, and serve.

NUTRITION INFORMATION: Per serving: 380 calories; 17 g fat (3.5 g sat); 175 mg cholesterol; 350 mg sodium; 27 g carbohydrate; 3 g fiber; 7 g sugars; 31 g protein

Ⓓ DOPAMINE BOOSTING RECIPE

Flank Steak Fajitas with Mango Salsa

Beef in small quantities is an excellent source of protein and a *dopamine* precursor.

FOR THE SALSA

1 cup cherry tomatoes, cut in quarters

1 mango, diced

¼ cup diced green pepper

❋ **¼ teaspoon red pepper flakes**

1 tablespoon plus 2 teaspoons lime juice

❋ **1½ teaspoons cumin**

FOR THE FAJITAS

❋ **1 teaspoon red pepper flakes**

❋ **1 teaspoon chili powder**

❋ **1 teaspoon cinnamon**

❋ **1 teaspoon cumin**

1 pound beef flank steak

½ cup low-sodium barbecue sauce

Olive oil spray

2 medium red peppers, cut into thick slices

2 medium onions, cut into ½" slices

4 (6-inch) whole wheat tortillas, warmed

Serves 4
440 calories per serving

Swap Box

- For more acetylcholine, substitute an equal amount of shrimp for the steak.

- For more GABA, serve with cooked spinach.

- For more serotonin, substitute an equal amount of turkey for the steak.

1. To make the salsa, toss cherry tomatoes, mango, green pepper, pepper flakes, lime juice, and cumin in a medium bowl. Cover with plastic wrap and let stand at room temperature until serving time.

2. To make the fajitas, in a separate bowl, mix pepper flakes, chili powder, cinnamon, and cumin; rub evenly onto both sides of steak.

3. Preheat broiler. Broil steak, turning every 5 minutes, to preference: 10 minutes total for rare, 15 minutes or more for well done. Each time you turn the steak, brush it with barbecue sauce.

4. Meanwhile, in a large sauté pan sprayed with olive oil, sauté red peppers and onions until soft, about 5 minutes.

5. When steak is done, let rest for 5 minutes. Cut steak across the grain into thin slices. Place meat and vegetables evenly down centers of tortillas; spoon 1 tablespoon of salsa on top of each, and roll up to enclose filling. Serve additional salsa on the side.

NUTRITION INFORMATION: Per serving: 440 calories; 15 g fat (6 g sat); 75 mg cholesterol; 450 mg sodium; 39 g carbohydrate; 6 g fiber; 11 g sugars; 36 g protein

Ⓖ GABA BOOSTING RECIPE

Sautéed Liver with Caramelized Onions

Liver is high in B vitamins, precursors for *GABA*. It is also packed with other nutrients, including zinc, iron, niacin, phosphorus, riboflavin, selenium, and vitamin A. However, it is high in dietary cholesterol.

1 cup green beans, trimmed

1 red pepper, sliced into strips

3 tablespoons safflower oil, divided

1 large red onion, thinly sliced

❋ **2 teaspoons ground cloves, divided**

❋ **2 teaspoons oregano**

❋ **2 teaspoons dried parsley**

❋ **Freshly ground black pepper to taste**

½ pound beef liver, thinly sliced

¼ cup white balsamic vinegar

Serves 2
430 calories per serving

Swap Box

- For a dopamine boost, add ½ teaspoon cayenne pepper or sugar-free hot sauce.

- For an acetylcholine boost, swap asparagus for the green beans.

- For a serotonin boost, add 1 teaspoon reduced-sodium soy sauce when sautéeing onion.

1. Steam green beans and red pepper strips for 5 minutes or until beans become dark and crisp. Drain and plunge vegetables into cold water (no more than 30 seconds) to stop them from cooking. Drain and and set aside.

2. Heat 1½ tablespoons oil in a skillet over medium heat. Add onion and sauté until golden brown, about 10 minutes. Add 1 teaspoon cloves, oregano, and parsley and sauté 1 minute longer. Season with black pepper. Transfer the cooked onion to a small bowl.

3. Heat remaining 1½ tablespoons oil in the same skillet over medium–high heat. Sprinkle liver with remaining 1 teaspoon cloves and a dash more pepper. Add liver to skillet and sauté until brown on outside but still pink in center, about 4 minutes per side. Transfer liver to serving plate.

4. Place onion back into the skillet and add vinegar. Simmer over low heat, stirring, for 1 minute. Spoon onion mixture on top of liver and serve with green beans and red pepper.

NUTRITION INFORMATION: Per serving: 430 calories; 26 g fat (4.5 g sat); 400 mg cholesterol; 100 mg sodium; 26 g carbohydrate; 4 g fiber; 12 g sugars; 25 g protein

D G DOPAMINE AND GABA BOOSTING RECIPE

Lamb Chops with Herbs and Tabouli

Lamb is a good source of protein, which is both a *dopamine enhancer* as well as a metabolism booster. The tabouli is an excellent and delicious *GABA enhancer.* Or, try other GABA-enriching grains like quinoa or whole wheat couscous.

❋ **2 tablespoons minced garlic**

❋ **2 tablespoons finely chopped fresh parsley**

❋ **¼ teaspoon freshly ground black pepper**

❋ **2 tablespoons rosemary**

2½ pounds (about 8) lamb loin chops, trimmed of fat

2 teaspoons safflower oil

FOR THE TABOULI

½ cup bulgur wheat

2 medium tomatoes, chopped

1 medium cucumber, peeled and chopped

❋ **2 tablespoons finely chopped fresh dill**

3 tablespoons lemon juice

> **Serves 4**
> **480 calories per serving**
>
> ## Swap Box
>
> - For more acetylcholine, serve with roasted or grilled asparagus.
> - For more serotonin, add 2 tablespoons basil to the rest of the spices.

1. In a small bowl, mash garlic, parsley, pepper, and rosemary together. Coat the lamb chops with garlic mixture, pressing hard so it adheres. Cover the lamb chops with plastic wrap and refrigerate until ready to cook.

2. For the tabouli: Prepare the bulgur according to package directions. Meanwhile, in a medium bowl, combine tomatoes, cucumber, dill, and lemon juice. Stir to combine.

3. When the bulgur is fully cooked, remove from the heat. Add to tomato mixture, and refrigerate for at least 1 hour before serving.

4. In a large nonstick skillet over high heat, heat the oil. Add the lamb chops and cook about 5 minutes per side, or until browned and internal temperature reaches 145° for medium rare. Serve with tabouli.

NUTRITION INFORMATION: Per serving: 480 calories; 19 g fat (6 g sat); 160 mg cholesterol; 150 mg sodium; 23 g carbohydrate; 6 g fiber; 4 g sugars; 55 g protein

Ⓓ Ⓐ Ⓖ Ⓢ TOTAL BRAIN CHEMICAL BOOSTING RECIPE

Moroccan Lamb Tagine with Cinnamon, Apricots, and Almonds

The vibrant mix of spices here will not only boost all of your brain chemistry, it will also effectively boost your metabolism. That's why I consider this dish to be a Younger (Thinner) You superfood.

Olive oil spray

2 pounds lean lamb, cut into 1½" cubes

❋ **1 tablespoon ras el hanout** (opposite)

3 cups chopped onions

5 carrots, cut into fourths, then sliced lengthwise into thin strips

❋ **3 cloves garlic, minced**

½ cup dried apricots, cut into ¼" strips

⅓ cup freshly ground almonds

½ cup tomato puree

2 cups low-sodium chicken broth

1 teaspoon minced lemon zest

1 tablespoon honey

❋ **1 cinnamon stick**

❋ **Chopped fresh mint**

> **Serves 8**
> **330 calories per serving**

1. Spray a large nonstick skillet with olive oil and heat to medium-high. Rub the lamb with the ras el hanout. Sauté lamb until browned, 6 to 8 minutes. Remove lamb to a plate.

2. Add onions and carrots to skillet and cook until tender, stirring frequently. Stir in the garlic, apricots, and almonds. Stir in tomato puree and cook 3 minutes, stirring occasionally.

3. Return the lamb to the skillet with the chicken broth, lemon zest, honey, and cinnamon stick. Bring to a boil. Reduce heat to low, cover, and simmer, stirring occasionally, for 1½ to 2 hours or until the meat is tender.

4. Remove cinnamon stick, garnish with chopped fresh mint, and serve.

NUTRITION INFORMATION: Per serving: 330 calories; 15 g fat (4 g sat); 65 mg cholesterol; 200 mg sodium; 24 g carbohydrate; 5 g fiber; 16 g sugars; 25 g protein

RAS EL HANOUT

❋ 2 teaspoons garlic powder

❋ 1 teaspoon cumin

❋ ½ teaspoon ground ginger

❋ 1 teaspoon turmeric

❋ 1 teaspoon cinnamon

❋ ¾ teaspoon freshly ground black pepper

❋ ½ teaspoon ground white pepper

❋ ½ teaspoon ground coriander seeds

❋ ½ teaspoon cayenne pepper

❋ ½ teaspoon cardamom

❋ ½ teaspoon allspice

❋ ½ teaspoon nutmeg

❋ ¼ teaspoon ground cloves

❋ 1 teaspoon paprika

❋ 1 pinch saffron

Combine all of the ingredients in a small bowl and stir until mixed. This spice mix will stay fresh in an airtight container at room temperature for up to 1 month.

G **S** GABA AND SEROTONIN BOOSTING RECIPE

Baked Sweet Potato Casserole with Pecans

Sweet potatoes are a *GABA-enhancing* food that is packed with important nutrients. Pecans are a terrific source of tryptophan, which supports *serotonin*. The serving sizes are for a main dish, but halve the amounts for a delicious and nutrient-dense side dish that can serve as many as twelve people.

6 large sweet potatoes, peeled

¼ cup honey

4 cups orange juice

1 tablespoon butter

❋ **¼ cup cinnamon**

❋ **1 teaspoon nutmeg**

1 teaspoon vanilla

❋ **½ teaspoon ground cloves**

❋ **½ teaspoon allspice**

½ teaspoon chopped orange zest

¼ cup pecans, toasted and roughly chopped

> **Serves 6**
> **360 calories per serving**
>
> **Swap Box**
>
> - For more dopamine, swap out the pecans for an equal amount of unsalted almonds.
> - For more acetylcholine, sprinkle 2 tablespoons of wheat germ into the potatoes before cooking.

1. Preheat oven to 350°F.

2. Boil sweet potatoes in a large pot of water. Drain, cool, and mash.

3. Place mashed sweet potatoes in a baking dish. Drizzle honey over potatoes.

4. Place orange juice, butter, cinnamon, nutmeg, vanilla, cloves, allspice, and orange zest in a saucepan over medium heat. Stir until it reaches a soft boil. Reduce heat and simmer 5 minutes; pour mixture over sweet potatoes. Top with pecans. Bake for 45 to 50 minutes, or until heated through.

NUTRITION INFORMATION: Per serving: 360 calories; 4.5 g fat (0 g sat); 0 mg cholesterol; 20 mg sodium; 77 g carbohydrate; 9 g fiber; 46 g sugars; 5 g protein

D G S DOPAMINE, GABA, AND SEROTONIN BOOSTING RECIPE

Sweet Potato and Chickpea Curry

This spicy curry is a nutrient powerhouse. Chili peppers are metabolism-boosting *dopamine* food, ginger and sweet potatoes support *GABA*, and cumin boosts *serotonin*.

2 medium red onions, quartered

1 clove garlic

1 small chili pepper (like Scotch bonnet), stem removed

❀ **3-inch piece ginger, peeled and sliced**

2¼ cups low-sodium vegetable broth

3 tablespoons safflower oil

❀ **1 teaspoon red pepper flakes**

❀ **2 teaspoons coriander seeds**

❀ **2 teaspoons cumin**

❀ **1 tablespoon turmeric**

❀ **3 cardamom pods, lightly crushed**

3 sweet potatoes, peeled and cut into 1" cubes

1¾ cups coconut milk

1½ tablespoons fresh lime juice

4 cups canned chickpeas

❀ **2 tablespoons chopped cilantro leaves**

> **Serves 6**
> **340 calories per serving**

1. In a food processor or blender, combine onions, garlic, chili pepper, and ginger. Pulse until finely chopped. Meanwhile, heat the vegetable broth in a separate saucepan.

2. Heat oil in a large sauté pan over medium heat. Add vegetable mixture and sauté until softened and onions are translucent, about 5 minutes. Add pepper flakes, coriander, cumin, turmeric, cardamom, and sweet potatoes. Add the coconut milk and stir until all the ingredients are thoroughly mixed.

3. Add lime juice to the heated broth, then add broth to the sauté pan. Bring to a boil and reduce the heat. Simmer, partially covered, until the sweet potatoes are just tender, about 25 minutes.

4. Add chickpeas and simmer until heated through, about 5 minutes. Transfer curry to individual serving bowls and garnish with the cilantro.

NUTRITION INFORMATION: Per serving: 340 calories; 11 g fat (1 g sat); 0 mg cholesterol; 430 mg sodium; 52 g carbohydrate; 11 g fiber; 11 g sugars; 13 g protein

G GABA BOOSTING RECIPE

Spicy Kale and Yams

This vegetarian medley can be served as a complete meal or a side dish. It is a perfect *high-GABA* meal. The sweet potatoes, kale, and cabbage are all GABA superfoods.

1 large head kale, chopped

2 sweet potatoes, diced

1 tablespoon safflower oil

1 large onion, chopped

❋ **1 tablespoon minced garlic**

❋ **1 tablespoon minced fresh ginger**

1 teaspoon diced seeded Serrano chili pepper

1 cup sliced purple cabbage

3 tablespoons reduced-sodium soy sauce

❋ **Freshly ground black pepper to taste**

❋ **1 teaspoon sage**

> **Serves 2**
> **390 calories per serving**

1. Rinse and drain kale well. Steam kale and sweet potatoes for about 20 minutes, or until kale is still colorful and sweet potatoes still have some firmness.

2. While kale and sweet potatoes are steaming, place oil in a large sauté pan and heat on medium heat. Add onion, garlic, ginger, and chili pepper and cook for 5 minutes, stirring frequently. Add cabbage and cook for 5 minutes, stirring frequently.

3. Transfer cabbage mixture to a large mixing bowl. Add kale and sweet potatoes, along with soy sauce, black pepper, and sage. Mix well and serve immediately.

NUTRITION INFORMATION: Per serving: 390 calories; 12 g fat (1.5 g sat); 0 mg cholesterol; 1010 mg sodium; 67 g carbohydrate; 11 g fiber; 18 g sugars; 12 g protein

Ⓓ DOPAMINE BOOSTING RECIPE

English Breakfast Tea Green Beans

This vegetarian medley can be served as a complete meal or a side dish. Cooking them in tea gives a *dopamine* boost.

1 cup brewed English breakfast tea

1 pound fresh green beans, trimmed

❋ **2 garlic cloves, minced**

1 teaspoon safflower oil

❋ **1 teaspoon marjoram**

❋ **1 teaspoon sage**

Toasted almond slices to taste

> **Serves 4**
> **55 calories per serving**
>
> ## Swap Box
>
> ● For more dopamine, make this with broccoli instead of beans.
>
> ● For more acetylcholine, make this with asparagus.
>
> ● For more serotonin, make with edamame (pods removed).

1. Steam green beans for about 3 minutes, or microwave until tender–crisp.

2. In a skillet, sauté garlic in oil until translucent, about 1 minute. Add tea, marjoram, and sage and simmer for 4 to 5 minutes.

3. Place beans in a large bowl and add tea mixture. Garnish with toasted almond slices and serve immediately.

NUTRITION INFORMATION: Per serving: 55 calories; 1 g fat (0 g sat); 0 mg cholesterol; 2 mg sodium; 11 g carbohydrate; 4 g fiber; 2 g sugars; 2 g protein

Nuts over Nuts

A quarter cup of nuts is a highly satisfying snack. Nuts contain roughly 2 grams of monounsaturated (heart-healthy) fat per serving. Choose unsalted nuts whenever possible. If you have salted nuts at home already, you can wash off the salt. Mixed nuts provide the greatest variety of nutrients. Create your own assortment with cashews, almonds, pecans, hazelnuts, peanuts, macadamias, and brazil nuts. Each has different oils that are filled with powerful nutrients to increase your nutrient calorie density.

SAUCES AND CONDIMENTS

D A G S TOTAL BRAIN CHEMICAL BOOSTING RECIPE

Yogurt-Cumin Marinade

Use this tangy, flavorful marinade to add zing to chicken, lamb, or pork.

½ cup fat-free plain yogurt

¼ cup prepared chutney

❋ **¼ cup finely chopped fresh mint**

2 tablespoons extra virgin olive oil

❋ **4 cloves garlic, minced**

❋ **2 tablespoons cumin**

> **Makes about 1 cup**

Combine all ingredients in a small bowl.

NUTRITION INFORMATION: Per teaspoon: 6 calories; 0 g fat; 0 mg cholesterol; 36 mg sodium; 1 g carbohydrate; 0 g fiber; 0 g sugars; 0 g protein

A Variety of Yogurts

There are some terrific natural, healthy yogurts out there. Some of my favorite brands include Axelrod, Dannon Light & Fit, Horizon Organic Fat-Free, and Stonyfield Farm.

D A G S TOTAL BRAIN CHEMICAL BOOSTING RECIPE

Garlic Lover's Rub

Perfect for grilling or broiling. This wet rub is so aromatic, so pungent and flavorful, and so versatile, it works with virtually any meat or vegetable. Try it on portobello mushrooms, onions, squash and zucchini, shrimp, salmon, chicken, pork, beef, and lamb.

❋ **16 cloves garlic, minced**

2 tablespoons extra virgin olive oil

❋ **4 teaspoons stone-ground mustard**

❋ **1 tablespoon rosemary**

❋ **1 tablespoon cumin**

❋ **1 tablespoon oregano**

❋ **½ teaspoon freshly ground black pepper**

1 teaspoon freshly grated lemon zest

> **Makes about ½ cup**

Combine all ingredients in a small bowl. Using your hands, spread the rub evenly onto your food of choice just before grilling.

NUTRITION INFORMATION: Per 2 teaspoons: 28 calories; 2 g fat (0 g sat); 0 mg cholesterol; TK mg sodium; 1 g carbohydrate; 0 g fiber; 0 g protein

Get Cracking over Weight Loss!

Whole grain crackers can make a light, delicious high-fiber snack, that, in many cases, has a reasonable amount of carbs. Do not eat them straight out of the box. Select one serving and put the box away. Then lightly spread them with a high-protein topping like cottage cheese, peanut butter, or hummus. Some of my favorite brands include Ry-Krisp, Ryvita, Wasa, Whole Foods 365 Baked Woven Wheats, and Trader Joe's Woven Wheat Wafers.

CHAPTER 11

Keep Track of Your Success

KEEPING A DETAILED record of your progress is the best way to determine how close you are to your weight loss goals. The process starts at the very beginning of the Younger (Thinner) You Diet.

KEEP A FOOD DIARY

If you've ever dieted before, you've already heard this advice. But this is one dieting truism: You don't realize what you eat all day unless you write it down. Several studies have shown that keeping a food diary greatly improves your chances of success. Doing so helps you gain better control of your intake, and it will also help minimize cheating (who wants to fess up to a handful of chocolate chips?). Sometimes you don't realize how much food you eat over the course of a day, but when you write it down, you're shocked to find out that you ate three pieces of cheese while you were making dinner. Often, this is exactly where unwanted calories add up, especially if you think that you already have good eating habits, or that you were "good" all day.

Within the Younger (Thinner) You Food Diary you'll be recording your weight every morning. I think this is important because knowledge is power: If you know what you weigh, you can tell if you are making progress. Check your weight every day on the scale. Record your weight at the same time each day. An ideal time to weigh yourself would be when you wake up and after you've emptied your bladder, because your body weight isn't yet affected by breakfast.

Throughout the day you'll record when you ate and what you ate. Include all the beverages you drank, including teas, as well as the nutrient supplements you took. Also, jot down how you feel each morning, or how you felt at the end of the day after following the eating plan. By recording your emotional state, you can see if you are making progress with your brain chemical imbalance.

The Younger (Thinner) You Diet is a 30-day plan that I recommend you stay on for at least three months. Photocopy these pages as often as you need to to keep track. Bind them up in a notebook so you can look back on your progress. You'll be amazed at how much will change in such a short time!

DAY ONE DATE: _____   **WEIGHT:** _____

Breakfast

_____

Lunch

_____

Dinner

_____

Snacks

_____

Supplements

_____

Mood

DAY TWO DATE: _____   **WEIGHT:** _____

Breakfast

_____

Lunch

_____

Dinner

_____

Snacks

_____

Supplements

_____

Mood

DAY THREE DATE: _____   **WEIGHT:** _____

Breakfast

_____

Lunch

_____

Dinner

_____

Snacks

_____

Supplements

_____

Mood

DAY FOUR DATE: _____   **WEIGHT:** _____

Breakfast

_____

Lunch

_____

Dinner

_____

Snacks

_____

Supplements

_____

Mood

DAY FIVE DATE: _____   **WEIGHT:** _____

Breakfast

_____

Lunch

_____

Dinner

_____

Snacks

_____

Supplements

_____

Mood

DAY SIX DATE: _____   **WEIGHT:** _____

Breakfast

_____

Lunch

_____

Dinner

_____

Snacks

_____

Supplements

_____

Mood

DAY SEVEN **DATE:**   **WEIGHT:**

Breakfast

Lunch

Dinner

Snacks

Supplements

Mood

TOTAL WEIGHT LOST THIS WEEK:

BMI

Record these numbers at the end of each week and circle your weight range:

	Normal range = 8.5–24.9	Overweight range = 25–29.9	Obese ≥ 30
Starting BMI _____	normal	overweight	obese
BMI After Week 1 _____	normal	overweight	obese
BMI After Week 2 _____	normal	overweight	obese
BMI After Week 3 _____	normal	overweight	obese
BMI After Week 4 _____	normal	overweight	obese
BMI After Week 5 _____	normal	overweight	obese
BMI After Week 6 _____	normal	overweight	obese
BMI After Week 7 _____	normal	overweight	obese
BMI After Week 8 _____	normal	overweight	obese
BMI After Week 9 _____	normal	overweight	obese
BMI After Week 10 _____	normal	overweight	obese
BMI After Week 11 _____	normal	overweight	obese
BMI After Week 12 _____	normal	overweight	obese

MONITOR CHANGES IN BODY FAT

Continuing to measure your body fat is a great way to monitor your progress on the Younger (Thinner) You Diet. Remember, less fat is better, and more muscle is better. Every two weeks, check your body fat percentage at your doctor's office or at the local gym, using the body fat assessment tools discussed in Chapter 2. Record your results here:

Body Fat Percentage at start of program: _____

Body Fat Percentage after week 2: _____

Body Fat Percentage after week 4: _____

Body Fat Percentage after week 6: _____

Body Fat Percentage after week 8: _____

Body Fat Percentage after week 10: _____

Body Fat Percentage after week 12: _____

EXERCISE LOG

Record here what type of exercise you did each day every week; the length of the workouts; and the size of the weights used. You should be exercising for at least 30 minutes every day, alternating between aerobic activity and resistance training.

	MONDAY	TUESDAY	WEDNESDAY
Week 1			
Week 2			
Week 3			
Week 4			
Week 5			
Week 6			
Week 7			
Week 8			
Week 9			
Week 10			
Week 11			
Week 12			

THURSDAY	FRIDAY	SATURDAY	SUNDAY

PART III

How to Personalize the Diet to Meet Your Health Needs

CHAPTER 12

Becoming Younger, Thinner, and Healthier

WEIGHT GAIN does not occur in a vacuum. In the first part of the book, I showed how your aging brain may be contributing to weight gain, or your inability to lose weight. But your brain isn't the only part of your body that can affect your health and your weight. In fact, your current health status may be part of your weight problem. When one system in your body isn't working properly, it can cause drastic changes that affect the rest of your body. In terms of your weight, your poor health can cause changes to your metabolism, your insulin levels could rise so that you can no longer process certain foods correctly, or you may develop specific food cravings. Just like an old brain leads to weight gain, an old body can create an unnecessarily heavy body. What's more, your aging brain chemistry is also directly linked to your aging body. Just as an unbalanced brain leads to weight gain, it can also lead to a host of conditions and symptoms, which then affect your weight.

It's also likely that your weight is affecting your health. If you have not had great results with other diets or previous attempts at weight loss—even if you were already eating healthfully and exercising regularly—and if you don't have food addictions, cravings, and your portions are reasonable, then your inability to lose weight is most likely connected to your declining health. The reason is twofold.

First, carrying excessive weight is an age accelerator: It speeds up the aging process, forcing the brain and the body to work harder and age faster. Being overweight affects the rest of your body more than any other single symptom or condition, and can create havoc with nearly every organ system. You may not realize that when you've gained a notch or two on your belt, your heart has had to work harder, your pancreas has to work harder, and your skin is stretched. The harder these organs work, the older they become. Eventually, one of them will give out and pull the rest of the body down with it. If you've been overweight at least three years, virtually every system in your body has suffered some age acceleration. So it stands to reason that if you can get your weight under control, you can stay trim, youthful looking, and healthy well into your golden years.

It doesn't matter if your weight is pushing you toward poor health, or if your poor health is causing you to gain weight, because the fix is the same: To reverse aging, lose weight and keep it off forever, you need to address your current illnesses and your weight at the same time.

The second part of the equation goes right back to your brain health. Each of the four primary brain chemicals governs specific aspects of your body's health. I describe this relationship in detail in my book, *The Edge Effect*, but for the purposes of this diet, you should know that the same way your brain chemistry governs your metabolism and cravings, it also governs the effectiveness of each of your body's systems and organs.

For example, the dopamine system is responsible for protecting the whole body against autoimmunity. As the dopamine system fails, the thyroid and all organs affected by the immune system fall victim to the development of autoantibodies and antibodies throughout the human body that attack body parts and cause them to age. When this happens, the dopamine system begins demanding more from other hormones it interacts with, such as GH, testosterone, cortisol, DHEA. These hormones are responding to the brain's cries for help. As the body starts to make more hormones to compensate, those hormone systems follow the same path as the original dopamine—fading out, leading to withered organs. This is similar to a sinking ship in a terrible storm sending out a cry for help, but each boat that responds starts to sink, too. The more the organ systems of the body fail, the harder it is to rebalance hormones and brain chemicals.

The hormones that interact with acetylcholine are: growth hormone, vasopressin, DHEA, calcitonin, parathyroid hormone, erythropoietin, and estrogen. As with dopamine, when acetylcholine fails, these hormone systems fall out of balance, leading to a host of effects including metabolic syndrome, depression, and osteoporosis. A GABA deficiency leads to anxiety, which we already know accelerates obesity and therefore every single hormone pause. The hormones that are affected by the serotonin system are: progesterone, growth hormone, pregnenolone, leptin, and aldosterone. When these systems fail, effects may include depression, hypertension, and dementia.

While you are following the Younger (Thinner) You Diet, you can also accurately diagnose your symptoms and conditions

Health Factors Contributing to Weight Gain

- Brain chemical imbalance
- Hormonal imbalances
- Metabolic disorders
- Inflammatory disorders
- Loss of bone density

before they become a medical catastrophe. What's more, I'll show you how to positively address the parts of your body that are aging you prematurely, and how they are linked to deficiencies in your brain chemistry. This part of the program is integral to becoming both younger and thinner. Without addressing the rest of your health, any diet, even the Younger (Thinner) You Diet, isn't worth your time. The reason is simple: Your body will be left in a diseased state even after you are thin. But if you follow this program, not only will you finally be able to lose weight, you will be turning back the clock to a younger, more vibrant self. You may find that when you follow the diet as prescribed for your brain chemistry, your overall health is likely to dramatically improve as well.

MEDICATIONS THAT MAY CAUSE WEIGHT GAIN

If you are taking any of the following medications, check with your doctor to see if there are alternatives that won't affect your waistline:

- **Antihistamines** thwart allergic reactions. They often can make you drowsy so you are not as physically active.
- **Anticonvulsants**, including Depakote/ Depakene/Divalproex, are used for anxiety and mood swings (mania and bipolar conditions) as well as migraine headaches. These medications can make you want to eat more. These medications are also known to cause depression, sleep problems, and anxiety, which are individually connected with obesity. Also causes you to retain water, which can make you gain weight.
- **Antidepressants** affect your serotonin and dopamine levels, which cause food cravings.
- **Diabetes agents** such as sulfonylureas cause hunger and thereby, weight gain. Rosiglitazone can increase cholesterol, and causes water retention. Pioglitazone can cause water retention.
- **Baclofen** is a muscle relaxer and an antispastic agent often used to treat MS. Baclofen can make you drowsy and constipated, which can lead to weight gain.
- **Carvedilol** is indicated in the treatment of congestive heart failure. It is known to cause weight gain in 10 to 12% of users, perhaps connected to the fatigue and edema (water retention) that it induces.
- **Danazol** is a synthetic hormone. It is used to treat pain, heavy menstrual flow, and infertility caused by endometriosis. It is also used in the treatment of fibrocystic disease in the breast. It is known to cause hypertension, depression, anxiety, sleep disorders, and constipation, each of which can lead to weight gain.
- **Diazoxide** is used in treating persistent hypoglycemia. Causes ileus (a blockage of the small and/or large intestine), anxiety, insomnia, fluid retention—all of which can lead to weight gain.
- **Estrogens/birth control pills** can cause water retention.

Can You Spot Illness and Aging?

If you really study our next quiz and fully understand what I've taught you in this book, eventually you will be able to walk into a room and see for yourself not only how your friends are aging, but if they are sick. The telltale signs are right in front of your eyes: Balding men with prostate problems; a pear-shaped figure with metabolic syndrome; both male- and female-pattern hair loss that's related to metabolic disorders; the arc around the iris of dementia patients; and the ear crease on the earlobe of those with heart disease.

- **Glucocorticoids** are hormones that predominantly affect the metabolism of carbohydrates and, to a lesser extent, fats and proteins.
- **Leuprolide** is used to treat hormone-responsive cancers such as prostate cancer or breast cancer, estrogen-dependent conditions (such as endometriosis or uterine fibroids), precocious puberty, and to control ovarian stimulation during *in vitro* fertilization. Causes depression, insomnia, fatigue, and edema, each of which can lead to weight gain.
- **Megestrol** is used to relieve symptoms caused by advanced breast cancer and advanced endometrial cancer. Causes hypertension, edema (swelling), insomnia, depression, fluid retention, each of which can lead to weight gain.
- **Minoxidil** is a vasodilator and was originally used as an oral drug to treat high blood pressure. It is commonly used for hair growth and reversing baldness. Can cause water retention, blood pressure decrease, anxiety, depression, each of which can lead to weight gain.
- **Neurontin** is used to treat seizures and nerve pain caused by the herpes virus. It can cause fatigue, water retention, depression, and constipation, all of which can lead to weight gain.
- **Prednisone** is a steroid medication used to fight inflammation. Steroids are known to cause increased hunger.
- **Progestins/gestagens** are used to treat the symptoms of endometriosis. Can cause fatigue, depression, water retention, and bloating, each of which can contribute to weight gain.

YOU'RE ONLY AS YOUNG AS YOUR OLDEST PART

Every time a single internal system changes, whether it is the brain, heart, skin, bones, or muscles, you age. The system that starts failing first becomes your oldest part. For some, it may start with aches and pains in their joints. For others, their hair may gray, or fall out. Still others begin to have problems with their memory. As your body weakens in any of these or countless other specific places, it speeds up the aging process all over the body, so that you become older than your chronological age. For

Meet Clarissa P.: She Lost Weight and Got Younger

Clarissa walked into my office for the first time when she was 62 years old. She handed me a list of the medications she was taking; the list was so long I had to sit down to read through all of them. Yet Clarissa was not feeling or looking well. She had already been diagnosed with depression and was taking Effexor to improve her mood. She couldn't sleep, so she was taking both Ambien and Lunesta. She'd been on and off the Weight Watchers program for the past twenty years, so her doctor prescribed Synthroid for a thyroid problem. Although Clarissa thought she had completed "the change," she was still experiencing breast lumps and cysts as well as frequent urinary tract infections, and had no real interest in sex. Clarissa also had high blood pressure, and was told she had a fatty liver—this pushed her over the edge, and she finally came to see me.

I touched Clarissa's hand and discovered her skin was as dry as parchment. Clarissa thought her medical issues were due to age, and to some extent she was right. But she I told her she didn't need to live with them anymore. While each of her other doctors was busy trying to fix one problem, I told her that with one program she could reverse aging in her entire body.

We then did BEAM testing, which concluded that Clarissa was low on dopamine, GABA, and serotonin. I started Clarissa on the Younger (Thinner) You Diet to get her brain chemistry back to normal levels. Immediately she began to lose weight. Then I began to address her health issues together, so the medications and supplements I chose would have a synergistic effect: They would work on more than one illness. I prescribed bioidentical hormone supplements that addressed her weight as well as her bone density and her menopausal conditions. I instructed her to take supplements including n-acetylcysteine and alpha lipoic acid, which cleaned out her fatty liver. Vitamin E improved her breast cysts and decreased her risk for future breast cancer. I also treated her brain chemical deficiencies more aggressively with nutrients, and now she sleeps like a baby without medicated sleep aids.

Clarissa is a classic example of someone who did not understand that aging wasn't inevitable. She didn't understand that menopause and its related hormonal losses were negatively affecting the rest of her health, including her mood and her weight. Now that she is under proper medical supervision, she feels younger than she has in years. Most, if not all, of her conditions have improved dramatically, and she has finally lost all the weight she wanted to. Clarissa is now well on her way to achieving full health.

It Doesn't Have to Be a Heart Attack to Bring You Down

Aging begins with one malfunctioning body part—a catastrophic illness, like a heart attack. It can also occur when there have been a series of problems with moderately old parts. It's like a sand castle that's made up of drippings: Your back hurts, your head hurts, your joints hurt, your liver's not so great, you've got gallstones, and all of a sudden—BOOM! You've got a pile of illnesses adding up.

example, if your chronological age is 40, it's not only possible but highly likely that you have the mind of a 30-year-old, while at the same time your heart is functioning like it's 60 years old, your skin appears to belong to a 50-year-old, and you have the sexual functioning of an 80-year-old. That's why I tell my patients all the time: You're only as young as your oldest part.

I refer to these failing systems as experiencing *pauses*: the time markers that identify the beginnings of wear and tear. During these pauses, the failing organ or internal system becomes older than the rest of your body. At the same time, its associated hormone levels drop, sending a signal or code to the rest of the body: Its purpose is to broadcast that the system is failing. This signal also begins the process whereby the whole body will begin to shut down. That's where death comes in.

Women are familiar with the term menopause, which is the model for this theory. We all know that menopause occurs when the ovaries no longer function and there is a decline in hormonal output, which leads to associated symptoms and conditions. For example, when Peggy started missing her regular menstrual cycle, she also noticed her hair lost its luster; her nails became brittle and weak; she was often depressed or irritable, and she put on weight. Originally she thought these symptoms were not linked, but they were. Her decline in estrogen, progesterone, and testosterone was causing each of these other systems to fail. Luckily, she came in and we began to reverse her menopausal symptoms. While we can't stop menopause from happening, there's no reason for you to look and feel older.

GOOD THING WE STARTED WITH THE BRAIN

Enhancing your brain chemistry through the Younger (Thinner) You Diet program, particularly with the emphasis on teas and spices, will go a long way to improving any symptoms and conditions that you may be experiencing. Brain function affects *every* illness and disease, so if you can restore your brainpower, speed, rhythm, and synchrony, even the most minor symptoms may disappear.

For example, loss of brainpower—or dopamine—allows the body to begin to oxidize, or burn up. When your brain is less powerful, you may experience fatigue. That's why we say we feel "burnt out" when we are tired. A loss of brain speed is a function of decreased acetylcholine, resulting in dehydration and atrophy of the rest of the body as well as the mind. Acetylcholine loss is directly related to lowered cognitive functioning/Alzheimer's disease (AD), and other degenerative brain diseases. The GABA-related loss of rhythm affects the structure of cells, the ossification or hardening of the human body and brain tissue, leading to chronic pain. Serotonin loss is related to sleep issues, depression, and phobias, and is known to cause inflammation throughout the body. Each of these symptoms or conditions becomes one of the pauses. But by following the Younger (Thinner) You Diet and addressing your brain chemistry imbalances, you can reverse some of this aging.

Just as you identified your brain/weight issue in Part 1, by identifying your brain/health issues now, you'll be ready to get back on track for better heath.

NAME THE PAUSES

The following are some of the different ways in which the body ages. Each of these pauses directly contributes to specific weight issues. Once you understand each of the pauses, the next step will be identifying which ones you may be experiencing, and then stopping them from making you prematurely old and unnecessarily heavy.

For a more extensive understanding of the pauses, see Appendix D, which lists all of them, as well as their typical onset age.

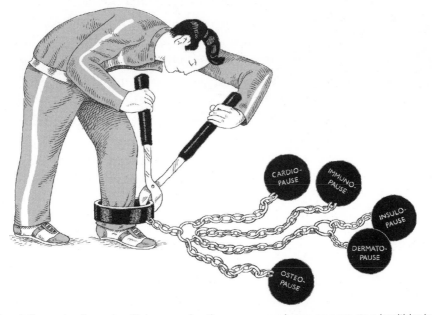

When you break the cycle of poor health by reversing the pauses, you're on your way to a healthier brain and a healthier, younger, and thinner body.

The Four Core Processes of Aging

Oxidizing→→→Dopamine→→→	Burning up
Dehydrating→→→Acetylcholine→→→	Drying up
Calcifying→→→GABA→→→	Turning to stone
Inflammation→→→Serotonin→→→	Swelling

My book, *Younger You*, discusses these pauses in detail.

Cardiopause/vasculopause represents an aging heart and vascular system, and is related to the brain chemicals dopamine and serotonin. Beginning around age 50, these pauses occur when changes in blood flow to and from the heart lead to coronary artery blockages, valve damage, enlargement of the heart, and decreased pumping action. Cardiopause can affect your weight because it reduces your metabolism, so you burn fuel slower, and the unused food taken in becomes body fat stored all over your body. High blood pressure and cholesterol issues are associated with cardiopause and vasculopause as well. Weight gain can begin premature cardiopause because the additional pounds you are carrying force the heart to work harder. This is the direct link between heart disease and obesity.

Immunopause occurs when the body's immune system is compromised, and is related to the brain chemical serotonin. The loss of immunity causes inflammation, followed at times by infection, which can occur anywhere in the body. Immunopause is also linked to developing certain cancers. Immu-nopause usually begins around age 30, but can start at any time if you were born with a compromised immune system, which covers everything from allergies to HIV. It takes a lot of brain work to fight infection and inflammation, which is why immunopause is so deadly: It ages brain chemistry rapidly. Once the brain is injured, it craves carbohydrates, leading to weight gain. Conversely, obesity causes inflammation and swelling all over the body, and is also linked as a risk factor for many types of cancer.

Insulopause affects our insulin resistance as well as our metabolism, and relates to the brain chemicals dopamine, acetylcholine, and serotonin. Changes in insulin and glucose tolerance result in carbohydrate cravings. That's why obesity and diabetes are integrally linked. Insulopause naturally begins around the age of 40, but childhood or earlier obesity can cause Type 2 diabetes at any age.

Dermatopause is the aging of your skin, beginning as early as age 30 when we start to naturally produce less growth hormone. Dermatopause is related to the brain chemicals acetylcholine and serotonin. It describes a decrease in the strength, subtlety, and luster of your hair and nails, your complexion, as well as various skin conditions. While dermatopause does not contribute to obesity, excess weight significantly affects your skin. Not only does it cause your skin to stretch, it is also linked to various skin conditions including psoriasis, scleroderma diabeticorum, vitiligo, acanthosis nigricans, fungal infections (candidiasis, tinea cruris), folliculitis, edema, lymphedema, gangrene, and leg ulcerations.[1]

Osteopause refers to the loss of bone mass that causes a decline in physical strength, and is related to the brain chemicals dopamine, acetylcholine, and serotonin. Osteopause can begin by age 30. When we are weak, we don't really feel like exercising, and often have a propensity toward making rash, and unhealthy food choices. An increase in parathyroid hormone, along with a loss of calcitonin, can affect bone density and result in a malnourished state where we crave unhealthy foods. Obesity puts added pressure on your bones and joints, causing osteoarthritis and contributing to osteoporosis.

Somatopause refers to the loss of growth hormone, which results in an increased ability of the body to convert muscle to fat, the loss of muscle and bone, and the loss of physical strength. Somatopause is related to the brain chemical acetylcholine and begins to kick in around the age of 30. Using muscles properly increases metabolism, which is why exercise is an important tool for weight loss. However, when we are overweight, we aren't likely to exercise, which makes our muscles weaker.

Menopause occurs in women with the loss of the body's sex hormones (estrogen, progesterone, and testosterone), and is related to all four brain chemicals. This directly results in roughly ten pounds of weight gain per decade beginning at about age 30. Conversely, obesity can wreak havoc on your immune system, increasing your risk for breast cancer, ovarian cysts, and growths, and send you into an early menopause.

Andropause is also known as male menopause, and is related to all four brain chemicals. Beginning at age 40 it occurs when there is a loss of testosterone, which can cause abdominal obesity initially, and then total body obesity as muscle turns to fat. Andropause also affects male sexual performance, which is directly affected by carrying additional weight.

Gastropause affects the stomach and GI tract and begins around the age of 30 and is related to the brain chemicals dopamine, GABA, and serotonin. The slowing down of nutrient absorption by the entire gastrointestinal tract results in digestive problems from GERD and irritable bowel syndrome to the development of a malnourished state. In some cases, even when we are overweight we can actually be suffering from

The AgePrint Identifies Whether or Not You Were Born Old

Your DNA or childhood illnesses may have preprogrammed you to have osteoporosis later in life. That is why an AgePrint is most useful when done at an early age; it allows you to identify weak links so you can work with your DNA and get younger. For example, if the proper treatments are implemented before osteoporosis sets in, we can prevent that pause from ever occurring, reversing the fact you were born old.

malnutrition because we choose foods that are nutrient deficient. When the body is hungry, it is actually craving nutrients; however, we often quench hunger and cravings with simple carbohydrates and other forms of junk food. Eating the wrong foods can exacerbate the problem by creating a constant state of dysnutrition. Gastropause can cause obesity when the stomach doesn't function properly, so you feel like you aren't full when in fact you are. Obesity can cause gastropause if you are constantly eating "bad for you" foods (and now you know what exactly that means) that upset your digestive tract.

KNOW YOUR AGEPRINT

I can't tell you how many patients are worried about the way their teeth look, spending thousands of dollars on veneers. They fix their teeth and all of a sudden they die from an aortic aneurysm that could have been detected by an echocardiogram. From age 30 on, almost every American is walking around with five silent diseases and abnormal brain chemistries that will contribute to health problems sooner rather than later. Yet everyone is focused on their clothes, their home, their bank account, instead of their internal body. They could be thin and fit and have the most amazing, abundant life if they took care of themselves instead of starting by fixing their teeth.

Your spiral to poor health often begins without you even realizing it. Virtually

every medical condition has a ten- to twenty-year antecedent—you don't just fall apart overnight. For example, if you have been overweight for twenty years, you can be certain your heart has not been optimally functioning the entire time you have been overweight; it's had to work two or three times harder than it normally would if you were of average weight. If your brain has been losing speed for twenty years, you are already becoming demented. If your bones have always broken easily, you are developing osteoporosis whether you have lost height or not.

When I can detect and begin to treat any illness early in its disease process, I find that my patients are more willing to change their behavior, which almost always leads to getting better results. For example, knowing your blood sugar is a little high when you don't have any symptoms, or understanding that your blood pressure is a little high may be all you need to start making lasting change. The goal is to reverse disease when it's called pre-hypertension, pre-dementia (mild cognitive impairment), pre-obesity (overweight), and prediabetes. Therefore, the first step is early detection of even the slightest change in your aging code.

That's why my program is so important: it's a lifetime bible for changing your weight and controlling your health. By assessing your health today, you can start reversing these signs of aging for a younger future. What's more, once you realize you may be developing a symptom or condition, you can accurately link it to your weight gain, instead of being frustrated and wondering why you can't lose weight no matter how hard you try.

The first step is to determine which parts or systems of your body are aging the most rapidly. The following quiz is called my AgePrint. It identifies the oldest parts of your body and sees which ones are affecting not only your health, but also your weight. Once we have this information, we can obtain the aging code of almost every part of your body—then break it.

That's why this unique program serves a dual role. It helps you lose weight *and* it helps you reverse aging. To best use this program, you'll want to individualize the diet to resurrect the parts of your body that are aging the fastest and affecting your ability to lose weight. Knowing the age of every part of your body and identifying your pauses will help you choose the right path toward better health and a more youthful body.

Diagnostic Blood Testing

How do you know you've identified the correct pause? The answer lies with multiple assessments. Aside from the AgePrint, there is advanced testing in the forms of blood work and computer imaging available to detect illness in every part of your body. Ask your doctor to run blood test gauge levels to see if you are currently experiencing any of the beginning stages of illness. These tests are listed in Appendix C.

THE AGEPRINT QUIZ: KNOW THE AGE OF EVERY PART

By completing this simple questionnaire, you are on your way to identifying your personal core markers of aging. You must first discover if any of the pauses have begun to affect your health and ability to lose weight already.

This quiz should not take more than fifteen to twenty minutes, but requires concentration. Try to take this quiz in one sitting. Find a time and a place that is as

Spices Make a Younger You

Spices make every part of your body younger. They enhance your brain chemistry, increase metabolism, and can improve your overall health. Here are the effects of some common ones:

- The anti-inflammatory power of rosemary and basil
- The dementia-fighting power of cumin and sage
- The obesity-fighting power of cayenne and cinnamon
- The sugar-regulating powers of coriander and cinnamon
- The calming affects of lemongrass, nutmeg, bay leaves, and saffron
- The cancer-fighting power of turmeric
- The fungus-beating power of oregano
- The heart-pumping power of garlic, mustard seed, and chicory
- The skin-saving power of basil and thyme

Ignorance Will *Not* be Bliss in 25 Years

Make sure you do a full AgePrint every year. Call it your *other checkup*. You may have to check some parts of your body more frequently than others, if for example, you know you have diabetes or another chronic condition. Having a better sense of the body causes people to work on their health, whether they have issues with glucose levels or bone density. In the words of Maya Angelou, "You did what you knew how to do, and when you knew better, you did better."

stress-free as possible, away from distractions, noise, or other activities. Check your physical state. Postpone taking the quiz if you feel particularly out of sorts, or if you're not well rested or well fed.

Each of the following questions can be answered as either True or False. Try not to think too long on any one question, and answer with regards to how you feel most or all of the time. There are no right answers to this assessment. Remember, we all have weak links, and we are all experiencing one pause or another.

If you want real insight into your health, answer the questions truthfully. It would be more astounding to find out you are not experiencing any pauses than if you discover you are. Some of the questions pertain to specific diagnoses you might have had. Make sure to check your medical records, and ask your physician or research via the Internet any terms you are unfamiliar with.

SCORING

Give yourself 1 point for every **True** response. Then, total your points at the end of each section. Multiply your total score of True responses by 10: This is your Age Code for that system. For example, if your score in the first section is 3, your Age Code for Cardiopause is 30. If your Age Code is younger than your chronological age, you're in good shape. If your Age Code is older than your real age, you need to carefully consider treatment. The earlier you treat each of your failing age codes, the better.

The section with the highest points will be your oldest part, which should be addressed first. After you've seen results by following a particular treatment regimen described in this book, take the test again to see what other areas of your health can be improved. You may see that when one Age Code is adjusted, other areas of your overall health may benefit as well. For example, by reversing aging in one area, you may find that you can finally lose the weight that you want without much further effort.

This version of the AgePrint quiz specifically relates to your weight issues. For an entire AgePrint, check out my website: www.youngeryoubook.com

GROUP 1: THE OVERWORKED CARDIOPULMONARY AND VASCULAR SYSTEMS

CARDIOPAUSE:

1. I have swollen legs.	T / F
2. I experience shortness of breath when I exercise.	T / F
3. I have experienced lightheadedness or have had episodes of loss of consciousness.	T / F
4. I have been told I have a heart murmur.	T / F
5. I have difficulty breathing when lying down.	T / F
6. I have a rapid heart beat.	T / F
7. I have been told I have an abnormal heart rhythm.	T / F
8. I have a cough that does not go away.	T / F
9. I have experienced pain, discomfort, heaviness and pressure in my chest.	T / F
10. My lips are often a bluish color.	T / F

Number of True Responses: _____ × 10 = **Cardiopause Age Code** _____

VASCULOPAUSE:

1. I have had blood clots.	T / F
2. I have cold hands and feet.	T / F
3. I see more veins on my legs than I used to.	T / F
4. My ankles, on occasion, swell.	T / F
5. I have had ulcers on my lower legs.	T / F
6. I have dry, thin, flaky skin.	T / F
7. My nails are soft and brittle.	T / F
8. The skin on my lower legs has turned to a darker or reddish shade.	T / F
9. I have lost hair on my lower legs.	T / F
10. I experience pain in my calves when I walk.	T / F

Number of True Responses: _____ × 10 = **Vasculopause Age Code** _____

GROUP 2: AGING METABOLISM AND IMMUNITY

IMMUNOPAUSE:

1. I have noticed more warts on my skin.	T / F
2. I have found many cysts on my body.	T / F
3. Cuts or bruises seem to take longer to heal.	T / F
4. I've gained weight only in the last three years.	T / F
5. I have a persistent cough that won't go away.	T / F
6. I have had frequent sinus or ear infections.	T / F
7. I have bloating or fullness in my abdomen that isn't related to food.	T / F
8. I have seen blood in my urine.	T / F
9. I never really feel hungry, but I eat anyway.	T / F
10. I often need to regulate my bowels with laxatives.	T / F

Number of True Responses: _____ × 10 = Immunopause Age Code _____

INSULOPAUSE:

1. I'm thirsty all the time.	T / F
2. I have to urinate frequently throughout the day and night.	T / F
3. I have a protruding belly.	T / F
4. My complexion is pale.	T / F
5. My fingers and/or toes tingle.	T / F
6. My sexual function has diminished.	T / F
7. I have low muscle tone: The skin on my upper arms is sagging.	T / F
8. I have cellulite on my thighs and/or buttocks.	T / F
9. I have frequent pain in my hips since gaining weight.	T / F
10. I have frequent lower back pain since gaining weight.	T / F

Number of True Responses: _____ × 10 = Insulopause Age Code _____

THYROPAUSE

1. I have an enlarged neck.	T / F
2. I feel weak and fatigued most of the time.	T / F
3. I have a greater sensitivity to cold.	T / F
4. I have delayed reflexes.	T / F
5. I have been told I am anemic.	T / F
6. I have a slow heartbeat.	T / F
7. My metabolism has slowed with age.	T / F
8. My menstrual cycle has changed to a heavier flow.	T / F
9. I have difficulty moving my bowels.	T / F
10. I am always hoarse.	T / F

Number of True Responses: _____ × 10 = Thyropause Age Code _____

GROUP 3: CHANGES OF THE SKIN

DERMATOPAUSE:

1. My skin is beginning to sag.	T / F
2. I have many wrinkles.	T / F
3. My skin does not appear as supple as it used to.	T / F
4. I have age spots.	T / F
5. I have skin discolorations. (Add one point for each type: cyst, lump, bump, spider vein, or red spot.)	T / F
6. My skin has lost its glow.	T / F
7. I have been diagnosed with skin cancer.	T / F
8. I have developed a "turkey neck."	T / F
9. I have jowls.	T / F
10. I believe I'm at a high risk for skin cancer because I spent much of my life in the sun without proper protection.	T / F

Number of True Responses: _____ × 10 = Dermatopause Age Code _____

GROUP 4: MUSCULOSKELETAL AGING

OSTEOPAUSE

1. I experience pain in my hips and knees.   T / F

2. I have been diagnosed with osteopenia or osteoporosis.   T / F

3. I have lost inches off my height over the years
   (take your height measurements now to find out, if necessary).   T / F

4. I have broken a bone in the past.   T / F

5. I have a history of either curved spine or
   hunchback/curved posture in my family.   T / F

6. I have weighed less than 126 pounds as an adult.   T / F

7. I abused recreational steroids in the past.   T / F

8. I've missed my period for more than a year.   T / F

9. I have suffered from an eating disorder that caused me to
   lose an excessive amount of weight.   T / F

10. I have fair skin and light eyes.   T / F

Number of True Responses: _____ × 10 = Osteopause Age Code _____

PARATHYROPAUSE:

1. My eyebrows are thinning.   T / F

2. I feel anxious more frequently.   T / F

3. I have blurry vision.   T / F

4. I have been told I have cataracts.   T / F

5. I fall often.   T / F

6. I feel sluggish most of the time.   T / F

7. I have been told my personality has changed.   T / F

8. My muscles twitch at times.   T / F

9. I often have yeast or candida infections.   T / F

10. My doctor has told me that my reflexes have diminished.   T / F

Number of True Responses: _____ × 10 = Parathyropause Age Code _____

SOMATOPAUSE

1. I am starting to get wrinkles.	T / F
2. My hair and nails are not growing as fast as they used to.	T / F
3. My friends have far fewer gray hairs than me.	T / F
4. My skin is thinning.	T / F
5. I am not as tall as I used to be.	T / F
6. I am not as agile as I used to be.	T / F
7. I am not as strong as I used to be.	T / F
8. I have problems opening jars or carrying heavy loads.	T / F
9. I have gained body fat, especially around my waistline.	T / F
10. I have been told that my cholesterol is high.	T / F

Number of True Responses: _____ × 10 = Somatopause Age Code _____

GROUP 5: AGING SEXUALITY

MENOPAUSE: FOR WOMEN ONLY

1. My nails are weaker and chip or split more often.	T / F
2. My vagina is drier than it used to be.	T / F
3. I lose lots of hair each week, and it feels more brittle than before.	T / F
4. My breasts have begun to sag.	T / F
5. I have hot flashes during the day.	T / F
6. I rarely feel like having sex.	T / F
7. My doctor has prescribed estrogen, progesterone, testosterone, or DHEA supplements. (Subtract one point if these substances are natural.)	T / F
8. I am experiencing the beginning stages of osteoporosis or height loss.	T / F
9. I can't remember details as well as I used to.	T / F
10. I have begun to have night sweats.	T / F

Number of True Responses: _____ × 10 = Menopause Age Code _____

ANDROPAUSE: FOR MEN ONLY

1. When I have sex, it takes me a long time to achieve an orgasm. T / F

2. I carry my excess weight on my abdomen. T / F

3. I have diminished sex drive. T / F

4. I have thin arms and legs. T / F

5. I have noticed that my ejaculate is diminished. T / F

6. I do not need to shave as often as when I was younger. T / F

7. I have lost hair on my body. T / F

8. My neck is getting wider and broader. T / F

9. My doctor has told me my testosterone level is diminished. T / F

10. My testicles have shrunk; my scrotum is sagging;
    my penis is smaller. (Add one point for each.) T / F

Number of True Responses: _____ × 10 = Andropause Age Code _____

GROUP 6: AGING DIGESTIVE SYSTEM

GASTROPAUSE

1. I often feel like I have to throw up after eating. T / F

2. I have to take antacids regularly. T / F

3. I feel full quickly. T / F

4. I have had gallstones. T / F

5. I have food intolerances to wheat. T / F

6. I am lactose intolerant. T / F

7. I have loose stools often. T / F

8. I have constipation. T / F

9. I have specific food allergies. T / F

10. I often experience heartburn after a meal. T / F

Number of True Responses: _____ × 10 = Gastropause Age Code _____

It's All about the Brain

When the brain goes haywire, it sets the whole body off in a confused, dizzying spin. Low dopamine drains your energy, and throws off your metabolism so you eat the wrong foods. Lack of acetylcholine throws off your mind. No GABA, and you're not stable, which throws off your health. And without serotonin you lack good sleep, which again throws off your metabolism. As soon as your brain chemistry falls out of rhythm, you can bet that your physical self will get sick.

YOUR PERSONAL AGEPRINT

Record your Age Codes in the chart below. After six months of treatment and following the Younger (Thinner) You Diet, take the test again, and see if your AgePrint has changed. By following the suggestions outlined in the rest of the book, you will be able to chart dramatic improvements in every aspect of your health.

If any one of your Age Codes is more than twenty years older than your actual age range, consider yourself in a severe health category and make an appointment to see your physician immediately.

APPLES VS. PEARS

How you carry your weight is another factor in modifying your diet to create a program that is specific to your individual needs. These instructions are most often

AgePrint Code Worksheet

A more extensive list of pauses can be found on my Web site: www.pathmed.com

	INITIAL AGE CODE	6 MONTHS LATER	9 MONTHS LATER	ONE YEAR LATER	18 MONTHS LATER
Cardiopause					
Immunopause					
Insulopause					
Dermatopause					
Osteopause					
Somatopause					
Menopause					
Andropause					
Gastropause					

applied to women, but men can learn from them as well. Those carrying extra fat around their middle section are considered apple-shaped. Their body fat is stored as visceral fat, putting them at a higher risk for heart disease, type 2 diabetes, breast cancer, stroke, and irregular menstrual cycles. A pear shape has a smaller waist and larger hips, and is at a greater risk for osteoporosis, eating disorders, varicose veins, and poor body image.

Depending on your shape, there are different strategies for losing weight. Regardless of the results of the AgePrint test, you'll need to determine if you are an apple or a pear, and then read the corresponding chapters. An apple-shaped should modify the Younger (Thinner) You Diet

Top Health Conditions Caused by Obesity and Foods That May Help

DISEASE	FOODS	CONTAINS
Heart Disease	Red & purple grapes; garlic, ginger, walnuts, pomegranate, turmeric	Polyphenols (e.g., catechins, oligomeric proanthocyanidins, resveratrol)
High Cholesterol	Avocado, blond psyllium, walnuts, macadamia nuts	Beta-sitosterol
Type 2 Diabetes	Coffee, blond psyllium, glucomannan	Chlorogenic acids and lignans
Hypertension	Pomegranate	Polyphenols (e.g., anthocyanosides and punicosides: cyanidin, ellagic acid)
Stroke (ischemic)	Fish oil, green tea	EPA/DHA
Gallbladder Disease	Artichoke, coffee, ginger	Phenolic acids (e.g., caffeic acid, chlorogenic acid) and polyphenols (e.g., cynarin, luteolin)
Sleep Apnea	Soy (protein forms)	Tryptophan
Breast Cancer	Broccoli	Indoles (indole-3-carbinol) and glucosinolates (e.g., isothiocyanates, sulforaphane)
Prostate Cancer	Garlic	S-allylmercaptocysteine
Colon Cancer	Carrots	Carotenoids (e.g., lutein and zeaxanthin)
Osteoarthritis	Pineapple, avocado, ginger	Bromelain
Fatty Liver Disease	Flaxseeds	Lignans (e.g., matairesinol, secoisolariciresinol)
Poor Wound Healing	Citrus fruit	Bioflavonoids (e.g., hesperidin, rutin)

with foods mentioned in Chapter 11 that will help protect you from heart disease. Pear shapes should review the chapter on maintaining a healthy frame (Chapter 12), which will strengthen bones and ward off osteoporosis.

GOING FORWARD

The remainder of the book will focus on some of the most common pauses and how they contribute to your current weight issues. You will learn what the most common symptoms or related conditions are, and all modalities of treatment. Within each of the chapters, I will provide specific food and spice suggestions that modify the general Younger (Thinner) You Diet for your unique health needs, as well as medical information for each of your issues.

You can begin by reading through the chapter that correlates to your oldest part. Then read through your next highest Age Code, until you have balanced each of them. Along the way, record your progress in the chart above and congratulate yourself on the changes you'll be making towards a Younger You!

CHAPTER 13

Your Health Controls
Your Metabolic Fire

METABOLIC SYNDROME and inflammation affect every organ and system in your body, including your heart, your vascular system, your metabolism, your immune system, and even the condition of your skin. That's why they are called age accelerators: These conditions make your parts older than your chronological age. What's more, both metabolic syndrome and inflammation are conditions that stem from problems with your brain chemistry.

As we learned in Part I, your brain voltage, which is controlled by dopamine, controls your entire metabolic fire. That's why people between the ages of 12 and 20 have the lowest rate of weight gain because their

dopamine and their hormones are at their peak. It was no surprise to me that Olympic swimmer Michael Phelps revealed that he can eat more than 12,000 calories a day and still look as thin as a rail. We could all eat this amount when we were younger, especially if we were aggressively exercising like Phelps does. But as we get older and our dopamine and hormone levels drop, we just can't burn off this amount of food, and then we gain weight.

If your AgePrint shows an increased Age Code in Groups 1, 2, or 3, you may find that by reversing these age accelerators, you can not only improve your health, but finally lose the weight you want. You'll learn how to use specific foods, teas, spices, nutrients, medication, and exercise suggestions with the general Younger (Thinner) You Diet so that you'll be personalizing your program to meet your specific needs. The general Younger (Thinner) You Diet will increase your metabolic fire, which will help to reverse both metabolic syndrome and inflammation.

Your Health Is in Your Hands

There aren't any medical conditions that you should "learn to live with." Illness and discomfort are usually reversible and treatable once you recognize that health and weight problems are interconnected.

DEFINING METABOLIC SYNDROME

Metabolic syndrome is the ultimate chicken/egg debate when it comes to health and obesity. This syndrome is actually a collection of risk factors that signify an increased risk for heart disease, stroke, and type 2 diabetes. First identified in the 1950s, it is estimated that roughly 47 million American adults have been told that they have metabolic syndrome. Women with metabolic syndrome have a three times higher risk of dying from a heart attack or stroke, compared with women who don't have metabolic syndrome. Additionally, they have a nine to thirty times greater risk of developing type 2 diabetes. Yet it's hard to tell which comes first: the weight gain that leads to metabolic syndrome, or an aging body that develops metabolic syndrome that leads to weight gain?

The exact cause of metabolic syndrome is still unknown, although it is most closely associated with insulin resistance (which is why it is often a precursor to type 2 diabetes) and stress. Advanced age and excessive weight automatically increases your risk for developing metabolic syndrome. Living a sedentary lifestyle, eating a high-carbohydrate diet, smoking, and being postmenopausal all increase your chances of developing the syndrome.

I define metabolic syndrome from a brain chemistry perspective. Metabolic syndrome is primarily a loss of metabolism: a low dopamine condition. The other brain chemicals are involved as well. Acetylcholine is linked

The Shape of Metabolic Syndrome

Most people with metabolic syndrome and insulin resistance are apple-shaped, meaning their concentration of body fat tends to be on their midsection, including breasts, stomach, and abdomen. This is true for both men and women.

to diabetes (see chapter 4). Most postmenopausal women are low in GABA: In fact, most people in general are low in GABA. And, without proper amounts of serotonin, your brain can't reboot during rest, leading to a greater decrease in brainpower.

If you have three of the following risk factors, you may be diagnosed with metabolic syndrome:

- Elevated waist circumference (abdominal obesity); men 40" or greater, women 35" or greater
- Elevated triglycerides (greater than 150 mg/dL)
- Reduced high-density lipoprotein cholesterol (HDL-C or "good" cholesterol); men less than 40 mg/dL, Women less than 50 mg/dL
- Elevated blood pressure (greater than or equal to 130/85 mmHg)
- Elevated fasting glucose (greater than 110 mg/dL)

Blood Pressure and Food

The cornerstone of lowering blood pressure is the reduction of salt and bad fats; the same prescription as the Younger (Thinner) You Diet.

AVOIDING—OR REVERSING—METABOLIC SYNDROME

The good news is that you can prevent or reverse the damaging effects of metabolic syndrome by making key changes to your lifestyle. By adapting a low-carb diet like the one I've outlined in the Younger (Thinner) You Diet, you'll lower your risk for metabolic syndrome and its related disorders.

Vitamin D is known to control metabolic syndrome and help you lose weight.[1] We can get all the vitamin D we need from daily exposure to the sun: All you need is twenty minutes outdoors. What's more, there's plenty of vitamin D available in a well-balanced diet, like the one featured in this book. If you aren't getting outside much, you can choose to supplement with vitamin D as well.

Medications are often needed to control the individual diseases associated with this syndrome. For example, if you have been diagnosed with hypertension, your doctor may be treating you with diuretics or ACE inhibitors. Cholesterol drugs may be used as well if increased cholesterol is present. Diabetes is the ultimate presentation of metabolic syndrome's result.

DIABETES

If you have been diagnosed with diabetes, you need to eat lots of lean proteins at each meal, and to restrict your sugar and starch intake. You also need to choose fiber-rich whole grains to release glucose in a steady stream to moderate blood sugar levels. The Younger (Thinner) You Diet has tons of food options to support these specific needs, including:

- Eggs
- Flaxseed oil
- Lamb
- Lean beef
- Low-fat cottage cheese
- Nuts and seeds (raw): almonds, sesame seeds, hazelnuts, cashews
- Poultry
- Soybeans and soy products
- Tuna
- Veal
- Yogurt: plain, fat-free, no sugar added

IMPORTANT NUTRIENTS FOR NORMALIZING BLOOD SUGAR

Review Chapter 7 for specific foods and spices that contain these nutrients:

- Psyllium and other fiber sources, guar gum, bilberry leaf extract: These slow glucose absorption and prevent blood sugar spikes
- Essential fatty acids prevent insulin resistance
- Chromium, potassium, zinc: These may help to prevent arrhythmias for diabetics
- Fish oil improves insulin sensitivity, optimizes blood lipids
- Lipoic acid supports healthy nerve function
- Bilberry fruit extract provides antioxidant and circulatory support
- Biotin, folic acid, inositol, vitamins A, C, D, E, may decrease insulin resistance

HIGH-GLYCEMIC FOODS: CAMOUFLAGED SUGAR

The glycemic index is an important tool for diabetics. It ranks foods on how they affect blood sugar levels. It concentrates on foods that are high in carbohydrates. Foods high in fat or protein don't cause your blood sugar level to rise much, but most packaged foods will.

A complete glycemic index includes fresh foods as well as packaged or manufactured products, and can be found on various Internet health sites, including www. glycemicindex.com.

FOOD	AMOUNT	GLYCEMIC LOAD
Strawberries	½ cup	1
Carrots	½ cup cooked	1.5
Peach	1 medium	3
Green peas	⅓ cup	3
Grapefruit	½ cup	3
Cashew nuts	¼ cup	3
Beets	¼ cup	3.2
Pumpkin	⅓ cup, peeled, boiled	4.5
Watermelon	½ cup	4.3
Apricots	½ cup	5
Oranges	½ cup	5
Split peas	⅔ cup, boiled	5.2
Apples	½ cup	6
Kiwi	½ cup	6
Table sugar	2 teaspoons	6.5
Parsnips	⅓ cup	7.5
Lentils	½ cup cooked	8
Mango	½ cup	8
Grapes, green	½ cup	8
Sweet potato, peeled, boiled	⅓ cup	8.6
Whole wheat bread	1 slice	9.6
Brown rice	½ cup cooked	16
Banana	1 medium	17.6
Dates	¼ cup, dried	42

Bananas Beat Stroke

Potassium supplements, or potassium-rich foods, like bananas, may help to reduce the incidence of stroke. Potassium can stimulate GABA production, naturally calming you down and lowering your risk for high blood pressure.

I've listed some of my favorite Younger (Thinner) You foods (page 245) so that you can see how they rate. Certain nutrient-dense foods may seem surprising that they are on the list of foods to avoid. For example, if you know that you have diabetes or metabolic syndrome, carrots should be eaten sparingly because they have a higher impact on blood sugar levels than other vegetables. Swap out carrots and other high-glycemic foods from the recipes to tailor the diet to your needs. However, eating carrots is still much better than eating junk food. They may have a higher glycemic rating, but they're still loaded with vitamins, minerals, antioxidants, and nutrients.

A Glycemic Load of 20+ is regarded as high.
A Glycemic Load of 11 to 19 is regarded as medium.
A Glycemic Load of 10 or less is regarded as low.

We Are All "In-flamed"

Inflammation, or swelling, can occur anywhere in the body. Just eating the wrong foods can make us bloated, or inflamed, everywhere: The fix is easy: By taking care of yourself with more sleep and following the Younger (Thinner) You Diet—which includes lots of spices from rosemary to basil—you can reverse the inflammatory processes.

INFLAMMATION

Inflammation is the body's natural defense again foreign objects, and can occur spontaneously in any organ or internal system. Like metabolic syndrome, inflammation is one of the primary sources of aging, leading to infections and autoimmune deficiencies, and even cancers. It is also one of the hidden triggers to cardiovascular disease, increasing your risk for a heart attack or stroke. And just like metabolic syndrome, inflammation is directly connected to weight gain. Research shows that eating large quantities of sugar and bad fats creates inflammation throughout the entire body. It makes sense that the more toxic or unnatural foods you put in your body, the more inflammation your body will produce and the faster you will age.

After only a few days of following an anti-inflammatory diet will you see results, some of which include increased energy and fewer wrinkles. Your skin will feel tighter and more youthful. Your mind will be sharper. You will no longer need that extra cup of morning coffee. And you will no longer crave junk food as your body begins to detoxify. Long-term results include increased stamina, improved immunity, better circulation, smoother digestion and elimination, stronger muscles and bones, better memory and attention, improved cardiovascular functioning, and an overall improved sense of well-being.

Viruses Can Cause Obesity

Recent studies have shown that certain viruses can cause obesity. The human adenovirus and hepatitis C viruses, and possibly other viruses as well, damage the brain's dopamine chemistry, resulting in chronic fatigue. Fatigue in turn is an age accelerator that contributes to obesity:[2] Who can exercise when you are tired all the time?

These studies provide even more evidence that obesity is not simply the result poor self-control, but is often caused by an underlying issue. When viruses are the culprit, the cause is really immunopause: inflammation that leads to infection. Whether the problem originated with a brain chemical imbalance, an endocrine issue, or a virus, the paradigm of obesity as a disease that is completely "brought upon by oneself" has to go. Discriminating against people with obesity makes as much sense as blaming a person for catching a cold.

FIGHT INFLAMMATION WITH YOUNGER (THINNER) YOU FOODS

If you have been diagnosed with any sort of inflammation or immune deficiency, modify the Younger (Thinner) You Diet by focusing on the following foods, and staying away from red meat. Many of the recipes in Chapter 10 include these ingredients:

- Almonds
- Avocados
- Beans
- Beef liver
- Blackberries
- Blueberries
- Bran
- Broccoli
- Brown rice
- Carrots
- Cranberries
- Flaxseed
- Garlic
- Ginger
- Green tea
- Hazelnuts
- Herbal teas
- Kale
- Mackerel
- Olive oil (room temperature only)
- Poultry (remove skin)
- Raspberries
- Red pepper
- Safflower oil (for cooking)
- Salmon
- Spinach
- Strawberries
- Sweet potatoes
- Tomatoes
- Tuna
- Vinegar
- Winter squash

GREEN TEA IS KEY TO REBUILDING YOUR METABOLIC FIRE

It's never too late or too early to start drinking green tea. Habitual tea consumption for more than ten years is associated with a

Other Foods High in ECGC

- Apples
- Berries
- Cocoa
- Onions
- Wine

smaller waist and a lower percentage of body fat. What's more, green tea can reduce the effects of metabolic syndrome, reduce inflammation, and improve cardiovascular health.

Green tea is packed with antioxidants; specifically the polyphenol catechin called epigallocatechin gallate (EGCG). In fact, green tea has more EGCG than any other plant. Several 2007 studies have shown that EGCG can significantly improve cardiovascular and metabolic health in both the short and the long term. One study from Boston University School of Medicine clearly linked increased consumption of EGCG with improved vascular functioning as well as reduced cardiovascular risk.

A second, multinational study connected green tea with metabolic improvement and a reduction of blood sugar levels in patients with impaired glucose tolerance. This study proved that drinking green tea (as well as taking green tea supplements) can increase fat oxidation at rest and during physical activity. It can also reduce body fat and prevent the accumulation of fat when combined with a healthy, balanced diet like the Younger (Thinner) You Diet.[3]

The key to success is to drink enough tea to make a difference. You may need as much as 5 to 6 cups a day for the best effect, depending on your current weight and amount of abdominal fat. Discuss these findings with your doctor to determine your exact daily intake of green tea to support your weight loss goals.

HELP YOUR HEART

Metabolic syndrome and inflammation are both linked to heart disease. If you are experiencing one or both of these issues, you may have a tough time losing weight. If you've been diagnosed with any type of cardiovascular disease, it's a sign your heart has been working harder than it's supposed to, using lots of your body's energy, which then depletes your metabolism. At the same time, you may be increasingly fatigued and too tired to exercise. These two scenarios directly contribute to weight gain. Stress, tension, and nervousness can contribute to hypertension. Yet a person can be calm and

Antioxidants Support Exercise and Reduce Inflammation

Antioxidants like vitamins A, E, and beta-carotene are well known as cancer-busting nutrients. A 2006 study published in the journal *Obesity* shows that they also reduce inflammation and oxidative stress during exercise. This means that if you supplement with these antioxidants, or eat any of the Younger (Thinner) You foods that are high in antioxidants (see chapter 7), you will be able to get more out of your workout.

Yo-Yo Dieting Hurts More Than Your Ego

Losing and regaining weight is not only frustrating, it's bad for your health. A study from the Fred Hutchinson Cancer Research Center in Seattle showed that women who had gained and lost weight more than five times had consistently damaged their immune system, while women whose weight had been stable were not compromised.[8] Because the Younger (Thinner) You Diet is a diet for life, you won't have to stop this eating plan once you've lost the weight you want, putting an end to yo-yo dieting for good.

relaxed and still have high blood pressure, especially if they are overweight.

However, you can reverse—and certainly prevent—your heart from aging. If your Age-Print for cardiopause is more than twenty years above your chronological age, you need to be seen by a physician at least once a year who will manage your weight loss as well as your cardiac health. Your condition should be carefully assessed with a complete battery of tests. Besides the ejection fraction test (which is typically conducted with a noninvasive ultrasound), other tests will include an EKG or twenty-four-hour continuous EKG to detect arrhythmias, CT angiography to monitor for coronary artery disease, and a complete blood workup, including C-reactive protein and interleukins, homocysteine, cholesterol and other blood lipids, atrial (ANP), and B-type (BNP) natriuretic peptides.

REVERSE YOUR AGING HEART WITH YOUNGER (THINNER) YOU SUPER FOODS

By following the Younger (Thinner) You Diet, which is rich in fruits, vegetables,

healthy whole grains, and lots of low-fat proteins, you may be able to get your heart disease under control so that you will have more energy and better metabolism. Losing as little as 10% of your current body weight is often enough to see significant health improvements.

Younger (Thinner) You foods are low in sodium, which will naturally reduce internal swelling and water retention. They also replace high-risk foods that create cholesterol with low-risk foods that are rich in omega-3 fats as well as bioflavonoids, which possess amazing medicinal powers that improve circulation and strengthen the walls of blood vessels.

If you know that you have issues concerning your heart, you'll also need to focus on GABA foods that include fiber-rich fruits, vegetables, and complex carbohydrates. Fiber is essential in reducing the risk

A Healthy Immune System Comes from a Balanced Brain

The brain controls the immune system. A high dopamine and acetylcholine brain suppresses autoimmunity. A high serotonin and GABA brain suppresses infection.

of heart disease (not to mention some types of cancer, gallstones, obesity, diabetes and intestinal disease). Not enough dietary fiber leads to a lack of bile/cholesterol binding, allowing cholesterol to be reabsorbed back into the bloodstream, where it can damage arteries.

Remember, there are two types of fiber: Insoluble fiber, from grains, legumes, fruits, and the outer surface of some seeds (insoluble fiber promotes food passage and adds bulk, which reduces food cravings), and soluble fiber, which acts as a filter to help prevent cholesterol and glucose and other substances from being absorbed into the blood. A complete list of high-fiber foods is found in Chapter 7.

Additionally, choose fruits and vegetables that are high in folic acid and other B vitamins. Folic acid is a B vitamin that helps the body make healthy new cells and prevents an increase in homocysteine, an amino acid in the blood. According to the American Heart Association, epidemiological studies have shown that too much homocysteine in the blood (plasma) is related to a higher risk of coronary heart disease, stroke and peripheral vascular disease.[4] A study conducted by the *New England Journal of Medicine* shows that those with high levels of homocysteine and low levels of folic acid were twice as likely have arteries that were clogged at least 25% of the time.[5] If your diet is rich in fruits, vegetables, legumes, and whole grains, you should be getting enough folic acid in your foods.

9 POWERHOUSE SPICES THAT HELP THE HEART

Specific spices have amazing antiaging effects on the heart and support weight loss at the same time. For example, turmeric has been shown to have both antioxidant and anti-inflammatory effects that combat heart disease. Other important herbs and spices include:

- **Cayenne** helps control heart disease risk factors including high blood cholesterol and blood platelet aggregation.[6]
- **Cinnamon** reduces blood sugar levels in type 2 diabetics, improves glucose metabolism and the overall condition of individuals with diabetes by improving cholesterol metabolism, removing artery-damaging free radicals from the blood, and improving function of small blood vessels.[7]
- **Garlic** reduces blood pressure, helps maintain the elastic properties of the body's main artery, the aorta, prevents blood from clotting, greatly reducing your risk for a heart attack or stroke. Garlic can also help disperse fibrin, reducing your chance of many heart problems. Garlic can also boost the immune system.[8]
- **Ginger** is an effective antiseptic for acute viral respiratory infections, stimulates the functioning of stomach, can help abate nausea and sea sickness, and gives a boost to metabolism and skin nourishment. It is believed to be a good remedy for enhancing the sex urge in males and helps to combat inflammation of the prostate gland.[9]

- **Mustard seed** is an excellent source of selenium and magnesium. Like selenium, magnesium reduces the severity of asthma, lowers high blood pressure, restores normal sleep patterns in women having difficulty with the symptoms of menopause, reduces the frequency of migraine attacks, and prevents heart attack in patients suffering from atherosclerosis or diabetic heart disease.[10]

- **Onion** lowers high cholesterol levels and high blood pressure, helping prevent atherosclerosis and diabetic heart disease, and reducing the risk of heart attack or stroke.[11]

- **Peppermint oil** has been used to help reduce heart palpitations, improves the heartbeat, improves circulation throughout the body, and keeps your blood pumping strong. In addition to peppermint oil, you may also find some benefit from peppermint tea.[12]

- **Rosemary** contains caffeic acid and rosmarinic acid, both potent antioxidant and anti-inflammatory agents. These two natural acids are effective at reducing the inflammation that contributes to asthma, liver disease and heart disease.[13]

- **Turmeric** contains antioxidant and anti-inflammatory effects that combat heart disease. Additionally, it helps prevent heart disease by lowering cholesterol and preventing the formation of the blood clots that trigger heart attack (and many strokes).[14]

RED AND PURPLE PROTECT YOUR HEART—NATURALLY

Eating red and purple (indigo and violet) foods keep your heart pumping. Phytonutrients like lycopene and anthocyanins are found in abundance in raspberries, cherries, tomatoes, and watermelon and reduce the risk of heart-related illnesses, including heart attacks. Review the red, indigo, and violet lists in Chapter 7 for a complete resource of great fresh red fruits and vegetables.

Red and purple grapes, including their seeds and skins, have a host of impressive nutrients. But you don't have to overindulge in red wine to get all of grape's benefits. A study from Greece showed that people with diseased arteries received the same benefits from a single glass of alcohol-free red wine as they did with a glass of the harder, more calorie-laden stuff. In other

Eat Nuts (Sparingly) for Heart Health

Researchers from Harvard Medical School and the Harvard School of Public Health[15] have examined the effect of eating nuts on cardiovascular health. They have found that nuts are a wise dietary choice, especially for men at risk for heart disease. Healthy men, and those who have already suffered a heart attack, can reduce cardiovascular risk by eating nuts regularly. Just watch your serving size: Nuts are nutrient dense but highly caloric. Don't eat more than ¼ cup (a single handful) of any nuts in one sitting.

Meet Michael R.: Younger and Thinner by Taking Care of His Heart

When Michael was 36, he came to see me, practically dragging himself through my door. He was 6' 2" and tipped the scales at 250 pounds. He immediately blurted out, "Doc, I have these scary chest pains and I think that I'm dying of heart disease." He already had three stents surgically implanted in his heart, but his doctors were telling him that they weren't doing enough. Michael wanted to know, "How can I save my life?"

I sat Michael down and told him that his problem was much bigger than just his heart. Then I performed a full workup to check out his health. Michael was a roly-poly, sweaty, beefy guy who looked like his skin belonged on a 70-year-old. I found that he had a mass on his thyroid, which was completely exhausting its hormone production. His muscle mass was that of a 70-year-old. His obesity seemed to point at a brain metabolism dopamine deficit. In fact, Michael told me that for most of his life he'd been using carbohydrates, salt, and sugar as stimulants.

What was most surprising, and probably a shock for Michael, was that he was not about to have a heart attack: The stents had been implanted to prevent vasospasms caused by anxiety attacks. However, his myocardium (the thick muscular layer making up the major portion of your heart) was inflamed. This was the likely culprit for his vague chest pain and abnormal heartbeat. But even with his weakened heart, Michael was still more at risk for stroke than heart attack; he was more at risk of dying from a broken bone.

Michael was stunned when we showed him his tests, including his brain map, a PET scan that revealed the thyroid nodule, and his low bone density. We showed him the changes in his carotid artery thickness, his damaged skin, and his fatty liver. What he saw was the crushing, unnecessary blow to his family, the devastation, the hole in their lives his death would cause.

I started Michael on the Younger (Thinner) You Diet along with the right nutrients, hormones, and medications to help his various problems. A natural thyroid treatment shrunk his thyroid nodule, his dopamine treatment cut his appetite. Sleep aids gave him the sleep that helped reverse his sluggish brain metabolism. Natural repair hormones strengthened his bones and muscles. N-Acetyl cysteine and lipoic acid cleaned out his liver. Within a year, Michael looked and felt significantly better. He dropped more than 50 pounds, and repeatedly thanked me every time he came into the office. He knew that we were able to show him his new future, one where he lived a healthy and happy life.

Put Eggs Back on Your Breakfast Plate

Eggs used to be off-limits because of their high cholesterol content. However, research has shown that foods such as eggs, which are high in dietary cholesterol, do not raise blood cholesterol levels by more than 2%. Rich in amino acids, eggs are a perfect protein, increasing your feeling of fullness so you won't overeat at your next meal. Choose eggs that are enhanced with omega-3s: They contain five times the omega-3s found in ordinary eggs. Then sprinkle your eggs with your favorite spices and create a Younger (Thinner) You superfood!

words, it's the red in the grape juice that's good for you, not the alcohol.

The latest findings show that whole grape extract is a calorie-free way to get all the benefits of eating grapes. Grape extract supports cardiac health and reduces inflammation, and encourages collagen growth, which is the underlying supporting structure of the skin.[16] This means using grape extract supports a Younger You both internally and externally.

NATURAL SUPPLEMENTS FOR A YOUNGER HEART AND A YOUNGER (THINNER) YOU

Cholesterol is the precursor to pregnenolone and DHEA: the miracle hormones that turn into nutrients that are critical to your heart's health. They help keep cortisol, the stress hormone, under control. Yet as we age the body loses its ability to convert cholesterol, so we need to supplement. Here are some other supplements to help your heart:

- Fish oil, to prevent blood clots
- Niacin, helps raise your "good" HDL cholesterol

- Taurine, to improve your heart's pumping action and reduce stress
- Inositol, to reduce stress
- Melatonin, to promote sleep
- B-complex vitamins to reduce homocysteine
- Policosanol is a mixture of eight solid alcohols extracted from sugar cane that has a remarkable ability to both lower "bad" LDL-cholesterol and increase "good" HDL-cholesterol

YOUR THYROID IS JUST AS IMPORTANT AS YOUR HEART

The thyroid is a gland in the neck that many people blame their weight issues on, and they are often right. The thyroid is an overrated but underdiagnosed gland that controls the rate at which your body burns the fuel necessary to keep you going. It does so by synthesizing the hormones thyroxine (T4) and triiodothyronine (T3). These thyroid hormones help regulate fat digestion, and increase intestinal absorption of carbohydrates. While metabolic syndrome is not associated with the thyroid per se, it is an important gland

Nutrients for Reversing Heart Disease

NATURAL TREATMENTS	SUGGESTED DAILY DOSAGE
CoQ10	25 to 1200 mg
Carnitine	500 to 5000 mg
Hawthorne	200 to 1000 mg
Magnesium	300 to 1000 mg
Potassium	3000 to 5000 mg
Fish oils (EPA and DHA)	500 to 3000 mg
Garlic	500 to 3000 mg
Policosanol	5 to 20 mg
Vitamin B_6, B_{12}	B_6: 10 to 500 mg, B_{12}: 100 to 5000 mcg
Folic acid	200 to 1000 mcg
Betaine	500 to 5000 mg
ISO flavonoids	200 mg
Taurine	500 to 10000 mg
Tocotrienols (Vitamin E)	50 to 200 mg
Niacin (Vitamin B_3)	50 to 3000 mg

that you need to be aware of, and learn how to manage for better health.

Thyropause marks the beginning of a metabolic disorder, which frequently begins between the ages of 30 and 40. The changes that occur are often so subtle that without taking an AgePrint, you may not know if you are experiencing thyropause. However, if you know that you have a dopamine deficiency, you are a likely candidate for experiencing thyropause sooner than you think. There is a distinct relationship between your thyroid and a dopamine deficiency. While you can augment your dopamine with foods and nutrients, the thyroid really needs more of its own stuff, namely natural, bioidentical hormones, to get it back in proper working order.

Your thyroid health may require bioidentical supplementation of the hormones T3 and T4. T3, or three iodine molecules on a thyroid hormone, is associated with a decrease in aging as it augments the functions of many nutrients. It can lead to an improvement in mood. Combined with T4 and iodine, it is the most effective way of sustaining a healthy thyroid throughout your life. When this happens, you'll see that it will be much easier for you to lose weight.

FOODS TO AVOID FOR A HEALTHIER THYROID

If your AgePrint shows you are experiencing thyropause, stay away from a group of foods known as goitrogens. These foods interfere with the function of the thyroid gland. They include all the cruciferous vegetables, including cauliflower, Brussels sprouts, broccoli, cabbage, kale, kohlrabi, mustard greens, rutabaga, and turnips. Soybeans and soy-related foods—peaches, strawberries, peanuts, radishes, spinach, and millet—are also goitrogens.

All of these foods are most dangerous in their raw states: Cooking seems to temper their negative properties. However, it's best to avoid them entirely.

GOOD NUTRITION WILL SAVE YOUR SKIN

Skin damage starts from the inside, not the outside. It is often linked to issues of inflammation or dehydration. Both of these are acetylcholine-related conditions. Without the proper amounts of water—which means neither too much nor too little—your skin will begin to age. Add weight gain to the equation, in which you are literally stretching your skin, and you are creating an unhealthy scenario: Poor skin not only looks bad, but will no longer function as a protective organ.

I know that creams and emollients are temporary fixes for your skin. If you want healthy, supple, vibrant skin, you need to work from the inside out, and eradicate the damage that you have caused. Research, not department stores, is on my side with this way of thinking. A team of researchers at Monash University in Melbourne, Australia, looked at whether food and nutrient levels are associated with skin wrinkling. The study surveyed over 400 adults living in Australia, Greece, and Sweden. Those who ate a diet high in vegetables, olive oil, fish, and legumes and low in butter, margarine, dairy, and sugar products had the least amount of skin wrinkling. The authors speculate that this may be due to the high levels of antioxidants found in the beneficial foods. To keep your skin healthy and young, you can start by controlling inflammation, using inflammation-fighting foods from the list on page 247.

HERBS AND SPICES THAT SOOTHE YOUR SKIN

Spices and herbs can help your skin from the inside out. They are also beneficial when applied topically, although they are not as effective. Use this list as a reference for when you shop for bath and body products. Read these suggestions and follow the packages' directions accordingly:

- **Basil** is a blood purifier that kills the bacteria that causes acne.
- **Bay leaf** (cook with but do not eat) added to bathwater relieves aching limbs.

- **Chamomile** is believed to rejuvenate skin and hair. Tea facials are soothing, and when applied at least three times a day can help with skin irritations and sunburns. Chamomile products are ideal for replenishing and enriching dry or sensitive skin. It is a bactericidal, anti-itching, soothing, antiseptic, refreshing to the skin, and reduces swelling. The herb can also soothe burns and scalds, skin rashes, and sores.
- **Clove oil** can be used in a cream or lotion, and can help heal leg ulcers and skin sores. Use in low dilution of less than one percent.
- **Hyssop**, used as a cream or lotion can help skin heal without permanent scarring. It can also be used to help disperse bruising.
- **Juniper berries** can help soothe itchy skin.
- **Lavender oil** is useful for all types of skin problems such as abscesses, acne, oily skin, boils, burns, sunburn, wounds, psoriasis. It is a powerful insect repellent that works against head or body lice, and can treat insect bites or stings.
- **Lemon balm** is an excellent mosquito repellant.

Don't Say No to Liver

Liver contains iron and copper, which can help to improve the glow of your skin and hair.

- **Rosemary** helps ease congestion, puffiness, and swelling and can also be used for acne, dermatitis, and eczema. It is beneficial for improving blood circulation and decongesting the skin. Use topically in cream or lotion form.
- **Thyme or mint** can help with itchy skin: Try adding to a bath, combining it with mint and basil for an even more effective salve. You can also brew thyme like a tea and dip a washcloth in it. Run the washcloth gently all over the body to ease itchy skin.

COLORFUL FOODS LEAD TO HEALTHY SKIN

Beautiful skin comes from being well hydrated, so it's very important to drink lots of water throughout the day. Fruits are filled with water, which will help hydrate your skin. The colorful foods I've been talking about throughout this book will naturally afford your skin some protection against the sun's damaging UV rays just by eating them. For the most sun protection, choose fruits and vegetables with a red or orange hue. Dark green and yellow-orange foods rich in vitamin A will improve the look and feel of your skin. Citrus fruits that are filled with vitamin C will increase your skin's collagen, making it feel and appear plumper. Red rooibos tea is packed with alpha hydroxy acid, known to promote healthy skin.

SUPPLEMENTS YOUR SKIN CAN'T LIVE WITHOUT

Vitamin C and lysine protect your skin against cancer. They are also essential for the production of collagen, which degrades with age, so consider adding both to your daily supplement regimen. Vitamin D also prevents and reverses skin aging. Zinc is nothing short of amazing; it promotes skin healing and is beneficial to skin and hair health.

COMMERCIAL SKIN TREATMENTS THAT REALLY WORK

With your skin being the largest organ of the body, it seems wise to try to preserve it. But most women find that wrinkle creams fail them. This is because for the most part, the nutrients in these creams that are the most vital to the skin cannot penetrate its deeper layers. Some products can help remove the dead outer layer of skin or hydrate the skin and plump it up, giving the appearance of reduced wrinkles. But once you stop using the product, the wrinkles return, so ongoing use of the product can become expensive.

Another issue is that we make decisions about skin-care regimens based solely on marketing. We often purchase the creams that are the most gloriously advertised, instead of looking at their key ingredients. Many supposed wrinkle remedies do little more than clog pores and leave skin feeling greasy.

With new research coming to light regarding the harmful effects of Botox use, I'm steering my patients away from injections and back to more natural Younger (Thinner) You treatments. The best approach to beautiful skin is three dimensional: incorporating proper diet, supplementing with antioxidants, and applying topical moisturizers containing peptides. Science has proven that it is possible to reverse skin damage and promote cell rejuvenation with antiaging peptides. Peptides regulate cell function and maximize collagen production by stimulating the growth of collagen cells resulting in the reduction of fine lines and wrinkles. Peptides are able to penetrate the skin, reaching the vital under-layers.

A special combination of peptides known as pentapeptides have yielded the best results. Researchers have found that this chain of amino acids works synergistically to increase skin thickness and improve texture. The key ingredient is palmityl pentapeptide (also known as Matrixyl); look for this ingredient when buying moisturizers. Add argeline to the mix and you have a topical Botox alternative. Argeline, also known as acetyl-hexapeptide-3, is another peptide that relaxes the muscles in the face. To date, no side effects have been reported from the use of moisturizers containing peptides.

CHAPTER 14

Protect Your Bones and Maintain Muscle Mass

WE ALL WANT to have a lean, athletic body that will support an active lifestyle now and long into the future. That is the intention of The Younger (Thinner) You Diet: to help you achieve the body you deserve so you will be healthy and full of life forever. But being thin is not enough when your frame isn't strong. Thin and weak does not equal lasting health. Neither does remaining obese with signs of osteoporosis. Looking thin and frail might be all the rage, but it's bad for your overall physical and mental health. Weak bones and muscles mean a more sedentary lifestyle that is bad for the knees and hips as well as the heart and the waistline. This chapter will teach you something amazing: You can be thin and still have significant bone density as well as a healthy muscle mass.

If you are having problems with your muscles or bones, you aren't in great shape. In fact, your aging frame may be exactly what is holding you back from losing the weight you want. If your AgePrint highlighted an aging code in Group 4, you may already be experiencing the symptoms and conditions of aging muscles or bones.

As we get older, our "frame" begins to degrade and wither. Our joints start feeling achy, our bones weaken, and our muscles become tense and painful. These conditions can be halted, and even reversed, with proper care and attention. And you have to start now. Preserving bone and muscle mass is absolutely vital for healthy aging and weight loss. You need strong bones for mobility, so you can preserve metabolism-boosting muscle through exercise. And as you'll see at the end of this chapter, working out supports your health as it helps your muscles, bones, and brain stay young.

BONES AND BRAIN CHEMISTRY

Your bones and muscles are affected by three separate pauses: osteopause, parathyropause, and somatopause. Each of these pauses is governed by particular brain chemicals and their hormonal counterparts.

All of these are related to the brain chemical acetylcholine and issues of internal dryness. If you have an acetylcholine deficiency, chances are that you may also be experiencing the symptoms and conditions of aging muscles and bones. That's because our bones and muscles require lots of moisture to remain flexible. Without the proper amounts of moisture, our bones will become weaker and more brittle, and our muscles will become tense and painful.

The aging acetylcholine deficient brain can also trigger the joint system to age prematurely, which manifests as arthritis. Without the right levels of acetylcholine, the brain then pulls on the body's calcium resources in the bones to add moisture to the system, thereby drying up the bones as well (osteoporosis). And while your body is crying out for more calcium, your brain responds, forcing you to replace your lost acetylcholine with fatty foods to add moisture to your dry bones and get the calcium you desperately need. You can guess what happens next: weight gain. In order to stop this cycle, you've already learned how to

Look Deeply into Your Soles

Do your shoes wear unevenly at the heels or toes? If so, you may be experiencing bone loss: As your body shifts disproportionately, your gait is compromised. If your closet is filled with lopsided shoes, get a bone density test, now!

balance your acetylcholine and increase it to more youthful levels. Now you'll take those recommendations and add these illness specific ideas to create a personalized Younger (Thinner) You program.

OSTEOPAUSE: YOU'VE GOT OLD BONES

Osteopause refers to the weakening of the bones, and is more commonly known as osteoporosis, or loss of bone density. Bone is living tissue that is composed of a soft, porous center encased in a hard outer surface. Osteoporosis occurs when the density of the porous center is much less than the outer surface, and the bone literally collapses on itself. When this occurs, the bones throughout the

Are You Aging Your Own Bones?

You may not realize you are causing the wear and tear of your frame. A "yes" to any of these questions means you are aging yourself:

1. Do you stand or walk on hard surfaces for more than four hours daily?
2. Do you participate regularly in any physical sport (basketball, baseball, tennis, golf, bowling, etc.)?
3. Have you ever injured your knee, back, or neck?
4. Are you not exercising at all?

Meet Sophia R.: Her Old Bones Made Her Gain Weight

Sophia, a 57-year-old mother and grandmother, came into my office complaining of annoying aches and pains. A bone density scan revealed significantly low bone density for a woman her age. This was surprising, given that she exercised frequently and maintained an active lifestyle taking care of her very active grandchildren. According to her DEXA scan, she was at a healthy weight and had relatively low body fat. Sophia was doing all the right things to keep her body healthy. Yet for some reason, her bones were failing her.

I wrote Sophia a prescription for bioidentical hormonal supplements, but when she left my office, she chose not to fill it. Instead, Sophia chose to alter her lifestyle. She began to step more softly, and she stopped caring for her grandchildren. Soon she noticed she was leaving her home less frequently, and gave up her daily walks. In a few weeks Sophia noticed that her aches and pains were dissipating, but so was her quality of life.

Sophia came back to see me a few months later, and I tested her bone density again. The results were the same. But what had changed was her weight. Sophia had gained the equivalent of 7% of her overall body weight and increased her body fat by 3%. After this startling news, Sophia decided that limiting her activity wasn't working, even though she was feeling better. This time, she agreed to medical treatment for her bones. I recommended that she start parathyroid treatment to lower her slightly elevated parathyroid hormone levels and to increase her calcium absorption. She also started taking Forteo, a bone-building medication I frequently prescribe to prevent osteoporosis.

After one year on the Forteo, Sophia had her bone density rescanned and there was significant improvement. And Sophia told me that she was once again walking daily and enjoying her grandchildren. The weight she gained came right off, and she told me that she felt younger than she had in years!

Remember, virtually all bone density loss can be reversed, though you won't regain the height you lost. In the most successful examples, we can reverse the first stages of osteopenia and first stages of osteoporosis.

Is Back Pain Due to Osteoporosis?

Not always. Back pain can be caused by many factors, including osteoporosis, an abundance of calcium (osteoarthritis), or tightening muscles around the spine. A good night's sleep, anti-inflammatory agents, and anxiety reduction have been proven to help. Finally, make sure you get a DEXA scan (see page 28) or an MRI to get the true AgePrint of your back.

body—but primarily within the spinal column—begin to weaken. Any change in your height or bone deterioration is considered abnormal, and certainly nothing that you should just "live with." Remember, you are only as young as your oldest part.

Your bone's age is affected by a host of variables, including hormone loss, vitamins, and minerals, as well as age, weight, drug use, and genetics. There are actually a host of genetic conditions that lead to aging bones. If you have ever been diagnosed with the following diseases, it may have caused your frailty, and your weight gain:

- Age-related loss of growth hormone, estrogen, testosterone, progesterone, pregnenolone, DHEA
- Cerebral palsy
- Crohn's disease
- Cystic fibrosis
- Diabetes
- Down syndrome
- Liver disease
- Neuromuscular diseases (Muscular dystrophy)
- Celiac disease
- Seizure disorders
- Sickle cell disease

ARTHRITIS

Arthritis is a three-part disease: An initial loss of moisture leads to dryness followed by inflammation and joint damage. Arthritis affects the cartilage that is supposed to protect the tips of our bones, separating them from one another. When this cartilage dries, it begins to wear thin, and eventually disintegrates. Without the cartilage that keeps your bones apart, they will begin to rub together. Rubbing is really an understatement: The bones actually grind against each other, causing pain and stiffness.

Arthritis is the number one cause of movement limitation, and may be your excuse for why you can't exercise. Almost everyone over the age of 50 has it to some degree, unless they've been smart and have been taking care of their bones all along. Arthritis in the hands is actually a predictor of later knee and hip problems. And while your arthritis is slowing you down, carrying extra weight will only make things worse. One type of arthritis, known as osteoarthritis, frequently affects individuals who are overweight.

But we do not have to suffer with painful joints: There are effective supplements I

Old Bones Are Fat Bones

By the time we're 30, more than half of our bone cells have turned to fat. Those of us with high osteopause Age-Prints have more fat in our bones than those with younger bones. Vitamin D$_3$ will help convert this type of fat back into bone, reversing the aging bone code.

prescribe all the time that give long lasting relief to my arthritis sufferers. Topical pain-killers, such as Zostrix are helpful, as well as the supplement glucosamine. Fish oils and other natural anti-inflammatory Younger (Thinner) You foods that are packed with vitamin D will help ease the pain.

REVERSE OSTEOPAUSE AND ARTHRITIS BY BALANCING YOUR BRAIN

Having enhanced brain chemistry automatically stimulates your bones to grow. Specifically, you can boost your bones by increasing your acetylcholine production. I have seen patients who have gone from crippling bed-bound lives to regaining full movement. This can be done starting with the acetylcholine program on the Younger (Thinner) You Diet. You may also want to add powerful nutrients and natural hormones to speed up the process. Growth hormone and para-thyroid hormone are the ideal treatments as they work synergistically to reverse the damage of old bones in both men and women.

Testosterone supplementation may help knee osteoarthritis for men. Testosterone is known to be an anti-inflammatory, and also seems to help build cartilage. As the testosterone to estrogen ratio changes, men appear to get more knee disease. I've used testosterone to reduce the progression of knee osteoarthritis in many of patients. When I've combined the protocol with an antidepressant, most patients get relief both physically and psychologically. Better still, these patients have been able to avoid knee surgery.

Once your bones are stronger, you will be able to have the strength and stamina necessary to exercise, which will in turn lead to weight loss. What's more, you'll look and feel younger and stronger.

PARATHYROPAUSE

Parathyropause refers to an increase of the parathyroid hormone, which also contributes to premature aging and a loss of bone density. Bioidentical parathyroid hormone supplementation is an increasingly popular option for treating osteoporosis. It is proven

Osteoporosis Is Not Only a Women's Health Issue

Two million of the ten million Americans afflicted with osteoporosis are men. Yet most men don't realize they are at risk for osteopause. A simple fifteen-minute DEXA scan can identify those at risk.

to increase spinal, hip, and total bone density because it directly mimics how the body's natural hormones work. I believe that it is more effective than drugs like Fosamax, Boniva, and Actonel.

SOMATOPAUSE: WHEN MUSCLE DISAPPEARS

Somatopause refers to the natural decline in growth hormone that occurs as we age, and affects our muscle mass. Over the course of a lifetime, 20 to 40% of total muscle can be lost, particularly if you do not exercise. The warning signs are subtle, and not exactly painful. Many are similar to a GABA deficiency. If you have identified a loss of GABA, you might be experiencing the following mental and physical symptoms as well, including weight gain:

- Cool hands and feet
- Decreased energy
- Decreased hair and nail growth
- Decreased insulin sensitivity
- Decreased strength
- Decreased sweating
- Depressed mood
- Impaired cardiac function
- Increased anxiety
- Increased body fat, particularly abdominal fat
- Poor social interaction
- Reduced sleep
- Thin skin and increased wrinkles
- Wounds take longer to heal

HORMONES REVERSE FRAILTY

You can supplement your hormone loss naturally, and reverse the symptoms of somatopause. Your hormones are needed to create the functional connection that links the spinal cord and skeleton with brain activity. They also control the receptors that are found throughout the entire brain, affecting memory, sleep, and your emotional well-being. So it's not just your bones that benefit from bioidentical hormone therapy, it's your whole body, brain, and mind.

REVERSING THE EFFECTS OF AGING ON YOUR MUSCLES AND BONES
Early Testing is Key

Catching any of the musculoskeletal pauses is easier than ever before. Using a new scanning technology, called micro-CT, doctors can now examine bone density with 100 times more detail, and can assess the effectiveness of drug and hormone therapies for restoring bone health, providing yet another weapon in the anti-aging arsenal.

Additionally, DEXA scans offer an effective screening tool for identifying bone density problems. As we discussed in Chapter 2, DEXA works like a full body X-ray except using minimal radiation; a DEXA scan offers half the radiation exposure of your average chest X-ray. Not only does it identify body fat percentages, it also measures bone density. This test is one of the most integral for keeping your health young.

Insurance companies often claim that bone density tests are medically unnecessary. Fight back and insist on these lifesaving tests. These companies are relying upon the drugging of the American public to make a profit, rather than promoting early intervention that can save lives and money. But you know better. Early knowledge and intervention is the key to reversing your present age code, and eliminating further decline.

BUILDING STRONGER BONES—TALK TO YOUR DOCTOR ABOUT THESE MEDICAL TREATMENTS

CONVENTIONAL TREATMENT	DOSAGE
Fosamax	70 mg per week
Actonel	35 mg per week
Boniva	150 mg once per month

HORMONES HOLD THE KEY TO YOUNGER BONES AND MUSCLES

Calcitonin is a hormone that inhibits bone resorption. It is proven to be a useful and safe therapy in male osteoporosis. Other important hormones supplements to consider are:

HORMONAL TREATMENT	DOSAGE—PER DAY
Estrogen	1 to 2 mg
Growth hormone	5 to 60 mg
Parathyroid hormone	20 to 40 µg
Progesterone	100 to 300 mg (up to 600 mg)
Testosterone	Men: 5 g of 1% (1 to 2 packets per day) Women: 2.5 to 10 mg daily
Calcitonin	200 IU daily

THE YOUNGER (THINNER) YOU DIET IMPROVES BONE AND MUSCLE MASS

You need to eat plenty of calcium-rich food to keep your bones strong. But did you know that some of the healthiest food choices may be working against you? A diet that is too high in animal protein washes calcium out of your blood so your bones don't get the chance to absorb this important nutrient. A purely vegetarian, high fiber diet isn't the answer, either. Too much fiber and not enough protein can bind important nutrients, so that they are excreted before they get absorbed.

If you have already been diagnosed with bone or muscle conditions (like arthritis, osteoporosis, or osteopenia) focus on Younger (Thinner) You Foods, such as fruits, vegetables, beans, nuts, seeds, salmon, and dairy products that are high in anti-inflammatory proteins called flavoproteins,

Look for Açai Berry Beverages

This Brazilian berry has been revered in the Amazon for its health-promoting properties for centuries. Today, researchers are regarding it as one of the world's top superfoods. This tiny fruit is rich in antioxidants, phytonutrients, omega-3 EFAs, amino acids, dietary fiber, vitamins, and minerals. Its unique combination of nutrients is necessary for healthy joint function. So if you have been diagnosed with arthritis, or just feel achy, try an açai blend beverage.

which prevent the degradation of body tissue. You also need to choose foods that support bone growth. Refer to the food lists throughout the book and focus on choices that are high in the protective nutrients you need: magnesium, calcium, potassium, vitamins K and D:

A diet high in vegetables promotes an optimal ratio of phosphorus to calcium. Leafy green vegetables such as kale, collard greens, bok choy, parsley, mustard greens and escarole are excellent sources of calcium, magnesium, vitamin K. Tofu (if produced with a calcium based coagulant) chickpeas, black-eyed peas, other legumes, most nuts, and many grains are excellent sources of calcium. Acidic foods such as lemon juice and vinegar help absorb calcium. Omega 3 essential fatty acids (fish oil, flax oil) increase calcium absorption from the gut, reduce urinary calcium excretion, increase calcium deposits in bone, and improve bone strength.

Foods to Avoid

If you are already suffering from arthritis or osteoporosis, make sure to take the following foods out of your diet ASAP:

- Foods that contain oxalates, which may bind with calcium and prevent it from being absorbed: spinach, chard, beet greens, and chocolate
- Foods with phytic acid will bind with calcium and prevent it from being absorbed: wheat and oats
- Limit your consumption of meat and dairy products (other than yogurt and kefir) because they increase urinary excretion (loss) of calcium. Milk and dairy foods are not the best sources of absorbable calcium.
- Foods high in refined sugar and sodium increase the loss of calcium in the urine. Soda contains excessive amounts of phosphorus, which leads to increased loss of calcium and magnesium in the urine.
- Caffeine from coffee increases loss of calcium in the urine.

Teas Are Good for Bones

A 2002 study from the University of Cambridge in England examined the tea-drinking habits and bone densities of over 1,200 elderly British women. They found that tea drinkers had stronger bones than non–tea drinkers. This may be due to the fact that tea is a leading source of quercetin, which inhibits bone loss. Just make sure to brush your teeth thoroughly at the end of the day: Strong teas will stain your teeth over time. And nothing says "old" like yellow teeth!

SUPPLEMENTS TO REVERSE AGING BONES AND MUSCLES

Although regular exercise is the best way to prevent the gradual decline of body tissue, especially muscle, there are supplements that can support the restorative process. These include calcium, magnesium, vitamin K_1, vitamin K_2, copper, manganese, zinc, boron, silica, vitamin C, strontium, omega-3, omega-6, and ipriflavone.

CHAPTER 15

Stay Sexy and Flatten Your Stomach

YOUR AGE CODE for Group 5 may have pinpointed specific symptoms or conditions that are making you look and feel old. If this is the case, and you are over 40 and having difficulty losing weight, chances are that your issues are hormonally related.

Regardless of gender, we all produce fewer hormones as we age. When women go through menopause, which is linked to estrogen loss, leading to hair loss and vaginal dryness, and progesterone loss, resulting in sleep problems, and men go through its male counterpart, andropause, linked to testosterone loss, resulting in a decline in libido, they also gain weight.

However, even though this excess weight is both distressing and frustrating, it doesn't have to be with you forever: You can lose these extra pounds by following the Younger (Thinner) You Diet and, if necessary, supplementing with bioidentical hormones, nutritional supplements, and even medications. It's also a good idea to incorporate an exercise program that takes your individual brain chemistry and other physical issues into account so you can increase your metabolism. Now you've created a personalized Younger You program!

The payoff is greater than just a younger, slimmer body. While the Younger (Thinner) You Diet knocks off pounds and keeps them from coming back, there's more you can achieve by following the recommendations in this chapter. I'm talking about restoring your libido and sexual function. Even moderate weight loss results in significant improvements in sexual functioning and satisfaction. And those who regularly exercise have higher levels of desire and enhanced ability to achieve orgasm. If you

The Big Three Sex Hormones

Estrogen is an intensive, energizing compound that works like dopamine to stimulate the brain and burn calories. **Progesterone** reduces anxiety and improves sleep, which diminishes craving for carbohydrates. **Testosterone**, like estrogen, is a calorie burning intensive hormone that both men and women create, although men have more.

are overweight, losing between 8 and 20 pounds will help you look and feel sexier, no matter what your age.

GOOD SEX BEGINS IN THE BRAIN

Youthfulness is identified with high sexual activity. This chapter will teach you how to keep your sex life at a healthy balanced state throughout your entire life. Outside of the brain, the next most important organs in terms of keeping the body young are the sex organs. Maybe that's why we often take them for granted, but we never stop thinking about them!

For both men and women, sexual hormone production is governed by your brain. When you are at the peak of your health, you will want to experience the joys of sex all the time. When your brain is experiencing a chemical deficiency in any of the four primary areas, sex won't seem so enticing and the physical act will leave you lacking. The four phases of sex can be directly correlated to the functioning of the four primary biochemicals:

- Desire is created in the brain by dopamine; when you are low on dopamine your energy for and interest in sex wanes, as well as your performance.
- Arousal is initiated by acetylcholine; when cognitive functioning and internal moisture goes awry and your acetylcho-

line becomes depleted, you will not be able to focus on sex, let alone keep up your attention and stimulation. You will also be uncomfortably dry.

- Orgasm is controlled by your levels of GABA. If GABA becomes depleted, you can't relax or let go, and hence, you can't have an orgasm.
- Resolution is related to serotonin. If serotonin becomes depleted, your timing is off. You're either coming to the party too early or too late.

WE MUST HAVE SEX TO BEAT THE PAUSES

Some people don't like the idea of combining food and sex, but the two are more intimately related than we think. Oddly, cholesterol is a precursor of all the sex hormones. Estrogen, progesterone, testosterone, pregnenolone, androstenedione, and DHEA all come from cholesterol. So, as we get older, and our cholesterol goes up, the ovaries and adrenal glands cannot make as much of their particular hormones, so estrogen, progesterone, and testosterone production slows. It should not be a surprise then that as our bodies produce less, we feel less sexy and less sexually motivated.

The goal for a Younger (Thinner) You is to maintain your best levels of hormone production. Why not start by sparking your sexuality?

GREAT EXPECTATIONS: A HEALTHY LEVEL OF SEXUAL FREQUENCY

Age 15 to 25	more than one time per day
Age 25 to 30	1 per day
Age 30 to 40	4 times per week
Age 40–50	3 times per week
Age 50–60	1 to 2 times per week
Age 60–70	1 time every two weeks
By age 80	0 to 1 time per month

Males and females have all the same sexual hormones in different quantities. When women have too much testosterone they develop weight gain and polycystic ovaries, leading to increased facial and body hair. When men have too much estrogen, they will have an increased risk of heart attack and stroke.

YOUNGER SEX IS FREQUENT SEX

Sexually speaking, men are generally "younger" than women and desire sex more often. But women can get younger: I see it all the time. I have had plenty of women that increased both their sexual desire and ability to have orgasms simply by taking bio-identical hormones including DHEA, growth hormone, estrogen, and progesterone. Their husbands, needless to say, are ecstatic. And, by the way, so are the women.

You don't need to have sex as frequently as you did in your twenties, but nor should you just try to get away with the minimum requirements either. Sexual frequency should never drop below once a week, though ideally it should be around twice a week. The effect an orgasm can have on your brain is like rebooting a computer. There are two ways to reboot your brain— by "turning it on" (like you do when you're exercising) or "turning it off" (like you do when you are relaxing). Sex reboots your brain both ways at the same time.

MENOPAUSE IS AN ULTIMATE AGE ACCELERATOR

Menopause is a natural stage of life that every woman must face. The onset of menopause does not have to be an awful experience, in fact, if you are mentally prepared for the challenge, it might be the best years of your life.

Menopause is not associated with any particular age: It simply marks the decline in production of progesterone and estrogen. Many of my female patients had been misinformed, thinking that menopause started during midlife, around the age of 50. But I tell them time and again that when you begin to experience symptoms, your pause is already in the middle of its course. Menopause actually begins around age 35 (now referred to as perimenopause), and can take as many as ten to fifteen years

There's Another Reason Why You Might Be Bloated

Gastropause, and its associated symptoms and conditions, are as much a part of aging as is menopause or andropause. As we get older, we simply can't digest some of the same foods we used to, leaving us bloated and uncomfortable. That's why greasy/fried foods, rich cheese sauces, and even hard alcohol can upset our stomachs now, even though we could tolerate these foods when we were younger. Some people also respond negatively to some of the Younger (Thinner) You superfoods. If you find that anything on this diet is difficult to digest properly, stay away from it: Its benefits can't outweigh your discomfort. Plus, you're not pulling nutrients out of the foods you can't digest.

If you suffer from gastropause, you might need to stay away from the following Younger (Thinner) You foods:

- Lemon
- Tomato
- Onion, raw
- Ground beef
- Coffee, decaffeinated or regular
- Tea, decaffeinated or regular
- Salad dressings

- Attention deficiencies
- Bone weakness
- Vaginal dryness
- Failure to ovulate
- Hair loss
- Hot flashes
- Loss of libido
- Mood swings
- Abdominal weight gain

WHAT HAPPENED TO MY STOMACH?

Increased body fat, loss of muscle tone, and gaining weight around your middle are all very common occurrences during menopause. The fall of estrogen and progesterone cause a cascade of rising blood sugars and lowered mental activity. Women begin to feel both hungry and tired: They eat more junk food to stay alert and exercise less. The good news is that we now have the ability to give low dosages of natural hormones that will transform not only the way you feel but the way you look.

HORMONE REPLACEMENT THERAPY CREATES A YOUNGER YOU

Most women have a menopause AgePrint of 100 by the time they are 55. If you take natural estrogen and other bioidentical supplements you can turn back the clock to age 40 to 45. The secret here is to trick your brain into thinking it is 45 forever.

before it is completed. Hormonal imbalances can start even earlier when brain stress is high.

The bottom line is this: Women in their thirties are already going into partial menopause. A loss of progesterone can make you cranky, moody, and increase the effects of PMS. By the time you reach 50, it is very likely you will be starting to feel the most obvious signs and symptoms, all due to estrogen loss. They include:

The only way menopause can be successfully treated is by imitating the body's own mechanisms, which means replacing the hormones that the body has naturally lost. By maintaining and increasing hormone levels, you can restore your health and even reverse the symptoms that have been affecting you. Natural hormones have been found to be capable of doing this with minimal negative side effects. You cannot mimic the bodies own natural hormone levels with horse urine-derived estrogen (such as Premarin) and you cannot mimic it with birth control pills.

This is the reason why I tell all of my patients that all hormones are not the same. Synthetic estrogens are made from horse urine and have been known for years to cause an increase in blood clots, heart attacks, stroke, and breast cancer. It has been scientifically determined that women taking estrogen derived from horses have an increased rate of cancer. Other complications associated with synthetic estrogen and progesterone include weight gain, heart disease, and stroke. It has also been shown that growth hormone from cadavers causes cancer.

I only prescribe bioidentical, natural hormones, which have the exact same molecular structure as those made in the human body. These natural preparations require taking only one tablet nightly, and their most common side effect is sleepiness. They have no effect on insulin resistance: If anything, they improve insulin resistance and the response to inflammation. Often, my patients become less arthritic because these natural hormones require smaller doses. These women will also see improvements in their health in multiple areas— they will have better concentration, thicker hair, smoother, more supple skin, as well as reduced inflammation, reduced insulin resistance, and an improved sex life.

Virtually all women need all three hormones (estrogen, testosterone, progesterone) to maintain a certain blood level of estrogen. If your doctor recommends hormone therapies called Biest or Triest, ask to choose again. Even though these supplements are bioidentical, they do not produce the same blood level results as estradiol. The patch is the best was to administer estrogen.

Women produce small amounts of testosterone themselves. The estrogen-to-testosterone ratio during some phases of the menstrual cycle at the age of 25 is 20:1. A typical menopausal woman at age 48 to 52 generally comes in with a 2:1, or occasionally a 1:1 ratio. However, some women should not take additional testosterone: If you are experiencing baldness, excessive facial or nasal hair, or have an imbalance of sex hormone–binding globulin.

Progesterone is a medical gift from the gods. It is a natural mood balancer, stress reliever, brain calmer, and it squashes cortisol. It is a natural diuretic, antidepressant, antioxidant, a precursor of cortisone, and necessary for survival.

WHO'S HOT IN HERE?

Hot flashes and other symptoms of menopause are no joke. While there is no medication that will stop menopause from occurring, many women experience such severe symptoms that medication may be needed to control them. If you are experiencing severe hot flashes (either in number or intensity), let your doctor know. S/he might prescribe estrogen-containing products, which are the most effective treatment. Prescription drug alternatives include progestogens, the antidepressants venlafaxine, paroxetine, and fluoxetine, as well as the anticonvulsant gabapentin. GABA and serotonin agents stop the "freak-outs" many women experience as a result of declining estrogen levels. This occurs because you're losing progesterone, the hormone that keeps you calm. Without progesterone many women experience a general "sinking" feeling. With the right medication, this feeling will go away.

VITAMIN D AND MENOPAUSE

You can strengthen your overall health by supplementing with vitamin D. The *American Journal of Clinical Nutrition* recently claimed that vitamin D made a big difference for those suffering during menopause. They found that women who were consuming at least 12.5 mg of vitamin D from either food sources or supplements had a 37% lower risk of hip fractures than women who took less than 3.5 mg. Neither milk nor a high calcium diet was associated with lowering the risks of these fractures.

MODIFY THE YOUNGER (THINNER) YOU DIET FOR BETTER HEALTH AND BETTER SEX

Weight gain is a very common side effect of menopause. By following the Younger (Thinner) You Diet, you'll be able to con-

CORE SEX HORMONES FOR WOMEN

HORMONAL TREATMENT	DOSAGE PER DAY	BRAIN CODE ACTION
Progesterone	100–200 mg	GABA, serotonin
Testosterone	2.5–10 mg	Dopamine
Estradiol (E2)	1–2 mg	Acetylcholine
Estriol (E3)	2–4 g	Dopamine
DHEA sulfate	50–100 mg	Acetylcholine
Pregnenolone	10–250 mg	GABA, serotonin
7-KETO	200 mg	Serotonin

trol your weight and tailor the meal plans to include lots of soy products and fish. Soy products are a healthy alternative to dairy, and can be found in choices that go far beyond tofu and tempeh. In most supermarkets you can find a wide selection of soy milks, soy cheeses (hard and soft varieties, even cream cheeses!), crackers, enriched whole grain breads, veggie burgers, and more. However, don't go on a soy binge: Watch the calorie content of these packaged goods carefully. Read labels for added sugars and salts. For example, soy milk is highly flavored with additional sugars, so it is not a great Younger (Thinner) You option. Tofu, tempeh, and edamame (cooked soy beans), are better, more natural ways of increasing your soy.

Fish is the number one anti-inflammatory protein. Fish oils lower risk of heart disease and help prevent osteoporosis, both conditions that increase when women reach menopause.

ANDROPAUSE: MEN GO THROUGH CHANGES, TOO

Men usually don't notice when their bodies are changing, except when it comes to sex. As men age, we turn into cantankerous old coots who throw temper tantrums. It's not that we've hit the wall: We are experiencing a decline in our hormone production that affects all the same parts as menopause. Andropause, the

male equivalent, affects our mood, memory, and thinking, sleep, and most of all, our health. Andropause typically begins for men at age 40 and is marked by a decline in production of the hormone testosterone.

Male menopause is different from female menopause in that men can cycle in and out of andropause. This occurs in cases of high stress, depression, excessive athleticism, drug use, war, and even divorce.

Luckily, there are many great treatments for andropause that go beyond traditional testosterone treatments. Using too much testosterone can lead to blood clots or pulmonary embolisms.

Instead, many of my patients use used pregnenolone, DHEA, nutrition (following the Younger (Thinner) You Diet), and stress-reduction techniques. Review the stress-reduction and meditation techniques in the GABA chapter (Chapter 5) before taking any medications to see if you can bring your andropause under control.

IT'S NOT ALL ABOUT THE ERECTION

There has been an explosion of erectile drugs on the market for men who need a little extra help getting it up. The tremendous volume of sales has demonstrated the magnitude of this problem. It's a shame that men have fallen into the pharmaceutical trap of believing that the only way to fix their problem is with a prescription. They are willing to risk serious side effects instead of seeking alternative methods.

The truth is that the majority of erectile dysfunction is due to a loss of testosterone. Male sexual dysfunction is therefore more effectively treated with testosterone supplementation. The loss of testosterone also results in low satisfaction, motivation and drive to do the activities they once found enjoyable—sex, exercise, and so forth.

THE MALE BRAIN CODE

Enhancing each of your brain chemicals will improve various aspects of your sex life. You may see from the following chart that your brain chemical deficiencies are causing issues in your sex life. By following the Younger (Thinner) You Diet that is modified by your deficiency, some of these issues might self-correct. However, if you notice that you still have issues after your brain chemistry is balanced, choose the area you would like to improve first, and continue following that particular diet:

Dopamine—>Libido—>Sexual reward
Acetylcholine—>Moisture—>Rapid
  erection
GABA—>Relaxation—>Better
  performance
Serotonin—>Fun—>Balanced
  ejaculation time

YOUR HEALTHY PROSTATE

Prostate cancer is not a sexually transmitted disease. In fact, the more ejaculations one has, the better. Frequent sex decreases the risk of prostate cancer by as much as 33%. Prostate cancer in some cases is genetic and is typically present in men with abnormal testosterone levels.

If your AgePrint showed that you were experiencing andropause, bring these results to your physician. He or she might recommend bloodwork and ultrasound testing with a prostate ultrasound and penile Doppler. Prostate, bladder and kidney health are all easily investigated using an ultrasound and tend to be more accurate than a manual exam (not to mention more comfortable).

There are many ways to treat the prostate, including natural and noninvasive options. Try using the spices in the chart on the opposite page.

KNOW YOUR RATIOS

For young men, testosterone-to-estrogen levels should be around 20:1. As we age, these levels do shift. Unlike women, however, when men's testosterone drops, they do not experience as drastic a fluctuation in hormonal levels. These ratios can fall to 6:1, which is one reason why the symptoms are less severe.

HERB	CONTAINS	HOW IT HELPS
Holy basil, a non-edible form of basil	1. Ursolic acid	1. A known inhibitor of COX-2 (an enzyme responsible for inflammation and pain).
	2. Eugenol, rosmarinic acid, apigenin	2. Antioxidant, anti-inflammatory agents
Ginger	22 molecules	Effective inhibitors of COX-2
Turmeric	Root	Inhibits COX-2
Green tea	1. 6 cups of green tea a day	1. Inhibits prostate cancer development and metastasis. Contains 51 anti-inflammatory phytonutrients.
	2. Contains the most antioxidants of any food	2. Has been found to down-regulate an enzyme called ornithine decarboxylase, which is overexpressed in cancer patients.
	3. Polyphenols	3. Inhibited prostate cancer growth in animal studies. Selectively inhibits COX-2.
Oregano	31 antioxidants	Have anti-inflammatory properties
Rosemary	Betulinic acid, caffeic acid, and its derivatives like rosmarinic acid and carsonic acid	Have antioxidant properties and COX-2 inhibiting properties.

THERE'S NOTHING FUNNY ABOUT ERECTILE DYSFUNCTION

. . . except those terrible television commercials. The majority of erectile dysfunction issues are due to a loss of testosterone. Male sexual dysfunction is therefore more effectively treated with testosterone supplementation than with Viagra or Cialis, no matter what you have seen on TV. Once you get your brain chemistry balanced, you will be able to enjoy longer, more frequent sexual relations entirely without the help of medications.

However, if you've been following the Younger (Thinner) You Diet for more than three months and still have trouble with sexual performance, the issue might lay in your vascular system. That's when medications such as Levitra, Cialis and Viagra can be helpful but should still remain a last resort. You can first try the natural supplement Arginine (500 to 2000 mg), which may be helpful for improving circulation to the penis.

CONVENTIONAL TREATMENT	DOSAGE
Levitra	5–20 mg
Cialis	5–20 mg
Viagra	25–100 mg

BREAK THE ANDROPAUSE CODE FOR A YOUNGER, SEXIER YOU

You can reverse a flagging sex drive and return your overall health to the same level as those younger boys. When you take a combination of bioidentical hormones, including testosterone, multiple pause areas begin to work better. You could happily and comfortably be 60 years old with a 40-year-old memory and a testosterone level of a 30-year-old.

Synthetic methyl testosterone has a black box warning now for liver cancer. Fortunately, there is no similar one on the natural, micronized testosterones. The natural testosterones treat hypogonadism by restoring testosterone to its normal range. I have been using testosterone and growth hormone replacement therapies for my male patients for more than ten years, which has enabled these men to maintain brain function as well as physical stamina and libido. A study reported in the *Journals of Gerontology* showed that men 65 to 87 who used testosterone transdermal patches for one year also improved their memory and concentration abilities.

There is a variety of natural testosterones available: pills, creams, patches, gels, and the AndroGel pump. AndroGel delivers natural testosterone in a gel that you simply rub into your skin—no patches or injections. Natural testosterone is now available in a patch. No longer do men have to endure the discomfort of an injection or pellets.

For example, Steven was 55 and both discouraged and depressed about his sexual dysfunction. I changed his antidepressant, put him on a CES device, and started him on my sexual-rejuvenation hormone program. He went from having sex with his wife once per month to six times per week!

HORMONAL TREATMENT	DOSAGE—PER DAY
Testosterone (bioidentical)	100 mg
DHEA	50–100 mg
Androgel (most effective form)	1% 5 g
Testim	1% 50 mg
Androderm	5 mg/d patch
Growth hormone	5–60 mg

DIABETIC SEXUAL HEALTH

Diabetic men often have difficulty with achieving orgasm, maintaining erections, and general sexual responsiveness. The overproduction of sugar damages the nerves, veins, and arteries, including those that flow to the penis. For example, any impaired venous and arterial flow problems

Meet Larry: He Tested Early and Fixed a Bigger Problem Before It Started

Larry came to see me when he was 50. He was recently divorced, and while he said his body was feeling fine, he told me that he was beginning to gain some weight, and was complaining of anxiety, tension, and lack of sexual activity.

His AgePrint and routine physical examination revealed that he was worse off than he believed: Larry's cardiopause was at 60 with mild hypertension. He was slightly overweight, but his EKG and pulmonary function test (PFT) were within the normal range. Larry's prostate was mildly enlarged; his Penile Brachial Index was within normal parameters, with the penis exhibiting normal circulation.

By any standards, Larry's health was borderline. Many doctors would send him home with just a pat on the back and a "wait and see" approach. But I knew that when overall health even minimally declines—especially with symptoms such as hypertension and obesity—sexual function may also be impaired. I also knew that tension and anxiety are symptoms of overall brain deterioration. So I had Larry go for further testing.

A full body Doppler ultrasound was performed to detect blockages of the arteries and veins. It turned out to be the best thing to happen to Larry. The ultrasound indicated a significant loss of circulation to the brain, originating in the left carotid artery. His BEAM revealed severe voltage suppression; his memory testing showed loss of verbal skills; and his personality profile indicated extremely high levels of anxiety. Blood testing revealed low testosterone, with normal levels of both DHEA and IGF-1.

Larry was treated with the testosterone patch; the antidepressant Paxil to address the anxiety, verbal memory loss, and overall brain function decline; I also prescribed DHEA supplementation. I put him on the Younger (Thinner) You Diet and monitored his vasculopause carefully. A few months into his treatment, Larry reported that he had started dating, and had improved sexual functions. Additionally, he lost ten pounds and felt as if he had calmed down. His AgePrint was down to 40 in every aspect of his health. He was literally ten years younger than when he first walked in my door.

Sexually Speaking, What's Holding You Back?

Great sex does not occur in a bubble: Your overall health and mental state directly affect your ability to enjoy frequent, long-lasting sex. Your weight gain may be on your mind, or it might be stress at work that stopping you from fully enjoying yourself. Other health issues may be affecting your sex life, as well as medications you may be taking. All of these are important considerations to think about, and discuss with your doctor.

or nerve damage can result in impotence. If you suffer from diabetes and have these issues, discuss them with your doctor, who may prescribe Levitra or one of the other ED medications.

For type 2 diabetes sufferers, the fix may be a little easier: Follow the Younger (Thinner) You Diet to reverse your adult-onset diabetes so that you can enjoy every aspect of your life. Your weight is directly affecting your sex life: isn't that reason enough to want to get into younger, healthier shape?

HERBS AND SPICES THAT BREAK THE ANDROPAUSE CODE

- Garlic
- Oregano
- Rosemary

Supplements for Andropause

Adding certain supplements to your diet can ensure that your brain chemical levels remain high—which helps reverse a flagging sex drive, enhances weight loss, and improves your overall well-being. Some supplements I recommend include DHEA, zinc, copper, and vitamin C.

YOUNGER (THINNER) YOU FOODS THAT LET YOU LOSE WEIGHT AND STILL EAT LIKE A MAN

You can increase your energy stores by boosting your dopamine, which will help create more testosterone and increase your metabolism so that you can lose weight and feel sexier. In order to do so, men need to beef it up, literally. Make sure you follow the traditional, high metabolism Younger (Thinner) You Diet that features lots of proteins, including lean meats, poultry, even eggs: Make sure to have animal proteins with each of your three main meals. The following tips will augment this particular eating regimen.

- Look for foods in Chapter 7 that are high in copper and zinc to aid hair growth: sources include barley, beets, garlic, nuts, pecans, soy, radishes, raisins, and seafood
- Fish provides essential fatty acids that keep hair healthy
- To improve stamina (circulation) eat vitamin C–rich foods such as beet greens, black currants, mangoes, sweet peppers, and pineapple

BEING IN SHAPE = MORE GREAT SEX

Even moderate weight loss results in significant improvements in sexual functioning and satisfaction. And those who regularly exercise have higher levels of desire and enhanced ability to be aroused and achieve orgasm. Remember: If you are overweight, losing between 8 and 20 pounds will help you look younger and feel sexier.

CHAPTER 16

Becoming Younger (and Thinner) Every Year

YOU'VE ALREADY taken many steps to improve your weight and your health. You've unlocked the secret of permanent weight loss, and discovered how your unique brain chemistry may be the primary reason why you have had difficulties losing weight in the past. By following the Younger (Thinner) You Diet, you are now able to reverse your brain chemistry to a younger, more vibrant state. You have learned how to boost your dopamine for more energy and greater metabolism, supporting your weight loss efforts, and redirecting your food addictions to different, more positive experiences. An increase in acetylcholine will keep your brain sharp and your attention focused so that you can continue to make good food decisions, and refuse to fill your body with bad fats. By boosting your GABA, you can finally calm down and stop worrying about your weight. You'll be able to set better boundaries for yourselves and others. And you'll be able to recognize when you've had enough to eat. Last, by increasing serotonin, you'll get the rest you need so that your brain can work at optimum levels, the next day, and every day.

I think that the best part about the Younger (Thinner) You Diet is that it is completely natural. The foods you eat and the supplements you'll take provide a framework to support better health that is completely free from chemicals or pollutants. You can feel good about the nutrient-packed foods that I've chosen because you now understand the importance of buying only the freshest ingredients for yourself and your family. You've learned to look at fruits and vegetables in terms of their color values, and have adopted a rainbow of favorite new foods: Each one is like taking a multivitamin with every meal. You can now easily cut out the foods you shouldn't be eating because you have so many new and delicious options to choose from. What's more, you have learned to use teas and spices to boost your metabolism as well as provide tons of additional nutrition. I'll bet that you'll never feel better than when you are following this diet.

You've also learned to identify exactly which aspects of your current health may be aging you prematurely and thwarting your weight loss efforts. My modified Age-Print is a simple way to evaluate your overall health. Remember, everything that happens within your brain and your body is directly related to your weight. In order to become thinner, you need to become younger. And that means that you need to become healthier overall. Whether you've targeted new medications or natural hormones to reverse your current symptoms, or if you've just recognized that your poor health may be the source of your weight gain, you are now operating from a position of power, because you have the knowledge to change your health today.

AN ADDITIVE EXPERIENCE

The combination of these lessons creates what I like to call an additive experience: Each time you fix one part of your health, it elevates everything else. When you fix your brain chemistry, your weight improves. When you lose weight, your health improves. And when your health improves, you get younger every year. That's why I know that you'll be able to stick to this plan, even if you haven't been able to follow other diets successfully before. I know that you will actually feel healthier and younger the longer you stay on the program.

I've had many patients who come back to me year after year for a youth checkup instead of a traditional annual physical. They aren't complaining of new aches and pains, and I'm happy to chart their progress. By sticking with the program, their metabolism gets stronger every year; they have successfully retrained their brain and body to burn fuel faster so not only are they able to keep off the weight they have lost, they continue to lose more weight each subsequent year. Their muscles and bones get stronger, and their skin looks younger each time they walk into my office.

Best of all, they all tell me the same thing: They don't feeling like they are dieting all the time. The Younger (Thinner) You Diet is not only a whole a new way of eating; it's a whole new way of living.

REJOICE AND REPEAT

Celebrate all of your hard work whenever you can. Set small goals, and when you achieve them, do something nice for yourself. You might need to do some clothes shopping, so go for it! Don't wait until you've lost "all your weight" before you reward yourself. Your efforts deserve to be recognized!

The first goal was to lose 10% of your body weight. Once you've hit the target, go back and retake the Younger (Thinner) You Diet Quiz as well as the AgePrint. See if there are changes that need to be made to your program, and adjust accordingly. Then, if needed, set the next goal to lose 10% of your new weight.

You will never need to take a break from the Younger (Thinner) You Diet. Keep following the diet, even after you've reached your final goals. By this time the eating plan should be second nature to you, and it won't feel like a diet at all.

Last, share the good news with the ones you love. Make the Younger (Thinner) You Diet a family experience, so that everyone benefits. There's no point in getting younger alone. My goal for you is to extend your life as long as possible, so that you will have numerous and wonderful experiences with your friends and your family, fully enjoying your future with vitality and a sharp mind. That's what a Younger You is all about.

APPENDIX A

SPICES AND BRAIN CHEMISTRY

NAME	POTENTIAL BENEFIT	CONTAINS	BRAIN CHEMICAL AUGMENTOR
Allspice	• Helps lower blood pressure • Prevents cardiovascular disease • Prevents neuro-degenerative conditions	• Lipids • Choline Antioxidants: Eugenol, methyleugenol, myrcene, proanthocyanidins, quercetin, salicylates, terpenes Others: Chavicol, cinnamaldehyde, limonene	Acetylcholine
Anise	• Alleviates cough • Helps relieve symptoms of menopause	Antioxidants: Caffeic acid, camphene, chlorogenic acid, eugenol, myristicin, rutin. Others: Bergapten, limonene, pinenes, terpinols	Serotonin
Basil	• Improves circulation • Improves digestion • Prevents cancer • Fights colds and viruses including herpes	• Carotenoids: Beta carotene • monoterpenes, the main constituents of essential oils • Calcium, magnesium • Polyphenols: Luteolin, an antioxidant and free radical fighter • Vitamin D Antioxidants: Apigenin, carophyllene, eugenol, geraniol, methyl eugenol, rosmarinic acid ursolic acid Others: Cineol, citral, linalool, methyl chavicol, methyl cinnamate	Acetylcholine and dopamine
Bay leaves	• Promotes perspiration • Increases the production of urine • Relieves high blood sugar • Relieves migraines and other headaches • Fights bacterial and fungal infections	• Calcium • Iron • Vitamin C • Potassium • Phosphorus	Dopamine

NAME	POTENTIAL BENEFIT	CONTAINS	BRAIN CHEMICAL AUGMENTOR
Black pepper	• Aids digestion • Relieves gas	• Vanadium • Piperidine • Piperolein A • Piperolein B • Piperanine • Piperine	Dopamine
Caraway	• Stimulates digestion • Alleviates indigestion	• Limonene	GABA
Cardamom	• Alleviates halitosis	• Pinene, limonene	GABA
Cayenne (aka Chile, Chilli, Chili Pepper, Hot Pepper, Red Pepper, Tabasco)	• Improves blood circulation • Helps prevent abnormal blood clots • Lowers blood pressure • Alleviates heartburn • Soothes stomach ulcers • Stimulates hair growth in men • Lowers cholesterol • Reduces fatigue • Stimulates the thyroid • Lowers triglycerides • Alleviates sinusitis	• Capsaicinoids • Vitamin C • Carotenoids: Capsanthin	Dopamine
Chamomile	• Stimulates digestion • Improves bladder health • Reduces fever • Alleviates arthritis • Alleviates muscle cramps • Can lessen anxiety • Alleviates pain	• Calcium phosphate, manganese, iron • Polyphenols: luteolin, quercetin • Terpenes: pinene • Vitamin A	serotonin
Cinnamon	• Lowers blood pressure • Alleviates heartburn • Alleviates nausea • Lowers blood sugar • Decreases LDL cholesterol levels • Prevents insulin resistance • Blocks inflammation that leads to diabetes	• Calcium, iron, zinc, phosphorus, magnesium, manganese Antioxidants: MHCP, vitamin B_1 • Vitamin B_2 • Vitamin B_3 • Vitamin B_6 • Vitamin C	GABA
Cloves	• Suppresses some forms of bacteria • Improves digestion • Alleviates pain	• Polyphenols • Volatile oils	GABA
Coriander/ Cilantro	• Alleviates indigestion • Alleviates colic • Lowers serum cholesterol • Increases HDL cholesterol levels • Lowers LDL cholesterol levels • Facilitates the removal of aluminum, lead, and mercury from the body	• Quercetin • ISO quercetin • Rutin • Chlorogenic acid • Caffeic acid • Coumarin • Alpha-linolenic acid	GABA

NAME	POTENTIAL BENEFIT	CONTAINS	BRAIN CHEMICAL AUGMENTOR
Cumin	• Lowers elevated blood sugar • Lowers cholesterol • Lowers elevated triglycerides • Alleviates intestinal cramps	• Iron, zinc, calcium, magnesium, phosphorus Antioxidant: Curcumin	Acetylcholine and dopamine
Dill	• Alleviates colic • Relieves heartburn • Alleviates insomnia	• Lipids • Volatile oils	Serotonin
Fennel	• Alleviates diarrhea • Alleviates indigestion • Improves kidney function • Improves liver function • Improves brain metabolism	• Amino acids: glycine, tyrosine, serine • Enzymes • Boron, cobalt, tin, calcium, zinc, • choline, B_2, A, C • Volatile oils	Dopamine
Fenugreek	• Alleviates sinus pressure • Improves digestion • Reduces lung congestion • Reduces inflammation • Reduces fever • Prevents breast and colon cancer	Iron Biotin Choline Vitamin B_1 Vitamin B_{12} Vitamin B_5 Vitamin B_6 Vitamin B_2 Vitamin D PABA Vitamin A Vitamin B_3 Inositol	Serotonin
Garlic	• Reduces the risk of heart attack • Helps prevent atherosclerosis • Helps prevent blood clots • Improves blood circulation • Helps strengthen blood vessels • Lowers blood pressure • Helps to prevent stroke • Eliminates intestinal parasites • May prevent several forms of cancer • Stimulates the immune system • Increases HDL cholesterol levels • Alleviates symptoms of rheumatoid arthritis	• Amino acids: cysteine, carnitine, leucine • Alliin, methiin • Alliinase, tyrosinase • Lipids: oleic acid • Calcium, germanium, iron, potassium, sulfur, copper, selenium, zinc, iodine • Adenosine, inosine, cytidine, • phytic acid , caffeic acid, quercetin, allixin, rutin • Ajoene • Biotin • Choline • Vitamin A • Vitamin B_1 • Vitamin B_2 • Vitamin B_3 • Vitamin C • Vitamin E	Dopamine

NAME	POTENTIAL BENEFIT	CONTAINS	BRAIN CHEMICAL AUGMENTOR
Ginger	• Improves blood circulation • Prevents atherosclerosis • Lowers blood pressure • Improves digestion	• Vitamin B_3 • Vitamin B_6 • Choline • PABA • Calcium • Iron • Magnesium • Phosphorus • Potassium • Sodium	Dopamine
Horseradish	• Improves colon function • Alleviates coughs • Alleviates pneumonia • Alleviates sinusitis	• Amino acids • Enzymes • Minerals • Vitamin C	Dopamine
Lemongrass	• Improves kidney health • Inhibits candida • Alleviates fevers	• Vitamin A • Vitamin C	GABA
Marjoram	• Alleviates intestinal cramps • Alleviates headaches • Alleviates insomnia	• Carvacrol • Thymol	Serotonin
Mustard seed	• Increases metabolism • Alleviates bronchitis • Alleviates the common cold	• Allyl isothiocyanate	Dopamine
Oregano	• Alleviates indigestion	• Monoterpenes, carvacrol, linalool, thymol • Calcium, iron, zinc, magnesium, copper, potassium, vitamin B_3 • Vitamin C	GABA
Paprika	• Alleviates diarrhea • Improves digestion • Alleviates toothache	• Capsorubin • Vitamin C	GABA
Peppermint	• Alleviates diarrhea • Alleviates colic symptoms • Prevents and dissolves gallstones • Alleviates indigestion • Relieves headaches • Alleviates nausea • Helps to clear sinuses	• Betaine • Alpha carotene, beta carotene • Acetic acid • Cobalt, magnesium • Vitamin C • Volatile oils	Serotonin
Poppy seeds	• May help prevent various forms of cancer	• Amino acids • Lipids • Polyphenols • calcium, zinc, copper, selenium, • Vitamin C, B_1, B_2, B_3, B_6, E	GABA

NAME	POTENTIAL BENEFIT	CONTAINS	BRAIN CHEMICAL AUGMENTOR
Rosemary	• Helps prevent atherosclerosis • Improves blood circulation • Lowers blood pressure • Alleviates halitosis • Increases the production of urine • Prevents cataracts • Helps prevent breast cancer • Alleviates allergies • Reduces inflammation • Alleviates gout • Helps to regulate menstruation • Alleviates the symptoms of asthma and emphysema	• Alpha-hydroxy acids: glycolic acid • Calcium, magnesium, phosphorus, sodium, potassium, Rosmarinic acid, ursolic acid • Polyphenols: diosmin, luteolin • Volatile oils: borneol, thymol, rosmanol	Dopamine
Saffron	• Alleviates depression	• Xanthophylls	Serotonin
Sage	• Prevents heart attacks • Prevents abnormal blood clotting • Reduces perspiration	• Carnosic acid • Labiatic acid • Rosmarinic acid • Ursolic acid	Acetylcholine
Savory	• Increases sexual desire • Increases production of adrenal and sexual steroid hormones	• P-cymene • Carvacrol • Tannin	Dopamine
Sesame seed	• Lowers blood pressure • Inhibits the absorption of dietary cholesterol • Lower LDL cholesterol	• Folic acid • Methionine • Cystine • Histidine • Glycine • Dietary fiber • Omega-3 • Alpha-linolenic acid	Dopamine
Spearmint	• Stimulates appetite • Alleviates hiccups and flatulence • Improves digestive health	• Monoterpenes • Polyphenols • Limonene • Rosmarinic acid	Serotonin
Tarragon	• Fights fatigue • Calms nerves • Works as a sleep aid	• Estragole • Ocimene	Dopamine
Thyme	• Suppresses some forms of harmful bacteria • Loosens congestion • Alleviates coughs • Alleviates laryngitis	• Caffeic acid • Ursolic acid, rosmarinic acid • Volatile oils: borneol, pinene	Acetylcholine
Turmeric	• Helps prevent and treat atherosclerosis • Inhibits abnormal blood clotting • Stimulates the immune system	• Monoterpenes, borneol, cineol • Potassium • Curcumin, curcumin II, curcumin III • Vitamin C • Volatile oils: turmerone, sabinene	Dopamine and acetylcholine

APPENDIX B

THE NUTRIENTS FROM COLOR FOODS

RED FOODS	NUTRIENTS	BRAIN CHEMICAL(S) IT MOST AFFECTS
Cranberry	Anthocyanidin, quercetin, resveratrol	Dopamine, serotonin
Red cabbage	Anthocyanins, glucosinolates, indole-3-carbinol, lutein	GABA
Red onions	Allyl propyl disulfide, fructooligosaccharides, glucosinolates, pectin, quercetin	GABA
Red peppers	Capsaicinoids, carotenoids	Dopamine, serotonin
Red potatoes	Catechols, chlorogenic acid	Dopamine
Tomatoes, all varieties	Beta carotene, chlorogenic acid, citric acid, fructooligosaccharides, lycopene, malic acid	Dopamine, GABA
Red apple, all varieties	Caffeic acid, chlorogenic acid, D-glucaric acid, ellagic acid, ferulic acid, pectin quercetin	Serotonin
Red bananas	Fructooligosaccharides, pectin, potassium	GABA
Raspberries	Anthocyanosides, ellagic acid	Dopamine, serotonin
Strawberries	Anthocyanosides, ellagic acid	Dopamine, serotonin
Red cherry	Anthocyanosides, ellagic acid, malic acid	Dopamine, GABA, serotonin
Red grapefruit	D-glucaric acid, lycopene, naringin	Dopamine
Red grapes	Ellagic acid, lycopene, oligomeric proantho-cyanidins, pectin, resveratrol	Dopamine
Watermelon	Cucurbocitrin, lycopene	Dopamine
Rhubarb	Anthraquinone, emodin, ferulic acid	Acetylcholine
Kidney beans	Galactomannan, lectins, protease inhibitors	Acetylcholine, serotonin

ORANGE FOODS	NUTRIENTS	BRAIN CHEMICAL(S) IT MOST AFFECTS
Carrots	Alpha carotene, beta carotene, lignin, lutein, lycopene, mannitol, pectin, xanthophyll	Dopamine
Spanish onions	Allyl propyl disulfide, fructooligosaccharides, glucosinolates, pectin, quercetin	GABA
Parsnips	Furocoumarin	Serotonin
Pumpkin	Alpha carotene, beta carotene, lutein, zeaxanthin	Dopamine
Sweet potatoes	Beta carotene, alpha carotene, chlorogenic acid, lutein, protease inhibitors	Dopamine
Apricots	Alpha carotene, beta carotene, cryptoxanthin, lutein, lycopene, zeaxanthin	Dopamine
Calimyrna figs	Furocoumarin, lignin	GABA, serotonin
Mangoes	Alpha carotene, anacardic acid, beta carotene, cryptoxanthin, ellagic acid, lutein, zeaxanthin	Dopamine
Casaba melon	Beta carotene, lutein, zeaxanthin	Dopamine, GABA
Crenshaw melon	Beta carotene, lutein, zeaxanthin	Dopamine, GABA
Nectarines	Beta carotene, cryptoxanthin, lutein, zeaxanthin	Dopamine, GABA
Oranges, all varieties	Beta carotene, cryptoxanthin, cyanidin, delphinidin, D-glucaric acid, hesperidin, tangeretin	Dopamine
Tangerines	Beta carotene, hesperidin, nobiletin, tangeretin	Dopamine
Peaches	Alpha carotene, lignin, lutein, zeaxanthin	GABA
Kumquat	Citric acid	GABA
Pumpkin seeds (unsalted)	Cucurbitin	Dopamine

YELLOW FOODS	NUTRIENTS	BRAIN CHEMICAL(S) IT MOST AFFECTS
Yellow snap beans	Alpha carotene, coumestrol, lignin, lutein, quercetin	GABA
Corn	Lutein, zeaxanthin	GABA
Cashew nuts (unsalted)	Anacardiol, fatty acids	GABA
Walnuts (unsalted)	Alpha-linolenic acid, linoleic acid, phytosterols	Dopamine
Peanuts (unsalted)	Isothiocyanates, resveratrol, saponins	Dopamine, acetylcholine, GABA
Chick-peas	Gamma tocopherol, protease inhibitors, saponins	Acetylcholine
Yellow globe onions	Allyl propyl disulfide, fructooligosaccharides, glucosinolates, pectin, quercetin	GABA
Pineapple	Bromelain, protease inhibitors	Acetylcholine, serotonin
Bell pepper	Beta carotene, capsaicin, capsanthin, capsorubin, cryptoxanthin, lutein, lycopene	Dopamine
Golden zucchini	Beta carotene	Dopamine
Butternut squash	Alpha carotene, beta carotene, lutein, zeaxanthin	Dopamine
Golden apples	Caffeic acid, chlorogenic acid, D-glucaric acid, ellagic acid, ferulic acid, pectin, quercetin	Serotonin
Grapefruit	D-glucaric acid, lycopene, naringin, naringin	Dopamine
Lemons	Citric acid, citronellal, limonene, P-coumaric acid	Dopamine, serotonin
Papayas	Ellagic acid, lutein, papain	GABA, serotonin
Jerusalem artichoke	Inulin	Dopamine
Soybeans	Alpha-linolenic acid, beta sitosterol, daidzein, gamma tocopherol, genistein, isothiocyanates, phosphatidylcholine	Dopamine, Acetylcholine
Pignoli nuts	Fatty acids	GABA
Macadamia nuts	Fiber, monounsaturated fatty acids	Dopamine, GABA
Bananas	Fructooligosaccharides, pectin, potassium	GABA

GREEN FOODS	NUTRIENTS	BRAIN CHEMICAL(S) IT MOST AFFECTS
Artichoke	Apigenin, caffeic acid, chlorogenic acid, cosmoside, cyanidine, cynarin, cynaropicrin, cynaroside, hesperiodoside, hesperetin, inulin, luteolin, maritimein, mucilage, pectin, quercetin, rutin, scolimoside	Dopamine
Asparagus	Asparagosides, zeaxanthin	Acetylcholine
Green snap beans	Alpha carotene, coumestrol, lignin, lutein, quercetin	GABA
Italian green beans	Alpha carotene, coumestrol, lignin, lutein, quercetin	GABA
Fava beans	Beta carotene, protease inhibitors, saponins	Acetylcholine
Lima beans	Alpha carotene, gamma tocopherol, lutein, protease inhibitors	Dopamine
Broccoli	Glucobrassicins, indole-3-carbinol, isothio-cyanates, quercetin, sulforaphane	Serotonin
Brussels sprouts	Alpha carotene, coumestrol, dithiolethione, isothiocyanates, lutein, protease inhibitors	Dopamine, acetylcholine, GABA, serotonin
Cabbage, all varieties	Glucosinolates, indole-3-carbinol, lutein	GABA, serotonin
Celery	Coumarin, lutein	GABA, serotonin
Cucumber	Protease inhibitors, silicon	Acetylcholine
Fennel	Beta-sitosterol, coumarin, limonene, pectin, stigmasterol, terpineol, urease, volatile oils	Dopamine, GABA, serotonin
Turnip greens	Vitamin C, calcium, iron, folacin, beta carotene	Dopamine, GABA, serotonin
Collard greens	Vitamin C, calcium, iron, folacin, beta carotene	Dopamine
Kale	Alpha carotene, beta carotene, indoles, isothiocyanates, lutein, quercetin, sulfora-phane, zeaxanthin	Serotonin
Dandelion greens	Lactucin, lactupicrin, taraxacin	Serotonin
Mustard greens	Isothiocyanates, lutein, zeaxanthin	GABA
Lettuces, all varieties	Alpha carotene, lactucarium, lutein, vitamin K, zeaxanthin	Dopamine, GABA, serotonin
Leeks	Allicin, allylic sulfides	Acetylcholine
Okra	Mucilages, pectins	Dopamine, GABA

GREEN FOODS	NUTRIENTS	BRAIN CHEMICAL(S) IT MOST AFFECTS
Green peppers	Beta carotene, cryptoxanthin, lutein, lycopene	Dopamine
Spinach	Alpha carotene, beta carotene, caffeic acid, coumestrol, ferulic acid, lutein, neoxanthin, zeaxanthin	Dopamine
Chives	Beta carotene, fumaric acid, sulfur	Dopamine
Zucchini	Beta carotene	Dopamine
Green apples, all varieties	Caffeic acid, chlorogenic acid, D-glucaric acid, ellagic acid, ferulic acid, pectin, quercetin	Serotonin
Avocado	Beta-sitosterol, glutathione, mannoheptulose	Dopamine
Plantains	Gums, mucilages	Dopamine, serotonin
Green grapes	Ellagic acid, pectin, resveratrol	Dopamine, GABA, serotonin
Kiwis	Actinidin, alpha carotene, beta carotene, lutein, zeaxanthin	Dopamine
Limes	Bioflavonoids, citral, citric acid, furocoumarins, nobiletin	Dopamine, GABA
Pears, all varieties	Citric acid, pectin	Dopamine, GABA
Mung beans	Protease inhibitors	Acetylcholine

BLUE FOODS	NUTRIENTS	BRAIN CHEMICAL(S) IT MOST AFFECTS
Black radishes	Diastase, gallic acid, methanethiol, pelargonidin, protease inhibitors, sulforaphane	Acetylcholine
Blueberries	Anthocyanidin, anthocyanosides, ellagic acid, myrtillin	Dopamine
Dark grapes, all varieties	Ellagic acid, lycopene, oligomeric proanthocyanidins, pectin, resveratrol	Dopamine
Currants	Anthocyanidin, anthocyanosides, ellagic acid	Dopamine
Black beans	Galactomannan, protease inhibitors	Acetylcholine
Black walnuts (unsalted)	Alpha-linolenic acid, linoleic acid, phytosterols	Dopamine
Brazil nuts (unsalted)	Alpha-linolenic acid, ellagic acid, lignin, selenium	Dopamine

INDIGO FOODS	NUTRIENTS	BRAIN CHEMICAL(S) IT MOST AFFECTS
Beets	Betaine, fumaric acid, glutamine, succinic acid	GABA
Blackberries	Anthocyanidin	Dopamine
Red cabbage	Anthocyanins, glucosinolates, indole-3-carbinol, lutein	GABA
Purple kale	Alpha carotene, beta carotene, indoles, isothiocyanates, lutein, quercetin, sulforaphane, zeaxanthin	Dopamine, GABA, Serotonin
Turnips	Glucosinolates, indoles, isothiocyanates, phenethyl isothiocyanate, sulforaphane	GABA
Red grapes	Ellagic acid, lycopene, oligomeric proanthocyanidins, pectin, resveratrol	Dopamine
Plums, all varieties	Alpha carotene, beta cryptoxanthin, lutein, malic acid, pectin, zeaxanthin	GABA
Prunes	Alpha carotene, beta cryptoxanthin, lutein, malic acid, pectin, zeaxanthin	GABA
Passion fruit	Anthocyanidin, harmala alkaloids	Acetylcholine

VIOLET FOODS	NUTRIENTS	BRAIN CHEMICAL(S) IT MOST AFFECTS
Purple broccoli	Glucobrassicins, indole-3-carbinol, isothiocyanates, quercetin, sulforaphane	Serotonin
Purple wax beans	Alpha carotene, gamma tocopherol, lutein, protease inhibitors	Dopamine
Chinese purple eggplant	Anthocyanidin, coumarin, gallic acid, protease inhibitors, saponins	Acetylcholine
Purple artichoke	Apigenin, caffeic acid, chlorogenic acid, cosmoside, cyanidin, cynarin, cynaropicrin, cynaroside, hesperiodoside, hesperetin, inulin, luteolin, maritimein, mucilage, pectin, quercetin, rutin, scolimoside	Dopamine, acetylcholine, GABA, serotonin

Appendix C

INDEX OF RECIPES

Recipes by Brain Chemical

RECIPE	PAGE NUMBER	BRAIN CHEMICAL	MEAL
Scrambled Eggs with Broccoli	162	Dopamine	Special Breakfasts
Pineapple Upside-Down French Toast	167	Dopamine	Special Breakfasts
Italian Omelet	163	Dopamine, serotonin	Special Breakfasts
Tuna–Stuffed Tomatoes	177	Dopamine, acetylcholine	Easy Lunches
Tofu Curry with Green Beans	181	Dopamine, serotonin	Easy Lunches
Flank Steak Fajitas with Mango Salsa	200–201	Dopamine	Delicious Dinners
Citrus Tuna	190	Dopamine, acetylcholine	Delicious Dinners
Blood Orange–Infused Salmon	192	Dopamine, acetylcholine	Delicious Dinners
Salmon and Tomato Stew	193	Dopamine, acetylcholine	Delicious Dinners
Lamb Chops with Herbs and Tabouli	203	Dopamine, GABA	Delicious Dinners
English Breakfast Tea Green Beans	209	Dopamine, GABA	Delicious Dinners
Mediterranean Turkey Legs	188	Dopamine, serontonin	Delicious Dinners
Salmon with Dill Crust and Tomato-Fennel Sauce	191	Dopamine, acetylcholine, serotonin	Delicious Dinners
Herb Frittata	161	Acetylcholine	Special Breakfasts
Salade Niçoise with Olives, Oranges, and Bell Pepper	174	Acetylcholine	Easy Lunches

RECIPE	PAGE NUMBER	BRAIN CHEMICAL	MEAL
Tuna Salad Pita Pocket	176	Acetylcholine	Easy Lunches
Navy Bean and Kale Soup	169	Acetylcholine, GABA	Easy Lunches
Spicy Black Bean Soup	170	Acetylcholine, GABA	Easy Lunches
Mahimahi with Ginger Glaze	197	Acetylcholine, serotonin	Delicious Dinners
Egg Bruschetta	164	GABA	Special Breakfast
Spinach and Strawberry Salad	171	GABA	Easy Lunches
Black Bean, Jicama, Corn, and Mango Salad	172	GABA	Easy Lunches
Asian Chicken Lettuce Wrap	175	GABA	Easy Lunches
Herb-Crusted Halibut	195	GABA	Delicious Dinners
Sauteed Liver with Caramelized Onions	202	GABA	Delicious Dinners
Spicy Kale and Yams	208	GABA	Delicious Dinners
Baked Sweet Potato Casserole with Pecans	206	GABA, serotonin	Delicious Dinners
Spicy Seared Tofu with Mandarin Orange Sauce	180	Serotonin	Easy Lunches
Middle Eastern Turkey Kebabs	187	Serotonin	Delicious Dinners
Rainbow Fruit Salad	165	All	Special Breakfast
Cinnamon Fruit Smoothie	166	All	Special Breakfast
Sprouted Pea Soup	168	All	Easy Lunches
Super Salad	173	All	Easy Lunches
Baigan Ka Bharta (Mashed Eggplant)	178–179	All	Easy Lunches
Tandoori Chicken	182	All	Delicious Dinners
Chicken with Prunes and Olives	183	All	Delicious Dinners
Lemon Garlic Rooibos Chicken	184	All	Delicious Dinners
Baked Chicken with Yogurt	185	All	Delicious Dinners
Rosemary Chicken with Broccoli	186	All	Delicious Dinners

RECIPE	PAGE NUMBER	BRAIN CHEMICAL	MEAL
Jasmine Tea–Infused Brown Rice with Sweet Peas and Duck	189	All	Delicious Dinners
Broiled Halibut with Yogurt-Dill Sauce	194	All	Delicious Dinners
Baked Tilapia	196	All	Delicious Dinners
Herb-Rubbed Mackerel with Snow Peas and Lemon	198	All	Delicious Dinners
Curried Shrimp	199	All.	Delicious Dinners
Moroccan Lamb Tagine with Cinnamon, Apricots, and Almonds	204–205	All	Delicious Dinners
Sweet Potato and Chickpea Curry	207	All	Delicious Dinners
Yogurt Cumin Marinade	210	All	Sauces and Condiments
Garlic Lover's Rub	211	All	Sauces and Condiments

Recipes by Meal

RECIPE	PAGE NUMBER	BRAIN CHEMICAL	MEAL
Herb Frittata	161	Acetylcholine	Special Breakfasts
Scrambled Eggs with Broccoli	162	Dopamine	Special Breakfasts
Italian Omelet	163	Dopamine, serotonin	Special Breakfasts
Egg Bruschetta	164	GABA	Special Breakfasts
Rainbow Fruit Salad	165	All	Special Breakfasts
Cinnamon Fruit Smoothie	166	All	Special Breakfasts
Pineapple Upside-Down French Toast	167	Dopamine	Special Breakfasts
Sprouted Pea Soup	168	All	Easy Lunches
Navy Bean and Kale Soup	169	Acetylcholine, GABA	Easy Lunches
Spicy Black Bean Soup	170	Acetylcholine, GABA	Easy Lunches
Spinach and Strawberry Salad	171	GABA	Easy Lunches
Black Bean, Jicama, Corn, and Mango Salad	172	GABA	Easy Lunches
Super Salad	173	All	Easy Lunches

RECIPE	PAGE NUMBER	BRAIN CHEMICAL	MEAL
Salade Niçoise with Olives, Oranges, and Bell Pepper	174	Acetylcholine	Easy Lunches
Asian Chicken Lettuce Wrap	175	GABA	Easy Lunches
Tuna Salad Pita Pocket	176	Acetylcholine	Easy Lunches
Tuna-Stuffed Tomatoes	177	Dopamine, acetylcholine	Easy Lunches
Baigan Ka Bharta (Mashed Eggplant)	178–179	All	Easy Lunches
Spicy Seared Tofu with Mandarin Orange Sauce	180	Serotonin	Easy Lunches
Tofu Curry with Green Beans	181	Dopamine, serotonin	Easy Lunches
Tandoori Chicken	182	All	Delicious Dinners
Chicken with Prunes and Olives	183	All	Delicious Dinners
Lemon Garlic Rooibos Chicken	184	All	Delicious Dinners
Baked Chicken with Yogurt	185	All	Delicious Dinners
Rosemary Chicken with Broccoli	186	All	Delicious Dinners
Middle Eastern Turkey Kebabs	187	Serontonin	Delicious Dinners
Mediterranean Turkey Legs	188	Dopamine, serontonin	Delicious Dinners
Jasmine Tea–Infused Brown Rice with Sweet Peas and Duck	189	All	Delicious Dinners
Citrus Tuna	190	Dopamine, acetylcholine	Delicious Dinners
Salmon with Dill Crust and Tomato Fennel Sauce	191	Dopamine, acetylcholine, serotonin	Delicious Dinners
Blood Orange–Infused Salmon	192	Dopamine, acetylcholine	Delicious Dinners
Salmon and Tomato Stew	193	Dopamine, acetylcholine	Delicious Dinners
Broiled Halibut with Yogurt-Dill Sauce	194	All	Delicious Dinners
Herb-Crusted Halibut	195	GABA	Delicious Dinners
Baked Tilapia	196	All	Delicious Dinners
Mahimahi with Ginger Glaze	197	Acetylcholine, serotonin	Delicious Dinners
Herb-Rubbed Mackerel with Snow Peas and Lemon	198	All	Delicious Dinners
Curried Shrimp	199	All	Delicious Dinners

RECIPE	PAGE NUMBER	BRAIN CHEMICAL	MEAL
Flank Steak Fajitas with Mango Salsa	200–201	Dopamine	Delicious Dinners
Sauteed Liver with Caramelized Onions	202	GABA	Delicious Dinners
Lamb Chops with Herbs and Tabouli	203	Dopamine, GABA	Delicious Dinners
Moroccan Lamb Tagine with Cinnamon, Apricots, and Almonds	204–205	All	Delicious Dinners
Baked Sweet Potato Casserole with Pecans	206	GABA, Serotonin	Delicious Dinners
Sweet Potato and Chickpea Curry	207	All	Delicious Dinners
Spicy Kale and Yams	208	GABA	Delicious Dinners
English Breakfast Tea Green Beans	209	Dopamine, GABA	Delicious Dinners
Yogurt Cumin Marinade	210	All	Sauces and Condiments
Garlic Lover's Rub	211	All	Sauces and Condiments

Appendix D

CORE AGE MARKERS OF EACH OF THE BODY SYSTEMS

PAUSE	DECLINE IN (MARKER)	TYPICAL ONSET AGE
Electropause	Electrical activity of brain waves	45
Biopause	Neurotransmitters	Dopamine: 30 Acetylcholine: 40 GABA: 50 Serotonin: 60
Pineal pause	Melatonin	20
Pituitary pause	Hormone feedback loops	30
Sensory pause	Touch, hearing, vision, and smell sensitivity	40
Psychopause	Personality health and mood	30
Thyropause	Calcitonin and thyroid hormone levels	50
Parathyropause	Parathyroid hormone	50
Thymopause	Glandular size and immune system	40
Cardiopause/vasculopause	Ejection fraction and blood flow	40
Pulmonopause	Lung elasticity and function with increase in blood pressure	50
Adrenopause	DHEA	55
Nephropause	Erythropoietin level and creatine clearance	40
Somatopause	Growth hormone	30
Gastropause	Nutrient absorption	40
Pancreopause	Blood sugar level	40
Insulopause	Glucose tolerance	40
Andropause	Testosterone in men	45

PAUSE	DECLINE IN (MARKER)	TYPICAL ONSET AGE
Menopause	Estrogen, progesterone, and testosterone in women	40
Osteopause	Bone density	30
Dermopause	Collagen, vitamin D synthesis	35
Onchopause	Finger and toe nails	40
Uropause	Bladder control	45
Genopause	DNA	40

Appendix E

Important Blood Work to Discuss with Your Doctor

ANEMIA

SMAC
Hemogram
Hgb electro
Ferritin (RIA)
Vitamin B_{12}
RBC Folate
Transferrin
Haptoglobin
Retic Count
Urinalysis
Vitamin B_6
Prealbumin
TIBC
Erythropoietin
Iron
% Saturation

CANCER SCREEN

CA 125
CA 15-3
CA 19-9
CA 27-29
ESR, CEA
CRP, AFP

hCG, Total, Quant
  (Tumor)
  Quest# 5140A
T help/T Supp Ratio
IPEP/SPEP
Br Ca 1, Br Ca 2

CELIAC DISEASE

Gliladin Abs IgG, IgA
Antiendomysial Abs
T help/T supp ratio
Total IgA deficiency
Reticulin Ab IgG, IgA
QUEST:
  tTG Ab, IgA
  Gliadin Ab, IgA
  Total IgA
  EMA Screen, IgA
  EMA titer
  tTG Ab, IgG

LIVER FUNCTION

LFTs
Hemogram
Protein EPH

Hepatitis A & B
Gastrin RIA
Apolipo-A
Apolipo-B
U/A
Prealbumin
Apo A1/B ratio

DIABETES

SMAC
Hemogram
Hemoglobin A1C
Insulin level
Urinalysis
Fructosamine
QUEST #10584N:
  GAD-65 Antibody
  IA-2 Antibody
  Insulin Antibody
Adiponectin
  899 (Nichols)
  Quest# 15060X
Erythropoietin
  Quest# 22376R

ENDOCRINE

LH
FSH
TSH—3rd Gen
Estradiol—Progesterone
DHT
Testosterone
  (free and total)
Prolactin RIA
Fract. Estrogen (F)
Androstenedione
Serum cortisol
DHEA
DHEA-S
Pregnenolone
IGF-1, IGF-BP3
  Quest# P3329
Sex Hormone Bind Globulin
Corticotropin RH
Plasma ACTH
Melatonin
PSA

HEALTH SCAN I

Chem Screen
  Quest# 18T
Hemogram
RPR
U/A

DIABETES II

C-Peptide
Serum Cortisol
ACTH Plasma RIA
Gastrin RIA
Insulin Level
Growth hormone
Zinc
Fructosamine

HEPATITIS

Hepatitis A Ab
Hep B Surface Ag
Hep B Surface Ab
Hepatitis B Core Ab
Hepatitis Be Ag
Hepatitis Be Ab
Hepatitis C
Hepatitis C Quant
Hepatitis C genotype
  Quest# 3711X
Hepatitis D (check if (+) HB
  surface Ag)
Hepatitis E

HYPERTENSION

SMAC
CBC with diff
Aldosterone
DHEA-S
BNP
Serum Cortisol
Renin
Urine Microalbumin
Cystatin C

GH

IGF-1, IGF-BP3
  Quest# P3329
Anti-GH antibodies
Leptin
IGF-II
  Quest# 24851P
  BR# 2474
IGF BP-II
  Quest# 127233P
IGF-BP 1

IMMUNE

ESR
CRP
IPEP
SPEP
T helper/T supp ratio
T-killer
TNF

LIPID

Lipo-pro Elect
Apolipo-A
Apolipo-B
Apo A1/B ratio
Triglycerides
Cholesterol
HDL Cholesterol
LDL Cholesterol
Fibrinogen
Homocysteine
Apolipoprotein E
  Genotype (BR# 1420)
VAP Cholesterol Test

PANCREAS/GB

Lipase
Amylase
Ionized Calcium
Trypsin
Leucine amino peptides
PT/PTT/INR
Chem Screen
H. pylori IgA, IgG, & IgM

OSTEOPOROSIS

Calcitonin
Ionized calcium
Osteocalcin
Parathyroid hormone

Urine telopeptides
Vitamin D, 1, 25 dihydroxy
  (Quest# 16493E)
Vitamin D, 25 hydroxy
  (Quest# 19893E)
24 hr Ca urine
Vitamin K1
Boron
  Alk Phos Isoenzymes
  BR# 5058
Boron urine
Strontium
  Quest only# 26508X

PANCREAS
Amylase
CA 19-9
Calcitonin
Gastrin
Insulin level
Lipase
Pancreozymine secretin test

HEALTH SCAN II
SMAC
Hemogram
RPR
ESR
Free T3
Free T4
Zinc
U/A

Apolipo-A
Apolipo-B
Apo A1/B ratio

RHEUMATOID
SMAC
RPR
Anti-Nuclear Ab
Anti-DNA Ab
CRP
ESR
RA Factor
LE Prep
U/A
Complement C3
Complement C4
Cardiolipin
Interleukin-1
Interleukin-2
Interleukin-6
Interleukin-8
TNF

SOFT TISSUE
SMAC
Hemogram
ESR
Adolase
  Quest only# 93310E
LD Isoenzymes
Haptoglobin

CRP
Serum lipase
Serum amylase
Complement C3

THYROID
SMAC
CBC with diff
T3
T3 Uptake
T4 Total
TSH
T7 Index
Ferritin RIA
Thyroid Auto-Abs

CLOTTING
CK Isoenzymes
ProteinC
Protein S
AT3
Plasminogen
Fibrinogen
Factor V
Factor VIII
Anticardiolipin Abs
EPP Free Erythrocyte
  Porphyrins

ENDNOTES

PART 1

Introduction

1. "Eating Disorders and Their Precursors." National Eating Disorders Association. http://www.nationaleatingdisorders.org/p.asp?WebPage_ID=286&Profile_ID=41138 2002.

2. "Poor Physical Performance in Adults, a Predictor of Future Disability." http://www.ndri.com/news/poor_physical_performance_in_adults_a_predictor_of_future_disability-295.html June 2007.

3. "How Foods Affect Triglycerides." Cleveland Clinic Heart and Vascular Institute. http://www.clevelandclinic.org/heartcenter/pub/guide/prevention/nutrition/triglycerides.htm April 2006.

4. Weinrauch L. "How do High Triglyceride Levels Affect Health?" http://www.healthcentral.com/heart-disease/c/77/11199/high-health

5. "Dementia/Alzheimer's." Food for the Brain. http://www.foodforthebrain.org/content.asp?id_Content=1634.

6. "Excess Weight and Obesity, Depression and Other Mental Disorders." Insulite Laboratories. http://weight.insulitelabs.com/Mental-Disorders.php.

7. Hilliard J. "Diet and Exercise can help Decrease Diabetes Risk." Medical College of Georgia. https://my.mcg.edu/portal/page/portal/News/archive/2007/Diet%20and%20exercise%20can%20help%20decrease%20diabetes%20risk January 31, 2007.

8. "Metabolic Syndrome." Natural Choices for You. http://www.naturalchoicesforyou.com/site/680805/page/219656.

9. "High blood cholesterol." All Health News. http://www.mtuchallengex.org/?p=4 December 31, 2007.

10. Smith S. "Heart research shifts to early detection." *The Boston Globe*. November 9, 2006.

11. "Age at the Onset of Menopause." Menopause Insight. http://www.menopauseinsight.com/menopause/age-at-onset.aspx.

Chapter 1

1. "New Food Addiction Link Found." Brookhaven National Laboratory. http://www.bnl.gov/bnlweb/pubaf/pr/2002/bnlpr052002.htm May 20, 2002.

2. Del Parigi A., Chen K., Salbe A.D., Reiman E.M., and Tataranni P.A. "Are We Addicted to Food?" *Obesity Research* 11:493–495 (2003).

3. Shamon M. "Thyroid Diet Secrets: Are You Eating Enough Calories to Lose Weight?" About.com. http://thyroid.about.com/cs/dietweightloss/a/eatingenough.htm?p=1 December 3, 2003.

4. "About Brain Waves/Alpha Brain Waves." The Biocybernaut Institute. http://www.biocybernaut.com/about/brainwaves/alpha.htm.

5. Taheri S. "Does the lack of sleep make you fat?" Henry Wellcome Laboratories for Integrative Neuroscience and Endocrinology. http://www.bristol.ac.uk/researchreview/2004/1113989409 December 20, 2004.

6. Balasubramanyan A. "Ghrelin and PYY: Rising Stars in Appetite Regulation." The Endocrine Society 2003 85th Annual Meeting.

7. Vanek C., and Connor W.E. "Do n–3 fatty acids prevent osteoporosis?" *American Journal of Clinical Nutrition*, Vol. 85, No. 3, 647–648, March 2007.

Chapter 2

1. Strauss E. "Wasting Away: Stress Response Keeps Aging Cells from Fattening Up (Fat Cell Formation)." *Sci. Aging Knowl. Environ.*, 27 February 2002, Vol. **2002**, Issue 8, p. nw25.

2. Grossman K. "Men's Belly Size Predicts Heart Disease." *About.com/The New York Times*. http://menshealth.about.com/cs/lifestyle/a/big_belly.htm?p=1 January 4, 2007.

3. Thomas D.B., Carter R.A., Bush W.H., Ray R.M., Stanford J.L., Lehman C.D., Daling J.R., Malone K., and Davis S. "Risk of Subsequent Breast Cancer in Relation to Characteristics of Screening Mammograms from Women Less Than 50 Years of Age." *Cancer Epidemiology Biomarkers & Prevention* Vol. 11, 565–571, June 2002.

4. "Ear Crease Early Warning Sign of a Heart Attack?" Universal College of Reflexology. http://www.universalreflex.com/article.php?story=20051027133133490.

5. Denmark-Wahnefried W., Schildkraut J.M., Thompson D., Lesko S.M., McIntyre L., Schwingl P., Paulson D.F., Robertson C.N., Anderson E.E., and Walther P.J. "Early Onset Baldness and Prostate Cancer Risk." *Cancer Epidemiol Biomarkers Prev.* 2000 Mar;9(3):325–8.

6. Peeters A., Barendregt J.J., Willekens F., Mackenbach J.P., Al Mamun A., and Bonneux L. "Obesity in Adulthood and Its Consequences for Life Expectancy: A Life-Table Analysis." *Annals of Internal Medicine* 2003 Jan;138(1):24–32.

7. "Overweight and Obesity, Frequently Asked Questions." Centers for Disease Control and Prevention. http://www.cdc.gov/nccdphp/dnpa/obesity/faq.htm.

8. "Defining Overweight and Obesity." Centers for Disease Control and Prevention. http://www.cdc.gov/nccdphp/dnpa/obesity/defining.htm.

9. "Classification of Overweight and Obesity by BMI, Waist Circumference, and Associated Disease Risks." Department of Health and Human Services. http://www.nhlbi.nih.gov/health/public/heart/obesity/lose_wt/bmi_dis.htm.

10. "A Mother's Obesity Can Harm Her Baby." http://www.virtualcardiacentre.com/news.asp?artid=2345.

11. Christakis N.A., and Fowler J.H. "The Spread of Obesity in a Large Social Network Over 32 Years." *N Engl J Med.* 2007 Jul 26;357(4):370–9. Epub 2007 Jul 25.

12. Kolata, G. "Find Yourself Packing It On? Blame Friends." *The New York Times*, July 26, 2007.

Chapter 3

1. Volkow N.D., Wang G.J., Telang F., Fowler J.S., Logan J., Childress A.R., Jayne M., Ma Y., and Wong C. "Cocaine Cues and Dopamine in Dorsal Striatum: Mechanism of Craving in Cocaine Addiction." *The Journal of Neuroscience*, June 14, 2006, 26(24):6583–6588.

2. "Scientists Find Link Between Dopamine and Obesity." Science Daily. http://www.sciencedaily.com/releases/2001/02/010205075129.htm February 6, 2001.

3. Wang G.J., Volkow N.D., Logan J., Pappas N.R., Wong C.T., Zhu W., Netusil N., and Fowler J.S. "Brain dopamine and obesity." *Lancet*. 2001 Feb 3;357(9253):354–7.

4. "Exposure to Food Increases Brain Metabolism." Science Daily. http://www.sciencedaily.com/releases/2004/04/040420014644.htm April 21, 2004.

5. Park, P. "Addiction: From Drugs to Donuts, Brain Activity May Be the Key." http://www.docshop.com/2007/08/09/food-addiction August 9, 2007.

6. "Scientists Find Link Between Dopamine and Obesity." Brookhaven National Laboratory. http://www.bnl.gov/bnlweb/pubaf/pr/2001/bnlpr020101.htm, February 1, 2001.

7. Volkow, N., and O'Brien, C.P. "Issues for DSM-V: Should Obesity Be Included as a Brain Disorder?" *Am J Psychiatry* 2007 May;164(5):708–10.

8. Pruessner J.C., Champagne F., Meaney M.J., and Dagher A. "Dopamine Release in Response to a Psychological Stress in Humans and Its Relationship to Early Life Maternal Care: A Positron Emission Tomography Study Using [11C]Raclopride." *J Neurosci*. 2004 Mar 17;24(11):2825–31.

9. Schatzberg A.F. "HPA Axis/Dopamine Interactions in Psychotic Depression." http://cogent.stanford.edu/hpa.asp.

10. Turner N. "Boost your Metabolism with Sleep." True Star Health. http://www.truestarhealth.com/members/cm_archives13ML3P1A19.html

11. "Depression and Addiction." Florida Detox. http://www.floridadetox.com/depression.asp.

12. Liu S. "Dietary Calcium, Vitamin D, and the Prevalence of Metabolic Syndrome in Middle-Aged and Older U.S. Women." *Diabetes Care*. 28:2926–32, 2005.

13. "Scientists Find Link Between Dopamine and Obesity." Brookhaven National Laboratory. http://www.bnl.gov/bnlweb/pubaf/pr/2001/bnlpr020101.htm February 1, 2001.

14. "Walking for Fitness: How to Trim Your Waistline, Improve Your Health." Mayo Clinic. http://www.mayoclinic.com/health/walking/HQ01612 December 22, 2006.

15. Parks R. "Phenylalanine Helps Control Symptoms of Chronic Pain." http://www.e-healtharticles.com/Detailed/2528.html Aug 30, 2006.

16. "Get the Skinny on Lean Beef." http://www.beefitswhatsfordinner.com/nutrition/leancuts.asp

17. "Dopamine—The 'Good Feelings' Neurotransmitter." http://www.pspinformation.com/medicine/medicine-other/dopamine.shtml, last modified 01/20/08.

18. Zemel M. "Calcium Modulation of Adiposity." *Obes Res.* 2003 Mar;11(3):375–6.

19. "Leptin." Colorado State University. http://www.vivo.colostate.edu/hbooks/pathphys/endocrine/bodyweight/leptin.htm November 7, 1998.

20. Ibid.

21. "Coffee is Number One Source of Antioxidants." Phys Org. http://www.physorg.com/printnews.php?newsid=6067.

22. Vetter M., and Gabel C. "What's Wrong with Caffeine?" Missouri Families. http://missourifamilies.org/features/nutritionarticles/nut82.htm.

23. Dzubow L. "The Latest Health Drink: Coffee." *O, The Oprah Magazine* 2007 Aug. 121:124,www.oprah.com/omagazine/200708/omag_200708_coffee_c.jhtml.

24. "The Trouble with Sugar Free.... How Sorbitol Causes Irritable Bowel Syndrome." http://www.foodintol.com/food_intolerance/hot_ibs.htm 25 Aug 2003.

Chapter 4

1. Shimabukuro M., Zhou Y.T., Levi., and Unger R.H. **"Fatty Acid-Induced Cell Apoptosis: A Link Between Obesity and Diabetes."** *Proc Natl Acad Sci U S A.* 1998 Mar 3;95(5):2498–502.

2. "Apoptosis." Http://users.rcn.com/jkimball.ma.ultranet/BiologyPages/A/Apoptosis.html.

3. Lauri H.T., Viljanen A., Parkkola R., Kemppainen N., Rinne J.O., Nuutila P., and Kaasinen V. "Brain White Matter Expansion in Human Obesity and the Recovering Effect of Dieting." *Journal of Clinical Endocrinology & Metabolism*, doi:10.1210/jc.2006–2495; *The Journal of Clinical Endocrinology & Metabolism* Vol. 92, No. 8 3278–3284.

4. "What is Myelin?" The Myelin Project. www.myelin.org.

5. Koudinov A.R., and Koudinova N.V. "Brain Cholesterol Pathology is the Cause of Alzheimer's Disease." *Clin Med Health Res* (2001) clinmed/2001100005.

6. "WAC: High-Fat Diet in Early Adulthood May Be Associated with Increased Risk of Alzheimer's." *Doctor's Guide: Global Edition.* www.pslgroup.com/dg/1d9536.htm July 12, 2000.

7 "National Diabetes Fact Sheet." CDC. http://www.cdc.gov/diabetes/pubs/ estimates.htm. December 20, 2005.

8. "The World's Healthiest Foods: Eggs." http://www.whfoods.com/genpage.php? tname=foodspice&dbid=92.

9. "Choline: Food for Thought." http://lowcarbdiets.about.com/od/nutrition/a/ choline.htm.

10. Xu J., Eilat-Adar S., Loria C., Goldbourt U., Howard B.V., Fabsitz R.R., Zephier E.M., Mattil C., and Lee E.T. "Dietary Fat Intake and Risk of Coronary Heart Disease: The Strong Heart Study." *Am J Clin Nutr.* 2006 Oct;84(4):894–902

11. "Is Saturated Fat Really as Bad as They Say It Is?" *Mercola.com.* http://articles. mercola.com/sites/articles/archive/2006/10/24/is-saturated-fat-really-as-bad-as- they-say-it-is.aspx October 2006.

12. "Health Effects of Fats: Heart Health." Fat of Life. http://fatsoflife.com/fatsoflife/ health-heart.asp.

13. Hu F.B. "The Mediterranean Diet and Mortality—Olive Oil and Beyond." *N Engl J Med.* 2003 Jun 26;348(26):2595–6.

14. "Trans Fatty Acids." AmericanHeart. http://americanheart.org/presenter.jhtml? identifier=3030450.

15. Coromega.com: Ingredient information for Coromega Omega-3 supplement. www.coromega.com/01What/a_Ingredients/a_Body.html.

16. "Fish and Omega-3 Fatty Acids." AmericanHeart. http://www.americanheart.org/ presenter.jhtml?identifier=4632.

17. "Mercury Contamination in Fish." http://www.nrdc.org/health/effects/mercury/ guide.asp

18. Zemel M. "Calcium Modulation of Adiposity." *Obes Res.* 2003 Mar;11(3):375–6.

19. "Lecithin." www.drdavidwilliams.com/c/daily_health_recs.asp.

20. "Turmeric." http://www.whfoods.com/genpage.php?pfriendly=1&tname= foodspice&dbid=78.

Chapter 5

1. Neimark N.F. "The Fight or Flight Response." http://www. thebodysoulconnection.com/EducationCenter/fight.html

2. Lemonick M.D. "How We Get Addicted." *Time.* http://www.time.com/time/ magazine/article/0,9171,1640436-1,00.html July 5, 2007.

3. Yoffe, E. "Stuffed!" *O, The Oprah Magazine* 2007 Aug. 135:136.

4. "Natural Complex Carbohydrates Food List." www.weightlossforall.com/complex-carbs.htm.

5. "Herbs at a Glance: Hoodia." Nccam.nih.gov/health/hoodia.

6. Mitchell, T. "Theanine: Natural Support for Sleep, Mood, and Weight." *Life Extension*, January 2006.

Chapter 6

1. "Salt, Sodium and High Blood Pressure." Dietician. www.Dietician.com/salt/html

2. "Causes of Sleep Deprivation." Sleep Deprivation, www.sleep-deprivation.com/articles/causes-of-sleep-deprivation.

3. Cappuccio F.P., Stranges S., Kandala N.B., Miller M.A., Taggart F.M., Kumari M., Ferrie J.E., Shipley M.J., Brunner E.J., and Marmot M.G. "Gender-Specific Associations of Short Sleep Duration with Prevalent and Incident Hypertension: The Whitehall II Study." *Hypertension.* 2007 Oct;50(4):693–700. Epub 2007 Sep 4.

4. Rosenberg E. "Carbs, Junk Food? Now Add Lack of Sleep to the Things That Can Make You Fat." jscms.jrn.Columbia.edu/cns/2006-02-14/Rosenberg-sleepdiet. February 14, 2006.

5. "Seasonal Affective Disorder." Family Doctor. http://familydoctor.org/online/famdocen/home/common/mentalhealth/depression/267.printerview.html.

6. Farooqi I.S., Bullmore E., Keogh J., Gillard J., O'Rahilly S., and Fletcher P.C. "Leptin Regulates Striatal Regions and Human Eating Behavior." *Science.* 2007 Sep 7;317(5843):1355. Epub 2007 Aug 9.

7. Gangwisch J.E., Malaspina D., Boden-Albala B., and Heymsfield S.B. "Inadequate Sleep as a Risk Factor for Obesity: Analyses of the NHANES I." *Sleep.* 2005 Oct 1;28(10):1289–96.

8. "Is It Depression or a Hormone Deficiency?" www.drmarinajohnson.com/Articles/Depression/tabid/117/Default.aspx.

9. Chamberlain A., Siegel R., and Saltzman E. "Medical Care of the Bariatric Surgery Patient." *Nutrition in Clinical Care.* Volume 7, Number 1, 2004 19–30.

10. "Serotonin Deficiency." http://www.nutritional-healing.com.au/content/articles-content.php?heading=Serotonin%20deficiency.

11. "Do You Have Serotonin Deficiency Syndrome?" http://www.smart-publications.com/depression/serotonin_deficency.php.

12. Hyland T. "Eating After Dark." *Penn Current*. May 12, 2005.

13. "Night Eating Syndrome." www.diagnose-me.com/cond/C303927.html.

14. Wilcox C. and Brizendine L. "Hormones May Prevent Addiction Relapse." www.jfponline.com/Pages.asp?AID=4311.

15. Tham D.M., Gardner C.D., and Haskell W.L. "Clinical Review 97: Potential Health Benefits of Dietary Phytoestrogens: A Review of the Clinical, Epidemiological, and Mechanistic Evidence." *J Clin Endocrinol Metab*. 1998 Jul;83(7):2223–35.

16. Tanskanen A., Hibbeln J.R., Tuomilehto J., Uutela A., Haukkala A., Viinamäki H., Lehtonen J., and Vartiainen E. "Fish Consumption and Depressive Symptoms in the General Population in Finland." *Psychiatr Serv*. 2001 Apr;52(4):529–31.

17. Zemel, M. "Calcium Modulation of Adiposity." *Obes Res*. 2003 Mar;11(3):375–6.

18. Hosokawa M, Kudo M, Maeda H, et al. "Fucoxanthin induces apoptosis and enhances the antiproliferative effect of the PPARgama ligand, troglitazone, on colon cancer cell." *Biochim Biophys Acta*. 2004 Nov 18;1675(1-3):113–9.

19. Rorie S. "Beating the Blues with Natural Antidepressants." www.healingwithnutrition.com/newsclips/blues.html. June 2000.

20. Warner-Schmidt J.L. and Duman R.S. "VEGF is an Essential Mediator of the Neurogenic and Behavioral Actions of Antidepressants." *Proc Natl Acad Sci U S A*. 2007 Mar 13;104(11):4647–52. Epub 2007 Mar.

PART II

Chapter 7

1. "The Overall Nutritional Quality Index (ONQI)." http://www.griffinhealth.org/Research/ONQI.aspx.

2. Nutrition Data Analysis. http://www.nutritiondata.com/help/analysis-help.

3. "Calories in Bagels, Plain, Unenriched." Calorie-Count.com. http://www.calorie-count.com/calories/item/18408.html.

4. Meyers, Steve. "The Organic Factor" 1/07/2008 http://www.naturalproductsinsider.com/articles/the-organic-factor.html.

5. Komatsu T., Nakamori M., Komatsu K., Hosoda K., Okamura M., Toyama K., Ishikura Y., Sakai T., Kunii D., and Yamamoto S. "Oolong Tea Increases Energy Metabolism in Japanese Females." *J Med Invest*. 2003 Aug;50(3-4):170–5.

6. Choo J.J. "Green Tea Reduces Body Fat Accretion Caused by High-Fat Diet in Rats Through Beta-Adrenoceptor Activation of Thermogenesis in Brown Adipose Tissue." *J Nutr Biochem.* 2003 Nov;14(11):671–6.

7. Wolfram S. "Effects of Green Tea and EGCG on Cardiovascular and Metabolic Health." *J Am Coll Nutr.* 2007 Aug;26(4):373S–388S.

8. Zemel M.B., Richards J., Mathis S., Milstead A., Gebhardt L., and Silva E. "Dairy Augmentation of Total and Central Fat Loss in Obese Subjects." *Int J Obes (Lond).* 2005 Apr;29(4):391–7.

9. Zemel M., Wilson B., Loan M., Teegarden D., Lyle R., and Matkovic V. "Role of Dairy Products in Modulation of Body Weight and Body Fat: A Meta-Analysis." Supplement to *Obesity.* Vol. 15, September 2007. Program Abstract Supplement— The Obesity Society 2007 Annual Scientific Meeting.

10. Woolston C. "How Much Sugar is Too Much?" AHealthyMe.com. www.ahealthyme.com/topic/toomuchsugar.

11. "The Health Effects of Drinking Soda: Quotes from the Experts." http://www.jupiterionizers.com/catalog/article_info.php?articles_id=71&tPath=.

12. "Vitamin C Depletion Reduces the Body's Ability to use Fat as a Fuel Source." MedicalNewsToday.com. http://www.medicalnewstoday.com/printerfriendlynews. php?newsid=40914, Apr 6, 2006.

13. Mynatt R., Zhang J., and Zvonic S. "Dietary Carnitine's Effect on Glucose Metabolism and Insulin Action." Supplement to *Obesity.* Vol. 15, September 2007. Program Abstract Supplement—The Obesity Society 2007 Annual Scientific Meeting.

14. "How does fruit juice compare to whole fruit?" TheWorld'sHealthiestFoods.com. http://www.whfoods.com/genpage.php?tname=george&dbid=24.

15. Miglio C., Chiavaro E., Visconti A., Fogliano V., and Pellegrini N. "Effects of Different Cooking Methods on Nutritional and Physicochemical Characteristics of Selected Vegetables." *J Agric Food Chem.* 2008 Jan 9;56(1):139–47. Epub 2007 Dec 11.

16. Galgano F., Favati F., Caruso M., Pietrafesa A., and Natella S. "The Influence of Processing and Preservation on the Retention of Health-Promoting Compounds in Broccoli." *J Food Sci.* 2007 Mar;72(2):S130–5.

Chapter 9

1. Tsanzi E., Light H.R., and Tou J.C. "The Effect of Feeding Different Sugar-Sweetened Beverages to Growing Female Sprague-Dawley Rats on Bone Mass and Strength." *Bone.* 2008 Feb 15.

2. Van der Heijden A.A.W.A, Hu F.B., Rimm E.B., and van Dam R.M. "A Prospective Study of Breakfast Consumption and Weight Gain Among U.S. Men." *Obesity.* 10 October 2007. Vol. 15. No. 10. 2463–68.

3. Taubert D., Roesen R., Lehmann C., Jung N., and Schömig E. "Effects of Low Habitual Cocoa Intake on Blood Pressure and Bioactive Nitric Oxide: A Randomized Controlled Trial." *JAMA.* 2007 Jul 4;298(1):49–60.

Chapter 10

1. Risérus U., and Ingelsson E. "Alcohol Intake, Insulin Resistance, and Abdominal Obesity in Elderly Men." *Obesity (Silver Spring).* 2007 Jul;15(7):1766–73.

PART III

Chapter 12

1. Gallagher S. "The Challenges of Obesity and Skin Integrity." *Nurs Clin North Am.* 2005 Jun;40(2):325–35.

Chapter 13

1. Pittas A.G., Lau J., Hu F.B., and Dawson-Hughes B. "The Role of Vitamin D and Calcium in Type 2 Diabetes. A Systematic Review and Meta-Analysis." *J Clin Endocrinol Metab.* 2007 Jun;92(6):2017–29. Epub 2007 Mar.

2. Dhurandhar N.V., Israel B.A., Kolesar J.M., Mayhew G.F., Cook M.E., and Atkinson R.L. "Increased Adiposity in Animals Due to a Human Virus." *Int J Obes Relat Metab Disord* 2000 Aug;(8):989–96.

3. Wu C.H., Lu F.H., Chang C.S., Chang T.C., Wang R.H., and Chang C.J. "Relationship Among Habitual Tea Consumption, Percent Body Fat, and Body Fat Distribution." *Obes Res.* 2003 Sep;11(9):1088–95.

4. "What is Homocysteine?" http://www.americanheart.org/print_presenter.jhtml;jsessionid=WWVQYG0HVMZLWCQFCXPSDSQ?identifier=535.

5. Hopkins P.N., Wu L.L., Wu J., Hunt S.C., James B.C., Vincent G.M., and Williams R.R. "Higher Plasma Homocysteine and Increased Susceptibility to Adverse Effects of Low Folate in Early Familial Coronary Artery Disease." *Arterioscler Thromb Vasc Biol.* 1995 Sep;15(9):1314–20.

6. Cayenne. Hyperhealth Pro Database.

7. Cinnamon. Hyperhealth Pro Database.

8. Garlic. Hyperhealth Pro Database.

9. Ginger. Hyperhealth Pro Database.

10. Mustard Seed. Hyperhealth Pro Database.

11. Onion. Hyperhealth Pro Database.

12. Peppermint Oil. Hyperhealth Pro Database.

13. Rosemary. Hyperhealth Pro Database.

14. Turmeric. Hyperhealth Pro Database.

15. "Benefits of Eating Nuts." http://www.health.harvard.edu/press_releases/ benefits_eating_nuts.htm.

16. Geopp J.G. "Protecting Cardiovascular Health with Whole Grape Extract." *Life Extension*, September 2007.

Index

Boldface page references indicate illustrations. Underscored references indicate boxed text.

M

Z

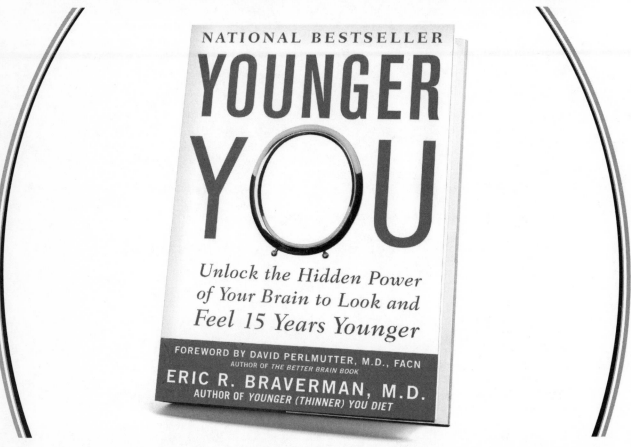